Primary and Ambulatory Care
of the HIV-Infected Adult

Primary and Ambulatory Care of the HIV-Infected Adult

Joseph R. Masci, M.D.

Director, AIDS Clinic;
Associate Director of Medicine,
Elmhurst Hospital Center,
Elmhurst; Associate Professor of Medicine,
Mount Sinai School of Medicine,
New York, New York

Illustrated

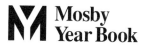
**Mosby
Year Book**

St. Louis Baltimore Boston Chicago London Philadelphia Sydney Toronto

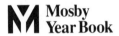
Mosby
Year Book
Dedicated to Publishing Excellence

Editor Stephanie Manning
Assistant Editor Jane Petrash
Project Manager Karen Edwards
Manuscript Editor Christine O'Neil
Designer David Zielinski
Production Assistant Ginny Douglas

Printed in the United States of America

Mosby–Year Book, Inc.
11830 Westline Industrial Drive
St. Louis, Missouri 63146

Library of Congress Cataloging-in-Publication Data

Masci, Joseph R.
    Primary and ambulatory care of the HIV-infected adult / Joseph R.
Masci.
        p.   cm.
    Includes bibliographical references and index.
    ISBN 0-8016-3159-9
    1. HIV infections. 2. Family medicine. I. Title.
    [DNLM: 1. Ambulatory Care. 2. HIV Infections—therapy.
    3. Primary Health Care.   WD 308 M395p]
    RC607.A26M363   1991
    616.97 92—dc20
    DNLM/DLC
    For Library of Congress   91-34897
                                                                            CIP

92 93 94 95 GW/MY/MY 9 8 7 6 5 4 3 2 1

To the nurses, social workers, physicians, and staff of the Elmhurst Hospital Center AIDS team and to our patients.

Preface

The acquired immunodeficiency syndrome (AIDS) epidemic has brought with it unique and well-chronicled challenges. Information about how the disease spreads and about the human immunodeficiency virus, type 1 (HIV), the virus that causes AIDS, has accumulated at a bewildering rate, yet progress toward effective therapy has been frustratingly slow. For the public, concerns about contagion as well as the prejudice of some toward homosexual men and intravenous drug users, the prime targets of the epidemic in this country, have contributed to an atmosphere of sensationalism, confusion, and irrational fear. Mistrust of the medical establishment by many who are infected with HIV and by their advocates has often served to polarize discussion about such vital issues as HIV testing, contact tracing, and the design of clinical trials of new therapies.

Often lost in this tangle of uncertainty and controversy, however, is the disease itself. Although unique in its range of clinical manifestations, HIV infection ultimately requires the same approach by the clinician to medical reasoning as other chronic multisystem diseases. Stripped of emotionalism, politics, and of its sometimes bizarre glamour, HIV infection can be recognized by the clinician as a disorder to be diagnosed, characterized, and treated. The simple humanity of an empathetic physician-patient relationship can transcend AIDS hysteria and differences in life-style and can permit effective care, while enriching both parties.

In this book an attempt has been made to examine and discuss care of the HIV-infected person from a number of clinical perspectives and to provide to the clinician a framework for care in the ambulatory setting. In addition to information regarding pathogenesis and clinical manifestations of HIV infection, practical strategies for the evaluation and care of patients at all stages of disease are provided. Because much of the challenge of primary care medicine is in the interpretation of clinical signs and symptoms, several sections of the text are devoted to the diagnostic evaluation of common HIV-related clinical syndromes. The unique issues of HIV testing and counseling and HIV infection and pregnancy are discussed in separate chapters. Case studies to illustrate major clinical points are provided in the final chapter.

The care of the HIV-infected patient requires a compassionate, informed, logical, and methodical approach. This is, increasingly, the mission of the entire medical profession. It is hoped that this book is useful to all who are a part of this mission.

Joseph R. Masci

Contents

CHAPTER 1

Overview of the AIDS Epidemic

1

In the decade since it was first described, the acquired immunodeficiency syndrome (AIDS) has had a profound impact on both the practice of medicine and our understanding of the pathogenesis of disease. Formerly obscure opportunistic infections that once were the exclusive province of the infectious disease specialist have been made commonplace by AIDS and are now routinely diagnosed and treated on general medical wards. The complex functions of the immune system have been greatly clarified through research into this new disease. Insights gained in the fight against AIDS have added to our understanding of such diverse disorders as cancer, collagen-vascular disease, and dementia.

Of equal or greater importance, the AIDS epidemic has focused attention on the means by which health care is provided and the interaction between physician and patient. In the course of the medical community's evolving response to AIDS, legitimate questions have been raised about basic public health strategies, how medical care is provided to disadvantaged groups, the adequacy of acute and long-term care facilities in inner-city areas, fears of contagion among health care workers, the importance of patient confidentiality balanced against the need to inform contacts, and the conduct of clinical trials of new drugs.

The profound impact of AIDS reflects its unique medical and social implications. The immunological abnormalities that characterize the disease are of a type and severity that had rarely been seen before. In fact, the concept that an infectious disease could lead to relentless, irreversible destruction of the human immune system was not even part of conventional medical thinking before the AIDS epidemic. The etiologic agent of AIDS, the human immunodeficiency virus (HIV, HIV-1), itself belongs to a class of viruses that had only recently been recognized as a cause of human disease when it was linked to AIDS. The extent of organ system involvement and the number of clinical syndromes associated with HIV infection are also unprecedented.

In human terms, the AIDS epidemic has had a devastating and far-reaching effect, magnified because AIDS is a disease of the young. In New York City more than 60% of AIDS victims have been under 40 years of age, and almost 90% have been under age 50.[89] By 1986, the annual incidence of AIDS was comparable to the combined incidence of all cancers among male homosexuals and intravenous drug users.[33] As of 1991, AIDS is expected to be one of the five most common causes of death in women of childbearing age in the United States.[24]

Even mortality statistics, however, do not fully reflect the magnitude of the human impact of AIDS. Disruption of families; discrimination in housing, employment, and education; and numerous individual tragedies also have accompanied the epidemic. The strikingly high rate of suicide reported among HIV-infected patients[84] suggests that the mortality of the disease may be even higher than national statistics indicate.

AIDS has presented a complex challenge to the world medical community. The areas in which substantial progress has been made include discovery of the human immunodeficiency virus and its effects on the immune system; development and widespread use of accurate diagnostic tests for HIV infection; and development and refinement of therapies directed against both the virus itself and AIDS-related opportunistic infections and malignancies. The positive impact of educational campaigns to reduce HIV transmission and of antiviral therapy also has become clear.

Despite these advances, AIDS remains an incurable disease, and the epidemic continues to expand on a worldwide scale. The development of new approaches to combating the disease and to reducing its impact on society will present formidable obstacles for the forseeable future.

THE HISTORY OF THE AIDS EPIDEMIC

Although AIDS seemed to appear abruptly as a rare syndrome affecting a small number of homosexual men in the United States, it was soon recognized as a worldwide epidemic. By August 1990 more than a quarter of a million cases had been reported to public health authorities worldwide, and it was estimated that an additional 350,000 cases had gone unreported since the beginning of the epidemic in 1981.[1] More than 85,000 of approximately 140,000 patients reported in the United States had died.

The immediate impact of AIDS was felt in urban areas in the United States, where it quickly became a major cause of death among young adults, and in certain underdeveloped areas of the world, particularly central Africa, where the disease joined a long list of uncontrolled and devastating infections.

AIDS was first recognized when unusual infections and malignancies indicating immune system impairment were diagnosed in a small number of otherwise healthy homosexual men in New York and California.[15] It soon became apparent that a similar disorder was occurring among intravenous drug users, as well as some individuals with hemophilia and other recipients of blood or blood products.[16] Epidemiological data suggested a transmissible agent spread by sexual contact or blood exposure. Heterosexual partners of infected individuals, both male and female,[60,98] and children born to infected mothers[107] also were found to be at risk of developing AIDS. The disease steadily increased in incidence, and cases eventually were reported from every state in the United States and from many other regions of the world, particularly central Africa.[26,93]

The cause of AIDS was identified as a lymphotropic retrovirus[8,14,47,52,95] belonging to the lentivirus family,[3] a type of organism that had not previously been known to cause human disease. This virus was initially designated the human T-cell leukemia/lymphoma virus type III (HTLV-III) by researchers in the United States and lymphadenopathy-associated virus (LAV) by researchers in France. After it was established that HTLV-III and LAV were variants of the same virus,[97] the current designation, human immunodeficiency virus type 1 or HIV (HIV-1[27]), came into use. A related virus, HIV-2, also capable of causing immunodeficiency, was later isolated from some individuals, most of whom appeared to have become infected in western Africa.[25]

Identification of HIV-1 as the primary etiologic agent of AIDS permitted two important advances: the development of blood tests to identify infected individuals and antiviral therapy.

Methods for screening donated blood for antibody to HIV-1 were rapidly developed[117,120] and went into widespread use in the United States in early 1985. These blood tests were also used to gather information about the prevalence of HIV-1 infection in various segments of the population so that the extent and nature of the epidemic could be better characterized.

It soon became clear that most patients infected with HIV-1 had no symptoms of disease and that the prevalence of asymptomatic infection was extremely high among male homosexuals and intravenous drug users living in certain geographical areas. On the basis of such serological surveys and prospective and retrospective clinical data, it was recognized that the natural history of HIV-1 infection typically spans a period of years,[80] during which cellular immunity is gradually eroded. AIDS was simply the culmination of this process, the so-called tip of the iceberg.

Efforts to identify drugs with potential activity against HIV-1 and to evaluate the effect of antiviral therapy at various stages of HIV infection have steadily intensified. In 1986 azidothymidine (AZT, zidovudine), a nucleoside analog previously shown to have antiviral activity in vitro, was found to improve survival and decrease the frequency of opportunistic infections in a subset of patients with AIDS[40] and was subsequently licensed for use. In nationwide clinical trials, AZT was also found to be beneficial for HIV-infected patients who had not yet developed AIDS.[41] Clinical trials of other antiretroviral compounds such as dideoxyinosine (DDI)[28,38] and dideoxycytidine (DDC)[13,66] are currently under way, and a variety of other therapeutic approaches are being investigated.[62,123]

Research into the development of vaccines against HIV-1 also had begun yielding optimistic results by early 1990.[11]

THE HUMAN IMMUNODEFICIENCY VIRUS TYPE 1

A great deal of information about the structure, genetic composition, and biological behavior of HIV-1 has been gathered since it was identified as the etiologic agent of AIDS.[78]

Like other viruses, HIV-1 has a simple structure—a protein core containing genetic material surrounded by a lipid envelope. Genetic information is encoded in ribonucleic acid (RNA) rather than deoxyribonucleic acid (DNA) as in most other organisms. Three genes, designated gag, pol, and env,[6,100] determine the structural properties of the virus. The gag gene codes for the core proteins p15, p17, and p24; the pol gene codes for viral enzymes, including reverse transcriptase; and the env gene codes for envelope glycoproteins designated gp41 and gp120. At least six other gene products that regulate steps in the life cycle of HIV-1 are encoded by the genome, which is complex compared to that of other retroviruses.[114] This genetic complexity enables the virus to adapt to a variety of host environments.

HIV-1 is classified as a retrovirus because its replication requires the reverse transcription of RNA into DNA. Much of the viral life cycle has now been clarified.[70] Infection begins with the attachment of the virus to a receptor on the surface of the host cell. One such receptor,[81] designated T4 or CD4, is present on the surface of T-helper/inducer lymphocytes and a variety of other cells. After attachment, the virus is internalized by the cell, sheds its coat, and reverse transcribes its RNA into DNA by means of the viral enzyme reverse transcriptase. This DNA is incorporated, by means of the viral enzyme integrase, into the host cell DNA, where it remains as a latent infection for a variable period of time. This DNA of viral origin (proviral DNA) codes for the synthesis of the viral structural proteins and RNA. The third viral enzyme, protease, is necessary for the assembly of new viruses. A variety of human cells other than the T-helper/inducer (CD4) lymphocyte may be infected by HIV-1.[78] The implications of viral infection of various tissues are discussed in subsequent chapters in the context of clinical syndromes associated with HIV-1 infection.

There is significant genetic diversity among isolates of HIV-1 from different individuals[58] and from the same individual over time.[59] This variability among HIV-1 strains has complicated vaccine strategies.[48]

THE PATHOGENESIS OF AIDS AND RELATED SYNDROMES

The disorders directly resulting from infection by HIV-1 have been classified into immunodeficiency, infection of the central nervous system (CNS), and abnormal proliferation of certain cell lines.[48]

Immunological Abnormalities

The immunological abnormalities associated with AIDS are complex and reflect impairment of both the cellular[37,110] and humoral[74] immune systems. Central to the immunological lesion that characterizes AIDS is the functional impairment[75] and progressive depletion[37] of the subset of T-helper/inducer lymphocytes (CD4 or T4). The consequent steady weakening and eventual destruction of the cellular immune system leave the host susceptible to an array of otherwise unusual infections, including *Pneumocystis carinii* pneumonia, cryptococcal meningitis, cerebral toxoplasmosis, progressive herpes simplex, disseminated mycobacterial infection, and others, and malignancies, including Kaposi's sarcoma and lymphoma.

Antibody responses also are impaired by CD4 cell depletion and by a polyclonal B-cell activation characteristic of the syndrome. Deficient or abnormal antibody production is manifested as increased susceptibility to infections,[105] inadequate antibody response to certain vaccines,[7] and production of unusual autoantibodies.[72]

Other components of the immune system whose functions are altered by HIV-1 infection include natural killer cells,[12] which normally are cytotoxic to tumor and virus-infected cells, and macrophages.[51,103]

Central Nervous System Involvement

The central nervous system is a common and sometimes very early site of involvement of HIV-1 infection.[54] Histological evidence of direct infection of the brain was found in 90% of AIDS patients in one autopsy series,[45] and HIV-1 itself has been identified in brain tissue by a variety of techniques.[50,63,113] Aseptic meningitis may be seen as a component of symptomatic acute HIV-1 infection,[63] and a characteristic histopathological and clinical pattern called the AIDS dementia complex[87,88] has been recognized as a manifestation of chronic infection. HIV-related syndromes involving the central and peripheral nervous systems are discussed in greater detail in Chapter 5.

Cells within the central nervous system that may be infected by HIV-1 include macrophages,[71] capillary endothelial cells, astrocytes, and neurons.[57] It is not known whether HIV-1 enters the central nervous system within infected macrophages[51] or invades directly.

For reporting purposes, a diagnosis of HIV encephalopathy can be made if (1) there are clinical signs of cognitive or motor dysfunction severe enough to interfere with daily living or, in a child, there has been a loss of behavioral developmental milestones,[19] and (2) there is laboratory evidence of HIV-1 infection. Other conditions that may cause these symptoms must be excluded through examination of the cerebrospinal fluid and either brain imaging (computed tomography [CT] or magnetic resonance imaging [MRI]) or tissue examination.

Abnormal Cell Proliferation

Abnormal proliferation of certain cell lines accounts for two common manifestations of HIV-1 infection: lymphoma and Kaposi's sarcoma. AIDS-related lymphomas are typically B cell in origin[77] and, some believe, may result from the effects of chronic antigenic stimulation or concomitant infection with the Epstein-Barr virus or other cofactors.[48] Evidence has accumulated that Kaposi's sarcoma, a tumor involving blood vessels, spindle cells, and other cell lines, may result from growth-stimulating substances released from HIV-infected lymphocytes.[48]

HIGH-RISK GROUPS AND MEANS OF HIV TRANSMISSION

Three routes of transmission of HIV-1 infection are recognized:
1. Inoculation of infected blood, blood products, or blood-containing material, either transdermally or onto mucous membrane surfaces
2. Heterosexual or homosexual intercourse
3. Perinatal transmission

Epidemiological data and clinical investigations have failed to implicate nonsexual personal contact[44] or insect vectors[90] in HIV-1 transmission, and there is no evidence indicating airborne, foodborne, or waterborne spread.

On a worldwide basis, HIV-1 infection is primarily a sexually transmitted disease, although the relative importance of heterosexual and homosexual transmission varies dramatically among geographical regions. In the United States and Europe, AIDS has been predominantly a disease of male homosexuals, and as a result females have accounted for fewer than 10% of reported cases.[21] In contrast, in central Africa[93] heterosexual intercourse is a far more common route of transmission, and the male-to-female ratio of cases is nearly equal.

In the United States, where the extent of the epidemic has been well characterized, male homosexuals and intravenous drug users have consistently accounted for over 90% of new AIDS cases reported annually.[21] In addition, serological studies have indicated a high rate of asymptomatic HIV infection among male homosexuals and intravenous drug users living in areas within the United States where the incidence of AIDS is highest.[69] This pattern has been attributed to relatively efficient transmission of HIV infection in these groups.

The importance of these primary risk groups is further illustrated by two other statistics:

- Approximately 80% of AIDS cases in women in the United States have resulted directly from intravenous drug use or from heterosexual contact with male intravenous drug users or bisexuals.[21]
- Approximately 60% of children with AIDS have been born to women who had a history of intravenous drug use or heterosexual contact with a high-risk male.[21]

During the first decade of the epidemic, the proportion of AIDS cases in the United States attributed to intravenous drug use steadily increased, whereas the proportion of new HIV infections among male homosexuals decreased.[9]

Male Homosexuals

The exact mode of transmission of HIV infection between male homosexual partners is not clear. However, the virus has been isolated from semen, and it is assumed that transmission results from the deposition of fluid containing viable virus on mucosal surfaces after anal and perhaps after oral intercourse.[10,91] Among homosexual men the likelihood of HIV-1 infection has been shown to correlate positively with the number of sexual partners[112] and to be highest in those who give a history of receptive rectal intercourse or douching.[112,121] A history of syphilis has been shown to be associated with an increased likelihood of HIV-1 infection in both homosexual and heterosexual men attending a clinic for individuals with sexually transmitted diseases.[96]

Heterosexual Partners

Heterosexual intercourse appears to be the most common mode of transmission of HIV-1 infection worldwide.[43] Nevertheless, the efficiency with which the infection is spread by this route is relatively low[64] when compared to other sexually-transmitted diseases.

In the United States, the vast majority of AIDS cases among heterosexuals has occurred in individuals belonging to established high-risk groups, such as intravenous drug users or recipients of blood transfusions. In approximately 5% of reported cases, however, heterosexual intercourse appears to have been the route of HIV transmission.[21]

The mechanism by which HIV is transmitted during heterosexual activity is not fully known, although the virus has been isolated from semen,[124] saliva,[56] and vaginal secretions.[122] Heterosexual spread occurs both from male to female[61,73] and from female to male.[98]

Several factors may increase the likelihood of HIV-1 transmission.[64] These include the presence of genital ulcers,[55,111] lack of circumcision in men,[108] the use of birth control pills, trauma during intercourse, and menstruation. Specific host properties such as human leukocyte antigen (HLA) haplotype and the presence of a CD4 receptor[64] are also factors.

Intravenous Drug Users

The prevalence of HIV-1 infection and the incidence of reported AIDS cases among intravenous drug users (IVDU) vary with geographical location, even within the United States.[43] The route of transmission of infection among intravenous drug users is presumed to be the mixing of blood that occurs when drug paraphernalia is shared, and the likelihood of infection has been shown to correlate with the number of injections with contaminated needles.[106] Neither the type of drug injected nor specific preparation and administration practices are known to affect HIV transmission.

Perinatal Transmission

Most pediatric AIDS cases result from transmission of HIV-1 infection from mother to child. Transmission potentially could occur before, during, or after birth, although only intrauterine infection[83] has been well documented. HIV-1 has been isolated from the breast milk of infected women,[115] and breast-feeding may have resulted in transmission in one reported case.[125] The risk of transmission of HIV-1 infection from mother to child has been reported to be as high as 65%,[17] although recent prospective data indicate that the risk may be substantially lower.[5] Studies have failed to demonstrate transmission of HIV-1 infection between infected young children and their household contacts.[101]

Transmission by Blood and Blood Products

Whole blood, packed red blood cells, platelets, clotting factors, and frozen plasma all appear to have served as vehicles for HIV transmission.[32,67,92] Patients with classic hemophilia receiving factor VIII replacement therapy from pooled donors were particularly at risk for HIV-1 infection in the early years of the AIDS epidemic.[34,65] The risk of transfusion-associated HIV infection has been substantially reduced in the United States since uniform screening of donated blood began in 1985, but AIDS cases attributed to transfusion continue to be reported because of the long incubation of the disease. In addition, HIV-1 transmission by this route has not been completely eliminated because of the false negative rate of current screening tests.[118]

DEFINITIONS

Much of the terminology used to describe and categorize HIV-1 infection came into use before the virus was discovered and therefore is somewhat arbitrary. Central to the disorder caused by HIV-1 is a gradual weakening of the immune system, culminating in the development of secondary infections and malignancies. Some of the infections, such as *P. carinii* pneumonia or cerebral toxoplasmosis, are almost never seen in immunologically normal hosts. Other infections, such as tuberculosis and herpes zoster, are more common in patients with impaired immunity but may also be seen with normal host defenses.

The following definitions reflect the fact that in the early stages of the epidemic, only individuals with secondary infections or malignancies strongly indicative of immune deficiency were recognized to be victims of the disease.

Acquired Immunodeficiency Syndrome

Acquired immunodeficiency syndrome (AIDS) is the most serious manifestation of infection with the human immunodeficiency virus. A diagnosis of AIDS is made when any of a number of infections or malignancies usually associated with impaired cellular immunity (so-called indicator diseases[19]) occurs in an individual who has no known immunocompromising disease and who is not receiving immunodepressing medications. This case definition, which was established before the discovery of HIV-1, has proven very effective in excluding unrelated conditions and has permitted accurate tracking of the epidemic.

It is anticipated that the case definition of AIDS may be expanded in early 1992 to include all adults and adolescents with proven HIV and CD4 lymphocyte counts less than $200/mm^3$. Indicator diseases diagnostic for AIDS are listed in the boxes on pp. 11 and 12.

It has long been clear, however, that most individuals infected with HIV do not meet even the expanded criteria for a diagnosis of AIDS, and a wide variety of other clinical syndromes associated with HIV-1 infection is now recognized. The terms AIDS-related complex (ARC), suspected AIDS, pre-AIDS, and lymphadenopathy syndrome (LAS) or persistent generalized lymphadenopathy (PGL) all have been applied to symptomatic patients infected with HIV who do not meet the clinical criteria for a diagnosis of AIDS.

AIDS-Related Complex (ARC)

The term "AIDS-related complex (ARC)" was coined shortly after the AIDS epidemic began, in order to characterize a combination of nonspecific signs

---

Surveillance Definition of AIDS (Adults): I. Indicator Diseases* Diagnostic of AIDS if HIV Antibody Status is Positive or Unknown[19]

Opportunistic infections

Candidal infection of the esophagus,† trachea, bronchi, or lungs
Extrapulmonary cryptococcal infection
Cryptosporidiosis with diarrhea lasting longer than 1 month
Cytomegalovirus retinitis with vision loss†
Cytomegalovirus infection involving sites other than the liver, spleen, or lymph nodes
Mucocutaneous herpes simplex infection with ulcer present longer than 1 month
Herpes simplex infection of the esophagus, lungs, or bronchi
Disseminated infection with *Mycobacterium avium-intracellulare* or *Mycobacterium kansasii* involving sites other than the lungs, skin, or cervical or hilar lymph nodes†
Pneumocystis carinii pneumonia†
Progressive multifocal leukoencephalopathy
Cerebral toxoplasmosis†

Malignancies

Kaposi's sarcoma in a patient under 60 years of age†
Primary lymphoma of the brain in a patient under 60 years of age

From Centers for Disease Control: Revision of the CDC surveillance case definition for acquired immunodeficiency syndrome, *MMWR* 1S-4S, 1987.
*Confirmed diagnosis in the absence of other explanation for immunodeficiency.
†Diagnosis may be presumptive.

---

and symptoms associated with HIV-1 infection that occurred without AIDS-defining opportunistic infections or malignancies.[4]

Clinical features associated with ARC include lymphadenopathy, fever, night sweats, or diarrhea occurring intermittently or continuously for at least 3 months, and fatigue and/or loss of at least 15 pounds or 10% of body weight. Laboratory abnormalities include decreased CD4 lymphocyte count, leukopenia, thrombocytopenia, anemia or lymphopenia, elevated serum globulins, abnormal skin tests of delayed type hypersensitivity, and/or laboratory evidence of decreased blastogenesis.[4]

The definition of ARC is thus broad, and the term encompasses a great spectrum of HIV-related illness ranging from mild fatigue and asymptomatic lymphadenopathy to severe diarrhea and profound weight loss. For this reason, the term led to diagnostic confusion, and it often is used as a nonspecific description of symptomatic HIV infection not meeting the case definition of AIDS. The term "ARC" has been rendered less applicable by the use of im-

Surveillance Definition* of AIDS (Adults): II. Additional Indicator Diseases Diagnostic of AIDS Only With Laboratory Evidence of HIV Infection[19]

HIV encephalopathy (see text)
HIV wasting syndrome (see text)

Opportunistic infections

Disseminated histoplasmosis at a site other than the lungs or cervical or hilar lymph nodes
Disseminated coccidioidomycosis at a site other than the lungs or cervical or hilar lymph nodes
Isosporiasis with diarrhea of more than 1 month's duration
Any atypical mycobacterial infection at site other than lungs, skin, cervical or hilar lymph nodes
Mycobacterium tuberculosis infection at any extrapulmonary site
Recurrent nontyphoid salmonella bacteremia

Malignancies

Kaposi's sarcoma at any age
Primary lymphoma of the brain at any age
Small noncleaved lymphoma
Immunoblastic sarcoma

From Centers for Disease Control: Revision of the CDC surveillance case definition for acquired immunodeficiency syndrome, *MMWR* 36:1S-4S, 1987.
*The definition may be expanded in early 1992 to include patients with CD4 lymphocyte counts of less than 200/mm³.

Surveillance Definition of Pediatric AIDS[19]

With laboratory evidence of HIV infection

Recurrent septicemia,* pneumonia, meningitis, bone or joint infection, or abscess of an internal organ or body cavity caused by *Haemophilus* or *Streptococcus* organisms or by other pyogenic bacteria
Herpes simplex infection of the esophagus, lungs, or bronchi†
Cerebral toxoplasmosis†
Cytomegalovirus infection of an organ other than the liver, spleen, or lymph nodes†
Any other condition listed in the box above

Without laboratory evidence of HIV infection

Lymphoid interstitial pneumonia and/or pulmonary lymphoid hyperplasia‡ (confirmed or presumptive diagnosis)
Any other condition listed in the box on p. 11

From Centers for Disease Control: Revision of the CDC surveillance case definition for acquired immunodeficiency syndrome, *MMWR* 36:1S-4S, 1987.
*Two or more episodes within 2 years.
†In a patient over 1 month of age.
‡In a patient under 13 years of age.

munological parameters to stage HIV infection more precisely. Nevertheless, since many HIV-infected patients have the clinical features of ARC, recognition of this complex may lead to an early diagnosis and permit therapeutic interventions before the onset of AIDS.

A diagnosis of HIV wasting syndrome (an AIDS-defining condition) may be made in cases of involuntary loss of more than 10% of the baseline body weight plus either diarrhea or weakness and fever for at least 30 days if there is laboratory evidence of HIV-1 infection.[19]

Persistent Generalized Lymphadenopathy (PGL)

Generalized, nonspecific enlargement of lymph nodes is a common sign of HIV-1 infection among individuals at risk and may be present for years before AIDS-defining opportunistic infections or malignancies develop. The term "persistent generalized lymphadenopathy (PGL)" currently is used to describe HIV-1–related lymph node enlargement lasting at least 3 months at two or more extrainguinal sites. The prognosis of patients with PGL who are otherwise asymptomatic appears to be similar to that of completely asymptomatic HIV-infected individuals. In prospective studies,[29] 10% to 15% of individuals with PGL progress to AIDS within 24 to 36 months.

Asymptomatic HIV-Positive Individuals

Individuals with documented HIV-1 infection but with no history of AIDS-defining opportunistic infections or malignancies and no signs or symptoms compatible with ARC are classified as asymptomatic. As will be discussed in subsequent chapters, a wide spectrum of HIV-related clinical disorders have been described that do not meet the criteria for AIDS or ARC. The relative prognostic significance of these disorders (e.g., seborrheic dermatitis, Reiter's-like syndrome, autoimmune thrombocytopenia) is not clear.

STAGING SYSTEMS

In recent years, efforts have been made to replace nonspecific terms such as ARC with clearly defined clinical and laboratory staging criteria for HIV-related illness and thereby improve diagnostic precision.

The recognition that HIV-1 infection causes a gradual deterioration of immune functions whose end point is AIDS has led to efforts to stratify patients according to their degree of immunodeficiency. Such stratification systems have proved valuable both in the practical management of HIV-infected patients and in designing clinical trials of new therapeutic agents. For example, it has been recognized that *P. carinii* pneumonia and other AIDS-related opportunistic infections are typically seen only in patients with laboratory ev-

TABLE 1-1.   The Walter Reed staging classification for HIV infection[98]

Stage	Characteristics
WR 0	Individuals at high risk of HIV infection without documentation of infection; CD4 lymphocyte count over 400/mm³; normal delayed hypersensitivity; no thrush or opportunistic infection
WR 1	Asymptomatic patients with documented HIV-1 infection; CD4 lymphocyte count over 400/mm³; normal delayed hypersensitivity; no thrush or opportunistic infections
WR 2	Documented HIV infection; chronic lymphadenopathy; CD4 count over 400/mm³; normal delayed hypersensitivity; no thrush or opportunistic infections
WR 3	Documented HIV infection; CD4 count under 400/mm³; normal delayed hypersensitivity; no thrush or opportunistic infections
WR 4	Documented HIV infection; CD4 count under 400/mm³; partial skin test anergy; no thrush or opportunistic infections
WR 5	Documented HIV infection; CD4 count under 400/mm³; complete skin test anergy or thrush; no opportunistic infections
WR 6	Documented HIV infection; CD4 count under 400/mm³; partial or complete skin test anergy; documented opportunistic infection

From Redfield RR, Wright CD, Tramont EC: The Walter Reed staging classification for HTLV-III/LAV infection, *N Engl J Med* 314:131-132, 1986.

idence of severe impairment of cellular immunity. This fact can be of great help to the clinician attempting to interpret symptoms of respiratory disease in a patient known to be HIV-infected if immunological staging has been carried out. In the development of new antiretroviral drugs and prophylactic therapy against opportunistic infections, immunological staging has permitted identification of patients at greatest risk of progression to AIDS, allowing quicker assessment of clinical benefit.

Several systems for staging HIV infection have been proposed. The two most commonly used are the Walter Reed staging classification[98] (Table 1-1) and the Centers for Disease Control classification system (Table 1-2).[18]

THE PROGNOSIS OF HIV-1 INFECTION AND AIDS

AIDS is the culmination and most severe manifestation of infection with HIV-1. It is estimated that AIDS occurs after 7 years in 50% of infected individuals and by 15 years in 78% to 100%.[9] Prospective studies have indicated that 10% to 15% of HIV-1–infected patients who are either asymptomatic or manifest only generalized lymphadenopathy and 40% of symptomatic patients will progress to AIDS within 36 months.[29]

Long-term survival after the onset of AIDS is rare. More than 55% of 82,674 AIDS patients reported in the United States since the beginning of the epidemic

TABLE 1-2. Centers for Disease Control staging classification[18]

Group	Definition
I	Acute infection (symptoms and documented seroconversion)
II	Asymptomatic infection
III	Persistent generalized lymphadenopathy
IVA	Chronic constitutional disease
IVB	Neurological disease
IVC1	HIV-related secondary infection (see infections listed in Table 1-1)
IVC2	HIV-related secondary infection (including oral hairy leukoplakia, multidermatomal herpes zoster, oral candidiasis, recurrent *Salmonella* bacteremia, tuberculosis, *Nocardia* infection)
IVD	HIV-related secondary malignancies (Kaposi's sarcoma, non-Hodgkins lymphoma, including small, noncleaved lymphoma and immunoblastic sarcoma, primary lymphoma of the brain)
IVE	Other HIV-related conditions

in 1981 had died of the disease by 1989.[9] The median estimated survival time among AIDS patients in New York City was 10.5 months by the end of 1985.[102] Mathematical projections indicate that 365,000 AIDS cases will have been diagnosed in the United States by the end of 1992, and that 263,000 (72%) of these individuals will have died.[21]

The poor prognosis of AIDS has also been illustrated in several prospective studies. The projected probability of survival at 6 months among AIDS patients not receiving antiretroviral therapy was 76% in an early clinical trial of the drug azidothymidine (AZT).[40] In a prospective cohort study, the median survival of patients with AIDS was found to be 11.2 months.[76]

The full impact of antiretroviral drugs and other therapeutic measures on the prognosis of AIDS is not yet clear, although improved survival has been demonstrated in some patients receiving AZT[31,40] and some forms of prophylaxis against *P. carinii* pneumonia,[39] the most common initial opportunistic infection in AIDS.

THE EXTENT OF THE HIV EPIDEMIC

The precise extent of the HIV-1 epidemic is not known. Although national and international surveillance efforts have provided some information, these studies have focused primarily on AIDS, the end point of HIV infection, rather than asymptomatic HIV infection or other earlier stages of disease. Estimates of the incidence of all forms of HIV infection have been made on the basis of seroprevalence studies of HIV infection in selected populations. Despite the lack of complete information, an increasingly clear picture of the magnitude

of the epidemic has emerged through calculations based on known seroprevalence data and mathematical models.

Reported AIDS Cases

In the United States, national surveillance of AIDS has been conducted, under
the auspices of the Centers for Disease Control (CDC), since shortly after the
epidemic began in 1981. This surveillance program that tabulates only cases
that meet the CDC definition of AIDS (see the boxes on pp. 11 and 12). Through
the end of 1988, both the number of AIDS cases reported and the rate of new
cases increased each year.[21] By August 1990 the total number of cases reported
in the United States since the beginning of the epidemic had reached approximately 140,000.[1] By the end of April 1991 the number of adult cases had
reached 171,865.[23a] (See Figures 1-1 to 1-3.)

Reporting of AIDS cases through this mechanism has not been complete,
however. Surveys have indicated that in some areas of the country, as few as
60% of known AIDS cases had been reported to public health authorities.[21]
Underreporting is particularly common in states with a low prevalence of HIV
infection.[21]

Throughout the first 10 years of the epidemic, most AIDS cases in the United
States had been reported among male homosexuals, although the proportion
accounted for by this group had fallen from 69% to 59% by 1991.[21,22,23a] Intravenous drug users accounted for 15% to 22% of reported cases, and an addi-

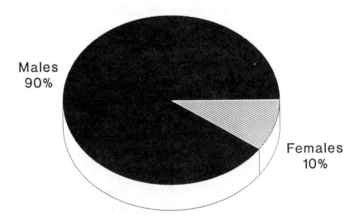

FIGURE 1-1. Adult U.S. AIDS cases by sex distribution. (Total U.S. cases: 171,865.)

From CDC HIV/AIDS Surveillance, May, 1991.

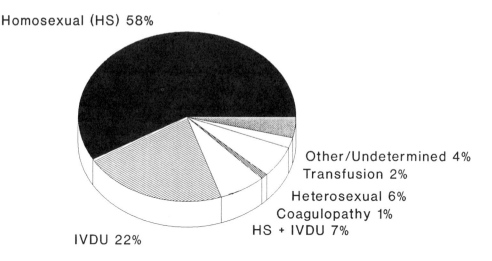

FIGURE 1-2. Adult U.S. AIDS cases: risk groups through April, 1991. (Total cases: 171,865.)

From CDC HIV/AIDS Surveillance, May, 1991.

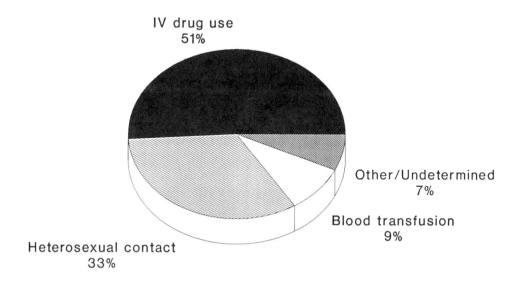

FIGURE 1-3. Adult female U.S. AIDS cases by risk group. (Total cases: 17,200.)

From CDC HIV/AIDS Surveillance, May, 1991.

tional group of males giving a history of both homosexuality and intravenous drug use accounted for 7% to 10%. The remainder of the distribution by risk groups through 1991 was as follows: recipients of contaminated blood, 1% to 2%; hemophiliacs, 1%; heterosexual contacts, 6%; individuals born in countries where HIV is transmitted predominantly by the heterosexual route, 1% to 3%; undetermined cause, 2% to 4%.[23a]

Number of Individuals Infected with HIV

A variety of methods have been used to estimate the number of individuals in the United States who are infected with HIV-1. Calculations performed in the 1980s based on the known seroprevalence of HIV-1 infection in some populations of high-risk individuals, particularly homosexual and bisexual men, intravenous drug users, and hemophiliacs, and on the background infection rates in blood donors, military recruits, and other large populations, led to estimates ranging from under 1 million to 1.5 million.[23] Currently the rate at which the number of HIV-infected individuals is increasing is unclear.[86]

Precise statistics are not available on the number of individuals who are infected with HIV-1, whether symptomatic or asymptomatic, but who do not meet clinical criteria for the diagnosis of AIDS. The size of this population must be estimated as described above, because HIV-1 testing is generally voluntary and because there is no uniform national reporting policy for cases of HIV infection not meeting the AIDS case definition.

Data reported by Polk and colleagues[94] give an indication of the proportion of HIV-infected individuals who do not have AIDS but who manifest HIV-related symptoms. Of 1,835 HIV-positive homosexual men enrolled in a prospective study, 35% were initially classified as asymptomatic, 60% had generalized lymphadenopathy, and 5% had symptoms of ARC. These proportions may not be applicable to individuals in other high-risk groups or to patients not enrolled in voluntary studies. It is important to note, nonetheless, that most patients had either no symptoms at all or only lymphadenopathy. National and New York City estimates in the 1980s indicated that there were sevenfold to tenfold more patients with ARC than with full-blown AIDS.[119]

A large proportion of HIV-1–infected patients who do not meet clinical criteria for the diagnosis of AIDS manifest significant degrees of immunosuppression on immunological profiling with lymphocyte subset analysis. It is estimated that more than half of all HIV-1–infected patients have abnormally low CD4 lymphocyte counts.[36] Two thirds of 72 asymptomatic HIV-positive patients identified at an anonymous testing site in New York City had evidence of significant immunodeficiency.[85]

Geographical Distribution of HIV-Infected Individuals in the United States

Cases of AIDS have been reported from each of the 50 states, although the incidence through 1988 varied from 0.6 cases per 100,000 persons in North Dakota to 81.2 cases per 100,000 in the District of Columbia.[21] This pattern of distribution has changed somewhat since the beginning of the epidemic. Before 1983, 63% of AIDS cases were reported from New York, New Jersey, or Pennsylvania; by 1988 only 32% of cases were reported from those states.[21]

Recent HIV-1 seroprevalence studies have provided a more complete picture of the regional patterns of HIV-1 infection. In the largest such study, the Sentinel Hospital Surveillance Project, conducted by the Centers for Disease Control, more than 89,000 blood samples from 26 hospitals in 21 states representing all regions of the country were screened.[104] Prevalence rates ranged from more than 5% at hospitals in Newark, New Jersey, and the Bronx, New York, to less than 1% in most hospitals in the Midwest and West. It is noteworthy, however, that HIV infection was detected among patients at every hospital surveyed.

Distribution of HIV-1 Infection by Sex

In the United States, more than 90% of AIDS patients reported through the end of 1988 were men; however, the proportion of women rose from 7% to 10% in annual statistics during the first 7 years of the epidemic.[21] Serological surveys to detect unsuspected HIV infection have indicated an overall male-to-female ratio of 7:1.[104] HIV-1 infection among women is most common in areas of the country with high overall seroprevalence, such as the Northeast.[104] In fact, the male-to-female ratio was as low as 2.4:1 among infected individuals between 25 and 44 years of age living in the inner city areas of highest prevalence in this survey.

Distribution of HIV-1 Infection by Race

In statistics compiled through the end of 1988, the incidence of AIDS was more than two-and-one-half times higher in Hispanics and more than three times higher in blacks than in whites in the United States.[21] Seroprevalence studies have demonstrated an overall ratio of HIV prevalence of 1.8:1 between blacks and whites,[104] with higher ratios in areas of the country reporting high proportions of AIDS cases related to intravenous drug use.

Distribution of HIV-1 Infection by Age

Through early 1991, 98% of AIDS cases had occurred in adults,[21,23a] most of them (68%) in men between 25 and 44 years of age. Serological surveys have shown a similar age distribution for HIV-1 infection, with 69% of HIV-infected patients being men in the same age group.

PREDICTED TRENDS IN THE AIDS EPIDEMIC

The future course of the HIV-1/AIDS epidemic will be dictated by a number of variables, some of which are not well understood at present. These variables include the number of individuals currently infected, the natural history of HIV-1–related illness, patterns of transmission, behavioral changes in response to the disease, and progress toward effective therapy and a vaccine.

It has been predicted that the annual incidence of AIDS cases in the primary risk groups (i.e., homosexual and bisexual men, intravenous drug users, their heterosexual partners, recipients of blood and blood products, and children born to infected mothers) will continue to increase through 1993 and that between 61,000 and 98,000 new cases of AIDS will be diagnosed in the United States during 1993.[23]

The annual incidence of new HIV-1 infections in the general population is unknown. Large, prospective studies of active duty military personnel[49,82] point to an incidence of between 0.28 and 0.77 new infections per 1,000 persons per year. However, the validity of applying these data to the general population is not clear. It has been pointed out that, since the military actively discourages homosexuality and intravenous drug use, these incidence rates may be somewhat lower than those of the general population.

The impact of antiviral drugs such as zidovudine (AZT) and other changes in therapy has been difficult to gauge. It has been noted that reported cases of AIDS began to fall below predicted levels among homosexual and bisexual men in the United States during 1987.[21] It appears that improvements in therapy account to some extent for this trend.[46]

THE IMPACT OF AIDS ON THE HEALTH CARE SYSTEM

The AIDS epidemic has had a profound impact on health care systems in regions of the United States where the incidence of AIDS is highest. By the mid-1980s, 5% of all acute care hospital beds in New York City were occupied by patients with AIDS.[119] A steadily increasing need for hospital beds can be predicted from seroprevalence data, which indicate that more than half of intravenous drug users in the borough of Manhattan[35] and as many as 20% of all male patients between 25 and 44 years of age in some inner city areas[104] are infected with HIV-1. Based on trends seen in the first 10 years of the epidemic, it is estimated that 40,000 AIDS patients will be living in New York City in 1991[2] and that hospital bed occupancy by patients with HIV-1–related illness will reach 25% to 50% in the 1990s.[119]

For many patients, particularly those with advanced disease, hospital stays may be frequent and prolonged. Early in the epidemic, it was estimated that the mean length of initial hospitalization was 31 days and that 35% of surviving patients were hospitalized more than half of the subsequent time.[60] The estimated lifetime cost of hospitalization for an individual with AIDS averaged $147,000.[60]

The health care crisis created by the AIDS epidemic goes beyond the increased demand for inpatient services, however. AIDS patients who recover during their initial hospitalization require ongoing ambulatory care. Since such patients remain at high risk for AIDS-related infections and malignancies and typically require several forms of potentially toxic maintenance therapy, their care necessitates frequent outpatient visits. In addition, as HIV-1 testing efforts have been expanded, an increasing number of infected individuals are seeking medical care in an asymptomatic or early symptomatic stage of the disease. Since therapy at an early stage may slow the progression to AIDS and prolong survival,[41] these patients also require sophisticated outpatient care.

As a result of these trends, improved ambulatory care services for patients at all stages of HIV-related illness have been proposed as a partial solution to the crisis the epidemic poses to the health care system.[42] Efficient outpatient care has been shown to decrease the frequency and cost of hospitalization of patients with advanced disease[68] and may provide an opportunity for effective early intervention in those with early disease.[42] However, questions remain about the means by which ambulatory care services are to be expanded.

Although the need for primary care physicians in the treatment of HIV-infected patients is clear, the source of such physicians is not.[30] Subspecialists trained in infectious diseases or oncology are frequently involved in the care of symptomatic patients, but the number of professionals in these fields is inadequate to provide for the primary care needs of patients at all stages of HIV infection. General internists and other primary care physicians often lack the necessary expertise to provide the complex care needed by HIV-infected patients with multisystem disease.[79,109] Recognition of these personnel and educational problems has led to calls for programs of specific training in HIV-related disease for primary care physicians.[30]

The major impact of the AIDS epidemic has been felt by groups who traditionally are disenfranchised and do not have ready access to the health care system. Homosexual and bisexual men, intravenous drug users and their heterosexual partners, and children continue to account for the majority of patients with AIDS and other forms of symptomatic HIV infection. Black and Hispanic members of these high-risk groups are disproportionately represented among the HIV-infected as well.[21] Patients who have been diagnosed with AIDS often lack personal support networks sufficient to deal with the numerous emotional and financial obstacles they face. They often do not have easy access to primary care when symptoms first appear and thus seek medical care only when the disease is far advanced. Coordinated care programs to address these problems[42] have been proposed and will be discussed in detail in subsequent sections of this book.

TRENDS IN THE MEDICAL APPROACH TO HIV INFECTION

The medical management of all stages of HIV-related disease is discussed in detail in subsequent chapters. Important trends in the approach to diagnosis and treatment are highlighted here.

Early Detection and Intervention

Although HIV infection currently is incurable, cogent arguments can be made for early detection.[42] Antiretroviral therapy has been shown to prolong survival in HIV-1–infected patients before the onset of symptoms,[41,116] and appropriate immunizations[20] and primary prophylaxis against certain HIV-related opportunistic infections are also beneficial.[39] Early detection of HIV infection may also make it possible to achieve an effective reduction in risk behavior and facilitate early contact notification.

Expanded Voluntary HIV-1 Testing

The benefits of early detection of HIV-1 infection have intensified calls for broad-based screening programs. The results of general and directed HIV-1 screening surveys of various segments of the population for HIV-1 infection are discussed in detail in Chapter 3.

Reporting Requirements and Contact Tracing

Shortly after nationwide surveillance of AIDS began in the United States, individual states began establishing reporting guidelines. Currently, all 50 states require that health authorities be notified of each case of AIDS as defined by the CDC case definition (see pp. 11 and 12).[53] In addition some states require that HIV-positive test results be reported.[53] Reporting requirements have changed in many states during the course of the AIDS epidemic. Local health authorities should be consulted for updated information in this area.

Clinical Trials

In the United States, a nationwide program of clinical trials of new therapeutic agents began during the 1980s under the auspices of the National Institutes of Health. Some investigational drugs have been made available through expanded-access programs for patients not enrolled in randomized trials. These programs are discussed in detail in Chapter 10.

Comprehensive Systems of Care

Dedicated inpatient and ambulatory units have been created in some centers to provide care for HIV-infected patients. Such units may allow for better coordination of medical, nursing, and psychiatric care and social services and may facilitate clinical trials of new therapeutic agents and other forms of research.

THE ROLE OF THE GENERAL INTERNIST IN THE CARE OF HIV-INFECTED PATIENTS

Since the AIDS epidemic entered its second decade, a myriad of clinical disorders reflecting opportunistic infections that were not initially recognized as related to HIV infection have been described. In addition, the direct effects of HIV infection on various organ systems, most notably the central nervous system, the kidneys, the skin, the gastrointestinal tract, and the cardiovascular system, have been increasingly appreciated. HIV-1 infection is now recognized as a multisystem disease that may manifest one or more end-organ syndromes long before the onset of true AIDS-defining opportunistic infections or malignancies. Therefore patients with a great many specific symptom complexes that are not initially recognized to be related to HIV infection may seek care from a general internist.

The ability to recognize clinical syndromes as potentially related to HIV-1 infection and the willingness and ability to elicit meaningful histories regarding HIV risk behavior before the onset of AIDS are becoming increasingly important skills for general internists. Although this is especially true of those practicing in areas where HIV-1 prevalence is high and those working with high-risk patients, a general familiarity with HIV-related disorders, as well as laws and policies regarding HIV testing, is important for all practitioners.

During the first decade of the epidemic, AIDS primarily affected young adults. As the number of symptomatic patients seeking medical care continues to grow and as antiviral therapy and other treatment strategies improve longevity, conventional medical problems not related to HIV-1 infection increasingly may be seen in this population. General internists may be called upon by their subspecialty colleagues to assist in the management of hypertension, diabetes mellitus, coronary artery disease, and the host of common and unusual general medical problems afflicting adults.

THE ROLE OF SUBSPECIALISTS IN THE CARE OF HIV-INFECTED PATIENTS

Because HIV-1 infection and its complications can affect any organ system, specialists working in areas of high prevalence may encounter HIV-infected patients in their practice. Practicing dermatologists, neurologists, hematologists, oncologists, gastroenterologists, gynecologists, and psychiatrists, in particular, may see increasing numbers of HIV-related disorders. In some cases they may be called upon to fulfill the primary care needs of these patients as well. Only through a general understanding of the breadth of HIV-related illness, which has been described, and of therapeutic options will they be equipped to offer their patients optimum care.

CONCLUSION

Ten years into the AIDS epidemic, a tremendous amount of information has been gathered about the human immunodeficiency virus and the clinical features, immunology, and epidemiology of HIV infection. Therapeutic agents are now available, some active against the virus and others effective in the treatment and prevention of AIDS-related opportunistic infections. The disease, however, remains fatal. HIV-1 infection continues to spread, despite increasing public awareness. Heterosexual spread, particularly to female sexual partners of male intravenous drug users, is becoming an increasingly important route of transmission, and the pediatric HIV-1 epidemic continues to parallel the adult epidemic. Progress toward a vaccine has been frustrated by the complexity of the virus and the host immune reponse that it elicits.

As the epidemic continues to expand, the number of symptomatic and asymptomatic patients in need of care is mounting. The impact on the health care system in areas of high prevalence has been formidable, and long-term solutions that would provide for adequate care of HIV-infected individuals from all socioeconomic backgrounds and at all stages of disease are not yet apparent.

REFERENCES

1. AIDS Clinical Care, 2:77-83, 1990.
2. Alderman MH et al: Predicting the future of the AIDS epidemic and its consequences for the health care system of New York City, *Bull NY Acad Med* 64(2):175-183, 1988.
3. Alizon M, Montagnier L: Lymphadenopathy/AIDS virus: genetic organization and relationship to animal lentiviruses, *Anticancer Res* 6(3B):403-411, 1986.
4. Allen JR, Curran JW: Epidemiology of the acquired immunodeficiency syndrome. In Gallin JI, Fauci AS, editors: *Advances in host defense mechanisms*, vol 5, New York, 1985, Raven Press.
5. Andiman WA et al: Rate of transmission of human immunodeficiency virus type 1 infection from mother to child and short-term outcome of neonatal infection: results of a prospective cohort study, *Am J Dis Child* 144(7):758-766, 1990.
6. Arya SK et al: Homology of genome

of AIDS-associated virus with genomes of human T-cell leukemia viruses, *Science* 225(4665):927-930, 1984.

7. Barkowsky W et al: Antibody responses to bacterial toxoids in children infected with human immunodeficiency virus, *J Pediatr* 110(4):563-566, 1987.

8. Barre-Sinoussi F et al: Isolation of a T-lymphotropic retrovirus from a patient at risk for acquired immune deficiency syndrome (AIDS), *Science* 220(4599):868-871, 1983.

9. Berkelman RL et al: Epidemiology of human immunodeficiency virus infection and acquired immunodeficiency syndrome, *Am J Med* 86(6 part 2):761-770, 1989.

10. Bernard J et al: HTLV-III in cells cultured from semen from two patients with AIDS, *Science* 226:449-454, 1984.

11. Bolognesi DP: Progress in vaccine development against SIV and HIV, *J Acquir Immune Defic Syndr* 3(4):390-394, 1990.

12. Brenner BG et al: Natural killer cell function in patients with acquired immunodeficiency syndrome and related diseases, *J Leukocyte Biol* 46(1):75-83, 1989.

13. Broder S, Yarchoan R: Dideoxycytidine: current clinical experience and future prospects: a summary, *Am J Med* 88(5B):31S-33S, 1990.

14. Brun-Vezinet F et al: Prevalence of antibodies to lymphadenopathy-associated retrovirus in African patients with AIDS, *Science* 226(4673):453-456, 1984.

15. Centers for Disease Control: Kaposi's sarcoma and *Pneumocystis* pneumonia among homosexual men—New York City and California, *MMWR* 30:3, 1981.

16. Centers for Disease Control: Acquired immunodeficiency syndrome (AIDS) update, United States, *MMWR* 33:309-311, 1983.

17. Centers for Disease Control: Recommendation for assisting in the prevention of perinatal transmission of HTLV-III/LAV and acquired immunodeficiency, *MMWR* 34:37-40, 1985.

18. Centers for Disease Control: Classification system for human T-lymphotropic virus type III/lymphadenopathy–associated virus infections, *MMWR* 35:334-339, 1986.

19. Centers for Disease Control: Revision of the CDC surveillance case definition for acquired immunodeficiency syndrome, *MMWR* 36:1S, 1987.

20. Centers for Disease Control: Recommendations of the Immunization Practices Advisory Committee for pneumococcal polysaccharide vaccine, *JAMA* 261(9):1265-1267, 1989.

21. Centers for Disease Control: AIDS and human immunodeficiency virus infection in the United States: 1988 update, *MMWR* 38(S-4):1-38, 1989.

22. Centers for Disease Control: Update: acquired immunodeficiency syndrome—United States, *MMWR* 39:81-86, 1989.

23. Centers for Disease Control: HIV prevalence, projected AIDS case estimates: workshop, Oct 31-Nov 1, 1989, *MMWR* 39:110-119, 1990.

23a. Centers for Disease Control: HIV/AIDS Surveillance, May 1991.

24. Chu SY et al: Impact of the human immunodeficiency virus epidemic on mortality in women of reproductive age—United States, *JAMA* 264(2):225-229, 1990.

25. Clavel F et al: Human immunodeficiency virus type 2 infection associated with AIDS in west Africa, *N Engl J Med* 316:1180-1185, 1987.

26. Clumeck N et al: Acquired immune deficiency syndrome in African patients, *N Engl J Med* 310:492-497, 1984.

27. Coffin JM et al: Human immunodeficiency viruses, *Science* 232:697-699, 1986.

28. Cooley TP et al: Once-daily administration of 2',3'-dideoxyinosine in patients with the acquired immuno-

deficiency syndrome or AIDS-related complex: results of a phase I trial, *N Engl J Med* 322(19):1340-1345, 1990.

29. Copper GS, Jeffers DJ: The clinical prognosis of HIV-1: a review of 32 follow-up studies, *J Gen Intern Med* 3(6):525-532, 1988.

30. Cotton DJ: The impact of AIDS on the medical care system, *JAMA* 260(4): 519-523, 1988.

31. Creagh-Kirk T et al: Survival experience among patients with AIDS receiving zidovudine: follow-up of patients in a compassionate plea program, *JAMA* 260(20):3009-3015, 1988.

32. Curran JW et al: Acquired immunodeficiency syndrome (AIDS) associated with transfusions, *N Engl J Med* 310:69-75, 1984.

33. Curran JW et al: The epidemiology of AIDS: current status and future prospects, *Science* 229:1352-1357, 1985.

34. Davis KC et al: Acquired immunodeficiency syndrome in a patient with hemophilia, *Ann Intern Med* 98:284-286, 1983.

35. Des Jarlais DC et al: HIV-1 infection among intravenous drug users in Manhattan, New York City, from 1977 through 1987, *JAMA* 261:1008-1012, 1989.

36. Dondero TJ, St Louis M, Anderson J: Evaluation of the estimated number of HIV infections using a spreadsheet model and empirical data. Paper presented at the Fifth International Conference on AIDS, Montreal, June 4-9, 1989 (abstract).

37. Fahey JL et al: Quantitative changes in T helper or T suppressor/cytotoxic lymphocyte subsets that distinguish acquired immune deficiency syndrome from other immune subset disorders, *Am J Med* 76:95-100, 1984.

38. Fauci AS: DDI: a good start, but still phase I, *N Engl J Med* 322(19):1386-1388, 1990.

39. Fischl MA, Dickinson GM, LaVoie L: Safety and efficacy of sulfamethoxazole and trimethoprim chemoprophylaxis for *Pneumocystis carinii* pneumonia in AIDS, *JAMA* 259(8): 1185-1189, 1988.

40. Fischl MA et al: The efficacy of azidothymidine (AZT) in the treatment of patients with AIDS and AIDS-related complex: a double-blind, placebo-controlled trial, *N Engl J Med* 317(4):185-191, 1987.

41. Fischl MA et al: The safety and efficacy of zidovudine (AZT) in the treatment of subjects with mildly symptomatic human immunodeficiency virus type 1 (HIV) infection: a double-blind, placebo-controlled trial, *Ann Intern Med* 112:727-737, 1990.

42. Francis DP et al: Targeting AIDS prevention and treatment toward HIV-1–infected persons: the concept of early intervention, *JAMA* 262(18): 2572-2576, 1989.

43. Friedland GH, Klein RS: Transmission of the human immunodeficiency virus, *N Engl J Med* 317:1125-1135, 1987.

44. Friedland GH et al: Lack of transmission of HTLV-III/LAV infection to household contacts of patients with AIDS or AIDS-related complex with oral candidiasis, *N Engl J Med* 314:344-349, 1986.

45. Gabuzda DH, Hirsch MS: Neurologic manifestations of infection with human immunodeficiency virus: clinical features and pathogenesis, *Ann Intern Med* 107:383-391, 1987.

46. Gail MH, Rosenberg PS, Goedert JJ: Therapy may explain recent deficits in AIDS incidence, *J Acquir Immune Defic Syndr* 3:296-306, 1990.

47. Gallo RC et al: Frequent detection and isolation of cytopathic retroviruses (HTLV-III) from patients with AIDS and at risk for AIDS, *Science* 224(4648):500-503, 1984.

48. Gallo RC: Mechanism of disease induction by HIV, *J Acquir Immune Defic Syndr* 3:380-389, 1990.

49. Garland FC et al: Incidence of human immunodeficiency virus seroconver-

sions in the US Navy and Marine Corps personnel, 1986-1989, *JAMA* 262(22):3161-3165, 1989.

50. Gartner S et al: Virus isolation from and identification of HTLV-III/LAV–producing cells in brain tissue from a patient with AIDS, *JAMA* 256(17): 2365-2371, 1986.

51. Gartner S et al: The role of mononuclear phagocytes in HTLV-III/LAV infection, *Science* 233:215-219, 1986.

52. Gelmann EP et al: Proviral DNA of a retrovirus, human T-cell leukemia virus, in two patients with AIDS, *Science* 220(4599):862-865, 1983.

53. Gostin LO: Public health strategies for confronting AIDS: legislative and regulatory policy in the United States, *JAMA* 261(11):1621-1630, 1989.

54. Grant I et al: Evidence for early central nervous system involvement in the acquired immunodeficiency syndrome (AIDS) and other human immunodeficiency virus infections: studies with neuropsychologic testing and magnetic resonance imaging, *Ann Intern Med* 107:828-836, 1987.

55. Greenblatt RM et al: Genital ulceration as a risk factor for human immunodeficiency virus infection, *AIDS* 2:47-50, 1988.

56. Groopman JE et al: HTLV-III in saliva of people with AIDS-related complex and healthy homosexual men at risk for AIDS, *Science* 226(4673):447-449, 1984.

57. Gyorkey F et al: Human immunodeficiency virus in brain biopsies of patients with AIDS and progressive encephalopathy, *J Infect Dis* 155:870-876, 1987.

58. Hahn BH et al: Genomic diversity of the acquired immune deficiency syndrome virus HTLV-III: different viruses exhibit greatest divergence in their envelope genes, *Proc Natl Acad Sci USA* 82:4813-4817, 1985.

59. Hahn BH et al: Genetic variation in HTLV-III/LAV over time in patients with AIDS or at risk for AIDS, *Science* 232:1548-1553, 1986.

60. Hardy AM et al: The economic impact of the first 10,000 cases of acquired immunodeficiency syndrome in the United States, *JAMA* 255:209-211, 1986.

61. Harris C et al: Immunodeficiency in female sexual partners of men with the acquired immunodeficiency syndrome, *N Engl J Med* 308(20):1181-1184, 1983.

62. Hirsch MS: Chemotherapy of human immunodeficiency virus infections: current practice and future prospects, *J Infect Dis* 161:845-857, 1990.

63. Ho DD et al: Isolation of HTLV-III from cerebrospinal fluid and neural tissues of patients with neurologic syndromes related to the acquired immunodeficiency syndrome, *N Engl J Med* 313:1493-1497, 1985.

64. Holmberg SC et al: Biologic factors in the sexual transmission of human immunodeficiency virus, *J Infect Dis* 160(1):116-125, 1989.

65. Jackson JB et al: Hemophiliacs with HIV antibody are actively infected, *JAMA* 260:2236-2239, 1988.

66. Jefferies DJ: The antiviral activity of dideoxycytidine, *J Antimicrob Chemother* 23(suppl A):29-34, 1989.

67. Jett JR et al: Acquired immunodeficiency syndrome associated with blood-product transfusions, *Ann Intern Med* 99:621-624, 1983.

68. Kaplowitz LG et al: Medical care costs of patients with acquired immunodeficiency syndrome in Richmond, Va: a quantitative analysis, *Arch Intern Med* 148:1793-1797, 1988.

69. Kelen GD et al: Unrecognized human immunodeficiency virus infection in emergency department patients, *N Engl J Med* 318:1645-1650, 1988.

70. Kieny MP: Structure and regulation of the human AIDS virus, *J Acquir Immune Defic Syndr* 3:395-402, 1990.

71. Koenig S et al: Detection of AIDS virus in macrophages in brain tissue

from AIDS patients with encephalopathy, *Science* 223:1089-1093, 1986.

72. Kopelman RG, Zolla-Pazner S: Association of human immunodeficiency virus infection and autoimmune phenomena, *Am J Med* 84:82-88, 1988.

73. Kreiss JK et al: Antibody to human T-lymphotropic virus type III in wives of hemophiliacs: evidence for heterosexual transmission, *Ann Intern Med* 102:623-626, 1985.

74. Lane HC et al: Abnormalities of B-cell activation and immunoregulation in patients with the acquired immunodeficiency syndrome, *N Engl J Med* 309(8):453-458, 1983.

75. Lane HC et al: Qualitative analysis of immune function in patients with the acquired immunodeficiency syndrome: evidence for a selective defect in soluble antigen recognition, *N Engl J Med* 313(2):79-84, 1985.

76. Lemp GF et al: Predictors of survival for AIDS cases in San Francisco. Paper presented at the Third International Conference on AIDS, Washington, DC, June 3, 1987.

77. Levine AM et al: Development of B-cell lymphoma in homosexual men: clinical and immunologic findings, *Ann Intern Med* 100:7-13, 1984.

78. Levy JA: Human immunodeficiency viruses and the pathogenesis of AIDS, *JAMA* 261(20):2997-3006, 1989.

79. Lewis CE, Freeman HE, Corey CR: AIDS-related competence of California's primary care physicians, *Am J Public Health* 77(7):795-798, 1987.

80. Lifson AR, Rutherford GW, Jaffe HW: The natural history of human immunodeficiency virus infection, *J Infect Dis* 158(6):1360-1367, 1988.

81. McDougal JS et al: Binding of HTLV-III/LAV to T4+ cells by a complex of the 110K viral protein and the T4 molecule, *Science* 231:382-385, 1986.

82. McNeil JG et al: Direct measurement of human immunodeficiency virus seroconversions in a serially tested population of young adults in the United States Army, October, 1985 to October, 1987, *N Engl J Med* 320(24):1581-1585, 1989.

83. Marion RW et al: Human T-cell lymphotropic virus type III (HTLV-III) embryopathy: a new dysmorphic syndrome associated with intrauterine HTLV-III infection, *Am J Dis Child* 140:638-640, 1986.

84. Marzuk PM et al: Increased risk of suicide in persons with AIDS, *JAMA* 259(9):1333-1337, 1988.

85. Masci JR et al: Immunological profiles of patients testing HIV+ at an anonymous testing site in New York City. Paper presented at the Sixth International Conference on AIDS, San Francisco, June 20-24, 1990.

86. Morgan M, Curran JW, Berkelman RL: The future course of AIDS in the United States, *JAMA* 263(11):1539-1540, 1990.

87. Navia BA et al: The AIDS dementia complex. I. Clinical features, *Ann Neurol* 19:517-524, 1986.

88. Navia BA et al: The AIDS dementia complex. II. Neuropathology, *Ann Neurol* 19:525-535, 1986.

89. New York City Department of Health: AIDS surveillance update, July 25, 1990.

90. Norman C: Sex and needles, not insects and pigs, spread AIDS in Florida town, *Science* 234:415-417, 1986.

91. Peterman TA, Curran JW: Sexual transmission of human immunodeficiency virus, *JAMA* 256:2222-2226, 1986.

92. Peterman TA et al: Transfusion-associated acquired immunodeficiency syndrome in the United States, *JAMA* 254:2913-2917, 1985.

93. Piot P et al: Acquired immunodeficiency syndrome in a heterosexual population in Zaire, *Lancet* 2:65-69, 1984.

94. Polk BF et al: Predictors of the acquired immunodeficiency syndrome developing in a cohort of seropositive homosexual men, *N Engl J Med* 316:61-66, 1987.

95. Popovic V et al: Detection, isolation, and continuous production of cytopathic retroviruses (HTLV-III) from patients with AIDS and pre-AIDS, *Science* 224(4648):497-500, 1984.

96. Quinn TC et al: Human immunodeficiency virus infection among patients attending clinics for sexually transmitted diseases, *N Engl J Med* 318:197-203, 1988.

97. Ratner L, Gallo RC, Wong-Staal F: HTLV-III, LAV, ARV are variants of the same AIDS virus, *Nature* 313:636-641, 1985.

98. Redfield RR, Wright CD, Tramont EC: The Walter Reed staging classification for HTLV-III/LAV infection, *N Engl J Med* 314:131-132, 1986.

99. Redfield RR et al: Heterosexually acquired HTLV-III/LAV disease (AIDS-related complex and AIDS), *JAMA* 254(15):2094-2096, 1985.

100. Robey WG et al: Characterization of envelope and core structural gene products of HTLV-III with sera from AIDS patients, *Science* 228(4699):593-595, 1985.

101. Rogers MF et al: Lack of transmission of human immunodeficiency virus from infected children to their household contacts, *Pediatrics* 85(2):210-214, 1990.

102. Rothenberg R et al: Survival with the acquired immunodeficiency syndrome, *N Engl J Med* 317:1297-1302, 1987.

103. Roy S, Wainberg MA: Role of the mononuclear phagocyte system in the development of acquired immunodeficiency syndrome (AIDS), *J Leukocyte Biol* 43(1):91-97, 1988.

104. St Louis ME et al: Seroprevalence rates of human immunodeficiency virus infection at sentinel hospitals in the United States, *N Engl J Med* 323(4):213-218, 1990.

105. Schlamm HT, Yancovitz SR: *Haemophilus influenzae* pneumonia in young adults with AIDS, ARC, or risk of AIDS, *Am J Med* 86:11-14, 1989.

106. Schoenbaum EE et al: Prevalence and risk factors among intravenous drug abusers in a methadone program in New York City. Paper presented at the Second International Conference on AIDS, Paris, June 23-25, 1986.

107. Scott GB et al: Acquired immunodeficiency syndrome in infants, *N Engl J Med* 310(2):76-81, 1984.

108. Simonsen JN et al: Human immunodeficiency virus infection among men with sexually transmitted diseases: experience from a center in Africa, *N Engl J Med* 319(5):274-278, 1988.

109. Somogyi AA, Watson-Abady JA, Mandel FS: Attitudes toward the care of patients with acquired immunodeficiency syndrome: a survey of community internists, *Arch Intern Med* 150:50-53, 1990.

110. Stahl RE et al: Immunologic abnormalities in homosexual men: relationship to Kaposi's sarcoma, *Am J Med* 73:171-178, 1982.

111. Stamm WE et al: The association between genital ulcer disease and acquisition of HIV infection in homosexual men, *JAMA* 259:1429-1433, 1988.

112. Stevens CE et al: Human T-cell lymphotropic virus type III infection in a cohort of homosexual men in New York City, *JAMA* 255:2167-2172, 1986.

113. Stoler MH et al: Human T-cell lymphotropic virus type III infection of the central nervous system: a preliminary in situ analysis, *JAMA* 256(17):2360-2364, 1986.

114. Terwilliger EF, Sodroski JG, Haseltine WA: Mechanisms of infectivity

and replication of HIV-1 and implications for therapy, *Ann Emerg Med* 19(3):233-241, 1990.

115. Thiry L et al: Isolation of AIDS virus from cell-free breast milk of three healthy virus carriers, *Lancet* 2:891-892, 1985.

116. Volberding PA et al: Zidovudine in asymptomatic human immunodeficiency virus infection: a controlled trial in persons with fewer than 500 CD4-positive cells per cubic millimeter, *N Engl J Med* 322:941-949, 1990.

117. Ward JW et al: Laboratory and epidemiologic evaluation of an enzyme immunoassay for antibodies to HTLV-III, *JAMA* 256(3):357-361, 1986.

118. Ward JW et al: Transmission of human immunodeficiency virus (HIV) by blood transfusions screened as negative for HIV antibody, *N Engl J Med* 318:473-478, 1988.

119. Weinberg DS, Murray HW: Coping with AIDS: the special problems of New York City, *N Engl J Med* 317:1469-1472, 1987.

120. Weiss SH et al: Screening test for HTLV-III (AIDS agent) antibodies: specificity, sensitivity, and applications, *JAMA* 253:221-225, 1985.

121. Winkelstein W et al: Sexual practices and risk of infection by the human immunodeficiency virus: the San Francisco Men's Health Study, *JAMA* 257(3):321-325, 1987.

122. Wofsy CB et al: Isolation of AIDS-associated retrovirus from genital secretions of women with antibodies to the virus, *Lancet* 1:527-529, 1986.

123. Yarchoan R, Mitsuya H, Broder S: Clinical and basic advances in the antiretroviral therapy of human immunodeficiency virus infection, *Am J Med* 87:191-200, 1989.

124. Zagury D et al: HTLV-III in cells cultured from semen of two patients with AIDS, *Science* 226(4673):449-451, 1984.

125. Ziegler JB et al: Postnatal transmission of AIDS-associated retrovirus from mother to infant, *Lancet* 1:896-898, 1985.

CHAPTER 2

The Natural History of HIV-1 Infection

After the discovery of human immunodeficiency virus type 1 (HIV-1) and its link to acquired immunodeficiency syndrome (AIDS), seroprevalence studies of various segments of the population demonstrated that most of those infected with HIV-1 did not meet the surveillance definition of AIDS and many, in fact, were completely asymptomatic. Subsequent longitudinal studies of infected individuals have indicated that HIV-1 infection is followed by a substantial asymptomatic period and that many patients develop nonspecific symptoms such as fever, weight loss, diarrhea, or lymphadenopathy or other clinical evidence of infection long before the onset of AIDS-defining opportunistic infections and malignancies. Such patients, as well as many asymptomatic HIV-infected individuals, can be shown to have defects in cellular immunity that are qualitatively similar to those seen in patients with AIDS, although generally less severe.

These observations have led to the current concept of HIV-1 infection as a slowly developing constellation of clinical and laboratory abnormalities that spans several years in most individuals and always or almost always, after a variable period of time, culminates in AIDS. Several important markers of disease progression and overall prognosis have been identified, and these play a major role in the staging of HIV infection for the purposes of antiviral therapy and prophylaxis of opportunistic infections.

Although the clinical and immunological features of AIDS have been well characterized, and the structure and life cycle of HIV-1 have been largely clarified, relatively little is known about the events that occur between initial infection with the virus and the onset of AIDS. However, several relevant facts have been established:

- HIV-1 causes a chronic infection with an asymptomatic latent period that lasts at least several years in most individuals.
- HIV-1 can be detected in the blood soon after infection and remains detectable for years.
- Antibody to HIV-1 can be detected in the serum of infected individuals several weeks to several months after infection and remains detectable in most individuals throughout the course of the disease.
- HIV-infected individuals may transmit infection indefinitely.
- Beginning in the latter phase of the latent period, progressive, irreversible depletion of CD4 (helper) lymphocytes develops, resulting in clinical immunodeficiency.
- Clinical manifestations of HIV-1 infection may become apparent before the onset of AIDS-defining opportunistic infections or malignancies.
- The risk of developing AIDS increases steadily with time after infection.
- Several clinical and laboratory abnormalities may predict progression to AIDS.
- Mathematical models indicate that virtually all HIV-infected patients eventually will develop AIDS, although latent periods appear to vary substantially.

The extent to which genetic, environmental, or infectious cofactors may influence the course of HIV-1 infection or the rate or likelihood of progression to AIDS currently is unclear, as is the impact of antiviral therapy.

The practitioner caring for HIV-infected patients must have a thorough understanding of the natural history of HIV-1 infection and its relationship to AIDS, for several reasons:

- Current strategies for antiviral therapy and prophylaxis against opportunistic infection depend on accurate clinical and immunological staging.
- Reasonable estimates of prognosis can be made only with a knowledge of typical rates of disease progression.
- Symptoms may be interpreted more accurately when patients can be stratified according to their risk of opportunistic infection.

This chapter reviews the immunological and clinical features of the natural history of HIV-1 infection and discusses the role of clinical and laboratory parameters in staging.

THE TIMING OF EVENTS IN HIV-1 INFECTION
Seroconversion after Primary Infection

Most patients experience a mononucleosis-like illness in association with seroconversion at the time of primary infection.[37] Antibody to HIV-1 usually can be detected in the blood by current testing techniques within 3 months of infection,[25] although intervals of longer than 6 months to seroconversion have been reported.[32] Experimental studies on a limited number of patients indicate that immunoglobulin IgM antibody is detected by sensitive assays at a mean of 5 days, peaks at a mean of 24 days, and disappears at approximately 3 months.[6] IgG antibody, on average, is first detected at 11 days, peaks at 3 to 6 months, and persists indefinitely.[6] Enzyme-linked immunosorbent assay (ELISA), the technique used for routine HIV-1 antibody testing, is somewhat less sensitive. Antibody is generally first detected between 17 and 90 days after infection by this technique (Table 2-1).[6]

Symptomatic Disease

HIV-related symptoms such as generalized lymphadenopathy, fever, weight loss, and diarrhea become prominent in a minority of patients, often several years before the onset of AIDS. In many patients other symptoms of HIV infection appear before the onset of AIDS-defining opportunistic infections or malignancies. Among these symptoms are oral thrush, oral hairy leukoplakia, seborrheic dermatitis, and herpes zoster.

AIDS

The rate of progression to AIDS after infection appears to vary and may change with time. Overall, AIDS is unusual within the first several years after seroconversion but it has been predicted that the disease will develop within 15

TABLE 2-1. Timing of events in natural history of HIV-1 infection (adults)

Event	Mean time after infection
Retroviral illness	2-6 weeks[25]
Detectable antibody*	6-24 weeks†
Symptomatic disease	1-10 years (?)
AIDS	7-11 years [3,25]

*By conventional tests.
†Delayed seroconversion has been reported.[32]

years in 78% to 100% of infected individuals.[3] Studies show that 10% to 15% of patients who are asymptomatic or who have only generalized lymphade-nopathy and 40% of symptomatic patients will progress to AIDS within 36 months.[7] Based on mathematical models, the mean interval from seroconver-sion to AIDS appears to be 8 to 11 years.[25] A much quicker progression appears to occur occasionally, however, and AIDS has been diagnosed as early as 2 months after primary infection.[19]

Immunological Derangements

The immunological abnormalities that follow HIV-1 infection have been ex-tensively characterized. Central to the disorder is progressive depletion of the population of lymphocytes designated CD4 and a resulting decrease in the ratio of CD4 to CD8 (suppressor) lymphocytes. Production of interferon gamma decreases in parallel to the fall in CD4 cell count,[30] and other indicators of cellular immunity, including response to skin test antigens, diminish.

Viral Studies

HIV-1 itself may be detected in the plasma of infected individuals before anti-HIV antibody.[36] This plasma viremia diminishes with the elaboration of IgG antibody,[36] but the virus remains detectable in the plasma and peripheral blood mononuclear cells at all stages of infection[17] if sensitive techniques are used.

FACTORS THAT MAY INFLUENCE THE NATURAL HISTORY OF HIV-1 INFECTION

Host Factors

Risk behavior and route of transmission. The natural history of HIV infection appears to be comparable in homosexual men, intravenous drug users, and hemophiliacs. In all three groups, acquisition of the virus is followed by a latency period that typically spans years before the onset of HIV-related symp-toms or frank AIDS. However, since the precise time of infection often is impossible to determine, subtle differences in the course of HIV-related disease between risk groups may be difficult to detect.

Age. Studies of hemophiliacs have indicated that the older an individual is at the time of primary infection, the quicker is the progression to AIDS.[11,15]

Pregnancy. Even under normal circumstances, pregnancy may be accom-panied by alterations in immune function. However, pregnancy-associated worsening of immunodeficiency in HIV-infected women appears to be un-usual.[34]

Genetic factors. Several human leukocyte antigen (HLA) types, including B35, CW4, DR2,[20] and DR1[26] appear to be associated with the development of AIDS among seropositive individuals. An association between AIDS-associated Kaposi's sarcoma and HLA DR5 also has been reported.[33]

Potential infectious cofactors. Both the herpes simplex virus (HSV) and cytomegalovirus (CMV)[35] have been shown in cell culture to increase replication of HIV. The clinical significance of this is unclear.

MARKERS OF DISEASE PROGRESSION

Several clinical and laboratory abnormalities (see the box below) may predict impending progression to AIDS; these markers include immunological abnormalities, viral studies, and clinical signs.

Immunological Abnormalities

Immunological profiling has become an indispensable tool in managing HIV infection. Two markers of cellular immune function, the absolute CD4 lymphocyte count and the ratio of CD4 to CD8 lymphocytes, show a progressive decline in infected individuals and allow reasonably reliable immunological staging. Prospective studies have demonstrated that a progressive decrease in CD4 lymphocytes is characteristic of HIV-1 infection and predicts progression to AIDS.[8,11,14,23] In a longitudinal study of more than 300 HIV-infected homosexual men, it was found that AIDS developed between 63 and 840 days (mean 466 days) after the CD4 lymphocyte count fell below $500/mm^3$.[8] A sudden decrease in CD4 cell count appears to be especially predictive of progression to AIDS.[11]

The relationship between a falling CD4 lymphocyte count and the development of AIDS was further demonstrated in a study of 100 HIV-infected

---

Markers of Disease Progression

Laboratory	Clinical
Falling CD4 lymphocyte count[11]	Oral candidiasis[22]
Rising β_2-microglobulin[2]	Oral hairy leukoplakia[16]
Rising antilymphocyte antibody[9]	Weight loss[25]
Thrombocytopenia (hemophilia)[11]	Fever[25]
Rising neopterin[12]	Severe herpes zoster[29]
Rising viremia[5]	Advanced age[11,15]

patients: 94% of episodes of *Pneumocystis carinii* pneumonia (PCP) and all episodes of pulmonary cytomegalovirus and cryptococcal infection occurred in patients with counts below 200/mm^3.[27] It has been pointed out, however, that PCP may occur even with a normal CD4 count.[21]

High circulating levels of antilymphocyte antibodies are also associated with a quicker progression to AIDS.[9]

Viral Studies

Techniques to measure the amount of circulating HIV-1, currently available in research laboratories, have shown a relationship between viral burden and the stage of disease. The highest levels of circulating virus are seen in patients at the most advanced stages of HIV-1 infection: that is, those with AIDS or AIDS-related complex (ARC).[17] Progression to AIDS is associated with the highest levels of plasma viremia.[5]

The predictive value of tests for viral antigen is unclear. The appearance of the antigen designated p24 has been associated with progression to AIDS in some series[1,8,28] but not in others,[27] and some question the clinical value of routine antigen testing.[24]

Clinical Signs

Lymphadenopathy. Although generalized lymphadenopathy in an individual with a history of high-risk behavior is strongly associated with HIV-1 infection, its prognostic significance is not clear. Lymphadenopathy was found in 70% of HIV-infected hemophiliacs who were seropositive for more than 3 years, but in only 10% of those seropositive for shorter periods.[10] However, lymphadenopathy was not found to predict the degree of immunodeficiency in a large study of homosexual men.[23] Regression of lymphadenopathy may predict the development of AIDS.[25]

Miscellaneous signs. Severe, painful herpes zoster, particularly if recurrent or involving cranial dermatomes, was correlated with a poor overall prognosis in one study,[29] and the appearance of oral thrush predicted progression to AIDS in an early clinical series.[22] In another study of homosexual men, the onset of oral hairy leukoplakia was associated with progression to AIDS within 16 months in 48% and within 31 months in 83%.[16] Unexplained fever, night sweats, and weight loss may also predict clinical progression.[25]

β_2-microglobulin. Serum levels of β_2-microglobulin often are elevated in patients with symptomatic HIV-1 infection[38] and generally are highest in patients with AIDS.[4] Longitudinal data indicate that high levels of this protein may predict rapid progression to AIDS regardless of the CD4 lymphocyte count.[2] However, in one series AIDS developed in more than 40% of individuals with normal levels over a 3½-year follow-up period.[31] The role of β_2-microglobulin assay in clinical staging of HIV-1 infection currently is being examined.

Neopterin. Serum and urine levels of neopterin, a substance produced by activated macrophages, may be elevated in association with HIV-1 infection and may correlate with the stage of disease.[12] Although longitudinal data suggest that high urinary levels may predict progression to AIDS,[13] the role of this test in clinical practice has not yet been defined.

Thrombocytopenia. Thrombocytopenia has been associated with quicker progression to AIDS in hemophiliacs[11] but not in homosexual men.[18]

THE PRACTICAL IMPLICATIONS OF THE NATURAL HISTORY OF HIV-1 INFECTION

If used wisely, an understanding of the natural history of the HIV-1 infection is a great advantage to the practitioner. Stratifying patients according to their degree of immunodeficiency and clinical parameters discussed above permits a more rational approach to several important issues, including:

- The timing of antiviral therapy and prophylaxis against *P. carinii* pneumonia
- The interpretation of symptoms and other clinical findings (e.g., opportunistic lung infection is substantially more likely to be the cause of a nonproductive cough in the patient with a CD4 lymphocyte count under $200/mm^3$ than in the patient with a count of over $500/mm^3$)
- The appropriate diagnostic evaluation of non-HIV–related disorders
- The likelihood of an adequate response to immunization
- The interpretation of diagnostic tests (e.g., tuberculin skin test) that may be influenced by immune deficiency

These areas are discussed in depth in later sections of this book.

It should be remembered, however, that the CD4 lymphocyte count provides only an approximation of the stage of disease and the risk of impending progression to AIDS. Opportunistic infection occasionally may occur in patients with normal counts, and in some cases other parameters, including the rate of fall in the CD4 count and the patient's clinical status, may be more important indicators of the short-term prognosis.

The clinician often is called upon to assess the overall prognosis. Such a request may come overtly, as when an HIV-infected patient or a family member asks about life expectancy. In addition to this, however, decisions about life-sustaining therapy and surgery and diagnostic evaluation for other medical conditions often are made on the basis of an implicit assessment of the patient's overall prognosis. Only the recognition that HIV infection is a chronic disorder and that many patients remain asymptomatic for prolonged periods after diagnosis allows for a rational approach to such issues.

REFERENCES

1. Allain J et al: Long-term evaluation of HIV antigen and antibodies to p24 and gp41 in patients with hemophilia: potential clinical importance, *N Engl J Med* 317:1114-1121, 1987.

2. Anderson RE et al: Use of beta-2 microglobulin level and CD4 lymphocyte count to predict development of acquired immunodeficiency syndrome in persons with human immunodeficiency virus infection, *Arch Intern Med* 150(1):73-77, 1990.

3. Berkelman RL et al: Epidemiology of human immunodeficiency virus infection and acquired immunodeficiency syndrome, *Am J Med* 86(6 pt 2):761-770, 1989.

4. Burkes RL et al: Serum beta-2 microglobulin levels in homosexual men with AIDS and with persistent, generalized lymphadenopathy, *Cancer* 57(11):2190-2192, 1986.

5. Coombs RW et al: Plasma viremia in human immunodeficiency virus infection, *N Engl J Med* 321:1626-1631, 1989.

6. Cooper DA, Imrie AA, Penny R: Antibody response to human immunodeficiency virus after primary infection, *J Infect Dis* 155(6):1113-1118, 1987.

7. Cooper GS, Jeffers DJ: The clinical prognosis of HIV-1: a review of 32 follow-up studies, *J Gen Intern Med* 3(6):525-532, 1988.

8. De Wolf F et al: Numbers of CD4+ cells and the levels of core antigens of and antibodies to the human immunodeficiency virus as predictors of AIDS among seropositive homosexual men, *J Infect Dis* 158(3):615-622, 1988.

9. Dorsett BH, Cronin W, Ioachim HL: Presence and prognostic significance of antilymphocyte antibodies in symptomatic and asymptomatic human immunodeficiency virus infection, *Arch Intern Med* 150:1025-1028, 1990.

10. Eyster ME et al: Development and early natural history of HTLV-III antibodies in persons with hemophilia, *JAMA* 253:2219-2223, 1985.

11. Eyster ME et al: Natural history of human immunodeficiency virus infections in hemophiliacs: effects of T-cell subsets, platelet counts, and age, *Ann Intern Med* 107:1-6, 1987.

12. Fuchs D et al: Neopterin levels correlating with the Walter Reed staging classification in human immunodeficiency virus (HIV) infection, *Ann Intern Med* 107(5):784-785, 1987.

13. Fuchs D et al: Neopterin as a predictive marker for disease progression in human immunodeficiency virus type 1 infection, *Clin Chem* 35(8):1746-1749, 1989.

14. Goedert JJ et al: Effect of T4 count and cofactors on the incidence of AIDS in homosexual men infected with human immunodeficiency virus, *JAMA* 257(3):331-334, 1987.

15. Goedert JJ et al: A prospective study of human immunodeficiency virus type 1 infection and the development of AIDS in subjects with hemophilia, *N Engl J Med* 321(17):1141-1148, 1989.

16. Greenspan D, et al.: Relation of oral hairy leukoplakia to infection with the human immunodeficiency virus and the risk of developing AIDS, *J Infect Dis* 155(3):475-481, 1987.

17. Ho DD, Moudgil T, Alam M: Quantitation of human immunodeficiency virus type 1 in the blood of infected persons, *N Engl J Med* 321(24):1621-1625, 1989.

18. Holzman RS, Walsh CM, Karpatkin S: Risk for the acquired immunodeficiency syndrome among thrombocytopenic and nonthrombocytopenic homosexual men seropositive for the human immunodeficiency virus, *Ann Intern Med* 106:383-389, 1987.

19. Isaksson B et al: AIDS two months after primary human immunodeficiency virus infection, *J Infect Dis* 158(4):866-868, 1988.

20. Jeannet M et al: HLA antigens are risk

factors for development of AIDS, *J Acquir Immune Defic Syndr* 2:28-32, 1989.

21. Kennedy CA, Goetz MB, Mathisen GE: Absolute CD4 lymphocyte counts and the risk of opportunistic pulmonary infection, *Rev Infect Dis* 12(3):561-562, 1990.

22. Klein RS et al: Oral candidiasis in high-risk patients as the initial manifestation of the acquired immunodeficiency syndrome, *N Engl J Med* 311:354-358, 1984.

23. Lang W et al: Clinical, immunologic, and serologic findings in men at risk for acquired immunodeficiency syndrome: the San Francisco Men's Health Study, *JAMA* 257(3):326-330, 1987.

24. Lelie PN et al: Clinical importance of HIV antigen and anti-HIV core markers in persons infected with HIV, *N Engl J Med* 318:1204-1205, 1988.

25. Lifson AR, Rutherford GW, Jaffe HW: The natural history of human immunodeficiency virus infection, *J Infect Dis* 158(6):1360-1367, 1988.

26. Mann DL et al: HLA antigen frequencies in HIV-1 seropositive disease-free individuals and patients with AIDS, *J AIDS* 1:13-17, 1988.

27. Masur H et al: CD4 counts as predictors of opportunistic pneumonias in human immunodeficiency virus (HIV) infection, *Ann Intern Med* 111(3):223-231, 1989.

28. Mayer KH et al: Correlation of enzyme-linked immunosorbent assays for serum human immunodeficiency virus antigen and antibodies to recombinant viral proteins with subsequent clinical outcomes in a cohort of asymptomatic homosexual men, *Am J Med* 83:208-212, 1987.

29. Melbye M et al: Risk of AIDS after herpes zoster, *Lancet* 1(8535):728-731, 1987.

30. Murray HW et al: T4+ cell production of interferon gamma and the clinical spectrum of patients at risk for and with acquired immunodeficiency syndrome, *Arch Intern Med* 148:1613-1616, 1988.

31. Murray HW et al: Progression to AIDS in patients with lymphadenopathy or AIDS-related complex: reappraisal of risk and predictive factors, *Am J Med* 86(5):533-538, 1989.

32. Ranki A et al: Long latency precedes overt seroconversion in sexually transmitted human immunodeficiency virus infection, *Lancet* 2:589-593, 1987.

33. Scorza Seraldi R et al: HLA-associated susceptibility to acquired immunodeficiency syndrome in Italian patients with human immunodeficiency virus infection, *Lancet* 2(8517):1187-1189, 1986.

34. Selwyn PA et al: Prospective study of human immunodeficiency virus infection and pregnancy outcomes in intravenous drug users, *JAMA* 261(9):1289-1294, 1989.

35. Skolnik PR, Kosloff BR, Hirsh MS: Bidirectional interactions between human immunodeficiency virus type 1 and cytomegalovirus, *J Infect Dis* 157(3):508-514, 1988.

36. Stramer SL et al: Markers of HIV infection prior to antibody seropositivity, *JAMA* 262(1):64-69, 1989.

37. Tindall B et al: Characterization of the acute illness associated with human immunodeficiency virus infection, *Arch Intern Med* 148:945-949, 1988.

38. Zolla-Pazner S et al: Quantitation of beta-2 microglobulin and other immune characteristics in a prospective study of men at risk for acquired immune deficiency syndrome, *JAMA* 251(22):2951-2955, 1984.

CHAPTER 3

HIV Testing: Methodology, Prevalence of HIV Infection, and Availability of Tests

Blood tests to detect antibody to human immunodeficiency virus type 1 (HIV or HIV-1) were developed and became widely available shortly after the discovery of the virus and its link to acquired immunodeficiency syndrome (AIDS). Such tests have made it possible to identify infected individuals before the onset of symptoms and, as a result, have led to three major advances:

1. *Protection of the blood supply.* Screening of donated blood for HIV antibody has dramatically diminished the risk of transfusion-associated AIDS.
2. *Determination of the extent of the epidemic.* Large-scale seroprevalence studies of various segments of the population have provided a more detailed picture of the epidemic and have provided a basis for focused HIV screening efforts. The risk of transmission of HIV infection to health

care workers and household and classroom contacts of infected individuals also has been quantified by studies using antibody screening tests.

3. *Identification of infected patients early in the natural history of disease.* Testing of patients at high risk for HIV infection has provided an opportunity for early therapeutic intervention and counseling to reduce the risk of further transmission. After the efficacy of early treatment of HIV infection with antiviral agents such as zidovudine was demonstrated in the late 1980s,[34,69,85,94] testing assumed a much more important role. Identification of infected individuals at the earliest stages of the disease could lead directly to therapeutic benefit.

For some infected individuals, however, HIV testing has had devastating social repercussions. Discrimination in housing, employment, entry to schools, and other areas has occurred. In many instances HIV testing became a requirement for obtaining life insurance. As recently as the late 1980s public opinion polls reflected substantial ignorance and fear concerning those infected with HIV. Confidentiality of test results, even when dictated by law, could not always be guaranteed. Such factors undoubtedly dissuaded and continue to dissuade some of those at high risk of infection from seeking testing.

Further complicating the situation has been the fact that many medical practitioners are unfamiliar with testing procedures and are not adequately informed about the legitimate medical uses of HIV testing, the means of obtaining testing, and the laws regarding confidentiality and informing a patient's sexual contacts.

In this chapter, testing methodology, as well as the results of HIV prevalence surveys of various segments of the population, is reviewed to provide a basis for a comprehensive approach to testing and counseling, which are presented in Chapter 4.

METHODS OF TESTING FOR HIV INFECTION

Although several methods of testing for HIV infection have been developed, routine testing is carried out on serum by means of the enzyme-linked immunosorbent assay (ELISA) for antibody to the virus. It is recommended that serum specimens testing positive by this technique be tested by the Western blot (WB) assay for confirmation (Figure 3-1).[18] Antibody to HIV usually can be detected in the blood by this procedure within 3 months of infection,[60] although intervals of longer than 6 months to seroconversion have been reported.[80] Although testing for HIV in this fashion has been shown to be quite accurate and reliable under most circumstances, there are two areas of potential concern about the technique—delay in diagnosis and the possibility of inaccurate results.

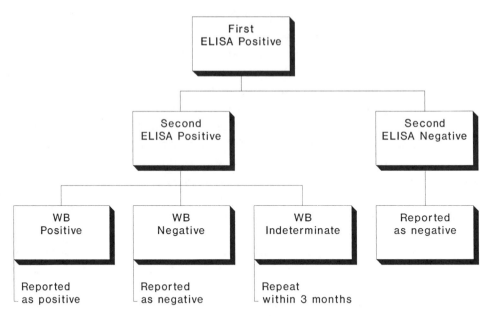

FIGURE 3-1. HIV antibody testing procedure.

Delay in diagnosis of HIV infection: Since antibody may not be detectable for weeks to months after infection has occurred, sequential testing often is needed to exclude infection in patients whose potential exposure occurred recently.

The possibility of inaccurate results: Concerns have been raised about the validity of ELISA and WB in screening patients at low risk of HIV infection and the potential for false positive results.[68,97] False negative antibody tests have also been reported.[47,95]

The following tests are the techniques currently available for detecting HIV in blood (see the boxes on p. 43).

Antibody Tests

As in other viral infections, IgM is the first antibody to appear after HIV infection. Although standard testing procedures (ELISA, WB) do not generally detect antibody for weeks to months after infection has occurred, IgM has been detected by highly sensitive assays in research settings within 5 days of the onset of symptoms of acute infection.[24] IgG appears at approximately 11 days and peaks between 70 and 189 days.[24] Antibody to the p24 antigen is almost universally present in HIV-infected patients and was detected in 96% of patients with AIDS or AIDS-related complex (ARC) in one series.[39] Anti-

---

HIV Testing Techniques: Antibody Assays

- Enzyme-linked immunosorbent assay (ELISA)*
- Western blot assay (WB)†
- Latex agglutination*
- Indirect immunofluorescent antibody (IFA)*
- Radioimmunoprecipitation assay (RIPA)†

*Screening.
†Confirmatory.

HIV Testing Techniques: Antigen Assays

- Viral culture
- P24 antigen
- Polymerase chain reaction (PCR)

---

bodies to p55, gp41,[39] and a variety of other antigens are also often present.[66] Loss of antibody to p24 may be a poor prognostic sign.[29]

Enzyme-linked immunosorbent assay (ELISA). Several kits employing the enzyme-linked immunosorbent assay (ELISA) technique for detecting antibody to HIV have been licensed in the United States. All use disrupted HIV as antigen on a solid phase, either beads or microtiter wells. Specimens of the patient's serum or plasma are incubated with the antigen preparation. If antibody to HIV is present, it binds to the antigen. Antibody bound in this fashion is then detected by the addition of an anti-globulin-enzyme conjugate followed by a reagent, which reacts with the enzyme to produce a color change. When measured spectrophotometrically, the degree of color change is proportional to the amount of anti-HIV antibody present. The sensitivity and specificity of ELISA are both greater than 99%.[17,39]

Western blot assay. Western blot (WB) is regarded as a more specific test for antibody to HIV than ELISA and is used as a confirmatory test on serum specimens testing positive by ELISA.

The technique, which is more laborious than ELISA, is as follows:

1. Disrupted virus is electrophoretically fractionated on gel.
2. Antigenic bands are then tranferred to nitrocellulose, which is then cut into strips and incubated with the patient's serum.

3. An antiimmunoglobulin reaction detects antibody bound to the nitro-cellulose strip.

Several different antibodies to HIV (e.g., against p24, p31, gp41, and gp120/gp160 antigens) typically are identified by WB, and interpretation of results may be somewhat subjective.

The criteria for a positive WB test are controversial.[22] Depending on which recommended criteria are used, a test may be reported as positive if bands are detected that include:

any two of p24, gp41 or gp120/gp160[18]

or

p24 or p31 plus gp41 or gp120/gp160[22]

or

one or more bands from each gene product group (gAG, pOL, eNV) (see Chapter 1).[18]

When antibody is detected in a pattern not regarded as positive, the result may be reported as inconclusive or indeterminate. Such indeterminate patterns, particularly isolated antibody to p24,[58] may be seen during seroconversion in patients who have recently become infected.[18] Indeterminate results were obtained in 15% to 20% of individuals at low risk of HIV-1 infection in early studies.[17] Such patients often are found to be uninfected on further testing.[48]

Other antibody testing techniques. Several other techniques not yet generally available are being evaluated for HIV antibody testing, including the following procedures.

Latex agglutination (LA). An antigen from regions of gp41 and gp120 is attached to polystyrene beads. When serum containing antibody to HIV is added, the beads agglutinate.[83] The validity of LA, which can be performed more rapidly that other antibody tests, was comparable to that of ELISA and the Western blot test in one series[78] but somewhat inferior in others.[44]

Indirect immunofluorescent assay (IFA). Serum is incubated on slides coated with HIV-infected cells.[59] After rinsing, fluorescein-labeled anti-human globulin is added so that immunofluorescence is detected if anti-HIV antibody is present. The sensitivity and specificity of IFA is comparable to that of the Western blot test.[9,59]

Radioimmunoprecipitation (RIPA). Radiolabeled virus or infected cells are incubated with serum and bind HIV antibody, if present. RIPA is cumbersome compared to other techniques but may be more effective at detecting some antigens than the Western blot assay.[21]

Miscellaneous. Other antibody assays have been developed but are not yet used in clinical practice. These include immunoassay with a cloned HIV envelope peptide,[5] indirect immunofluorescence,[59] autologous red cell agglutination,[51] and gelatin particle agglutination.[102]

Antigen Tests

Direct tests for HIV by viral culture or assay of viral structural or genetic components are available as research techniques and in some cases in commercial laboratories. It has been shown that HIV may be detected in the blood of patients with no detectable antibody.[65] In some cases antigen tests may provide evidence of HIV shortly after infection has occurred, before antibody is detected by ELISA, WB, or other techniques.[43]

P24 antigen assay. Assays to measure levels of p24 antigen, the major core protein of HIV, are available in some research and commercial laboratories. Such antigen testing may be useful in evaluating patients whose antibody tests repeatedly yield inconclusive results, although p24 may not be detected in most patients early in the course of HIV infection.[4,32,81] Detectable levels of p24 antigen,[32] as well as loss of antibody to p24,[35] have predicted progression to AIDS in some series. Persistent antigenemia early after initial infection may also indicate a poor prognosis.[84]

Polymerase chain reaction. Polymerase chain reaction (PCR) is a technique by which minute amounts of viral ribonucleic acid (RNA) or incorporated proviral deoxyribonucleic acid (DNA) from HIV may be detected in clinical specimens.[30,87] PCR currently is available as a research tool, but it is hoped that the technique will prove valuable in the diagnosis of HIV infection, particularly among recently infected individuals with no detectable antibody. The extreme sensitivity of PCR has raised concerns about possible false positive test results caused by cross-contamination of specimens.[54]

Viral culture. Techniques for culturing HIV are available in research laboratories. Because these techniques are laborious and require a high degree of technical expertise, as well as containment facilities, they are impractical for screening purposes, but they occasionally may be useful in evaluating individuals with indeterminate results on antibody studies. In research laboratories, culture of plasma or peripheral blood mononuclear cells may be more senstive than antibody or other antigen tests for the diagnosis of HIV-1 infection,[23] and the level of viremia may correlate with the clinical stage.[45]

Home Test Kits

Home HIV test kits have been under development by several manufacturers[1]; none currently are licensed by the U.S. Food and Drug Administration (FDA). A saliva test kit is also under evaluation.[10]

THE LIMITATIONS OF CURRENT TESTING TECHNIQUES
Validity

Because of the far-reaching implications of HIV-1 test results, some experts
have expressed reservations about the accuracy of current testing procedures.[68]
Particular concern has arisen over the false positive rate of ELISA when used
to screen low-risk populations. Even the high specificity of this test (99.8%,
as cited by the American Red Cross Blood Services)[17] yields a positive predictive value of only 83% in populations with a 1% prevalence of infection. Despite
these concerns, ELISA followed by WB confirmation of positive test results
was found to have a false positive rate of only 1 in 135,187 in a screening
program of applicants for service in the U.S. military, a low-risk population.[6a]

Quality Control

As with all laboratory tests, the reliability of HIV tests is highly dependent
on the quality of the laboratory. Unlicensed WB tests are used in some laboratories.[17] The College of American Pathologists conducts a proficiency testing
program for laboratories offering HIV-1 testing, and the choice of laboratory
should be guided by proven standards of reliability.[17] The practitioner should
bear in mind the possibility of inaccurate test results, particularly when those
results are unexpected.

THE PREVALENCE OF HIV INFECTION

Public health authorities have recommended that programs be designed to
offer HIV testing and counseling to individuals most likely to be infected.[15]
From studies conducted in recent years, an increasingly clear picture of the
HIV/AIDS epidemic has emerged. The likelihood of infection varies dramatically among various segments of the population (Table 3-1) and among geographical regions. The results of major seroprevalence studies are reviewed
here to provide a basis for testing strategies.

The number of individuals infected with HIV in the United States is not
known, although estimates of prevalence in the late 1980s ranged from 1.3 to

TABLE 3-1. Reported prevalence of HIV infection among various groups in
the United States

Population	Size of cohort	Prevalence
Blood donors[88]	868,000	0.038%
Applicants for military service[6]	306,061	0.15%
Applicants for a marriage license (Illinois)[93]	70,846	0.011%

3.0 per 1,000 individuals. Screening of large cohorts of blood donors from the general population in the mid-1980s indicated that approximately 1 in 2,500 were infected.[88] Serological surveys of various segments of the population, both those in known high-risk groups and those at lower risk, have yielded valuable information.

Geographical Distribution of HIV Infection in the United States

Considerable information about the nationwide prevalence of HIV infection and the geographical distribution among low-risk individuals has come from studies of volunteers for military service and follow-up of military personnel. Although young men are disproportionately represented in this population, such data have led to a better understanding of the distribution of HIV cases by geographical areas, ethnic background, educational level, and other parameters. In the absence of universal HIV testing, the information derived from military testing is of unique value in developing strategies to target testing efficiently.

Burke and colleagues[6] reported the results of HIV testing of more than 300,000 individuals from all 50 states and the District of Columbia who volunteered for military service between October 1985 and March 1986. Several important observations emerged from this study. The overall prevalence of HIV infection was found to be 1.5 per 1,000 individuals. Men were more than twice as likely as women to test positive, and prevalence increased with age, particularly among black males, to the age of 27. The geographical distribution of HIV infection in this population was comparable to that of the AIDS epidemic, that is, applicants from areas of the country where the incidence of AIDS is highest were most likely to test positive. The highest prevalence rates were seen among applicants from the District of Columbia (10.13 per 1,000), followed, in descending order, by New York (4.21), Maryland (3.71), New Jersey (3.54), Nevada (3.52), Delaware (2.33), and California (2.10). No applicants from Alaska, Maine, Montana, North Dakota, Rhode Island, Vermont, or Wyoming tested positive.

The Sentinel Hospital Surveillance Project, conducted by the Centers for Disease Control (CDC), has also provided data about geographical patterns of HIV infection. Testing of more than 89,000 blood specimens from hospitals in 21 states[86] revealed prevalence rates ranging from greater than 5% in Newark, New Jersey, and parts of New York City to less than 1% in most hospitals in the Midwest and West.

Trends in Geographical Distribution of HIV Seropositivity

An updated analysis of trends in seroprevalence data from military recruits during the first 2 years of testing, 1985 through 1987, revealed that HIV infection was spreading geographically from the urban areas of highest prevalence into adjacent suburban and rural areas.[37] During the study period, prevalence rates increased among applicants in nonepidemic areas adjacent to epidemic areas; this was particularly true in Florida, California, Texas, Illinois, and Ohio. The increase in the number testing HIV positive was greatest for black applicants but was seen among whites as well. Within the original high-prevalence areas, prevalence rates were seen to increase exclusively among young black applicants during this period.

Prevalence of HIV Infection Among Various Segments of the U.S. Population

High seroprevalence rates in some subsets of the population (e.g., those attending sexually transmitted disease clinics[77]) suggest that voluntary HIV testing and counseling should be systematically offered in some settings even to patients who deny high-risk behavior or who are not aware of exposure to the virus. Conversely, the low prevalence rates seen in surveys of more general populations indicate that universal testing is not likely to identify any substantial additional number of infected individuals.

Prevalence Within High-Risk Groups (Table 3-2)

Homosexual and bisexual men. Homosexual and bisexual men, taken as one group, were the first to be recognized as being at high risk for AIDS.[11] Since shortly after the AIDS epidemic was first appreciated, attempts have been made to define the prevalence and natural history of infection within this population and to clarify the specific sexual practices associated with HIV transmission. Although HIV-1 has been isolated from the semen of infected men,[3] and various studies have pointed to specific behavioral risk factors for transmission during homosexual encounters, the precise mode of transmission has not been defined. Most researchers believe that the deposition of virus-containing semen on traumatized mucosal surfaces during anal and perhaps

TABLE 3-2. Prevalence of HIV infection among some groups at highest risk*

Risk group	Prevalence	Year
Male homosexuals (San Francisco)[99]	48.5%	1984
Intravenous drug users (New York City)[28]	55%-60%	1984-1987
Individuals with hemophilia A receiving factor VIII concentrate[57]	78%	1984
Heterosexual partners of intravenous drug users with AIDS[42]	48%	1985

*Data cover studies done on a selected series of cases.

oral intercourse is particularly likely to result in transmission.[75] It has been proposed that other viruses that commonly infect homosexual men (specifically cytomegalovirus and Epstein-Barr virus) may influence the risk of infection with HIV.[79]

Valuable information has been obtained from the San Francisco Men's Health Study, begun in 1982.[99] This prospective study has followed more than 1,000 men living in an area of San Francisco that had the highest incidence of AIDS early in the epidemic. Enrollment in the study was voluntary, and the population studied was relatively well educated and affluent.

Rates of new infection and their correlation with changes in behavior aimed at reducing risk have been monitored.[99] In this cohort of men, who were between 25 and 54 years of age, the rate of HIV infection in 1984 was 48.5% among homosexual and bisexual men. No heterosexual men were found to be infected. Individuals who admitted to sharing needles were excluded from the analysis.

The infection rate was highest (70.8%) among those homosexual or bisexual men who had had 50 or more sexual partners within the 2 years before testing and lowest (17.6%) among those who had abstained from sexual contact for those 2 years. The vast majority of the homosexual or bisexual men (95.7%) had practiced anal or oral-genital sex, or both, within the preceding 2 years. Receptive anal intercourse and the use of dildos or douches were associated with the highest risk of HIV seropositivity.

The rate of new infection in this group fell from 18.4% per year from 1982 to 1984 to 4.2% in early 1986. This decline in the rate of spread correlated with a substantial decrease in high-risk sexual behavior.[99]

Intravenous drug users. Shortly after techniques were developed to detect antibody to HIV, several studies were conducted to determine the prevalence of infection among intravenous drug users. In this group, infection rates varied widely among individuals in different geographical areas. Studies conducted in some areas of New York City and northern New Jersey indicated that more than 50% of intravenous drug users tested positive for antibody to HIV, whereas the prevalence among similar populations in other areas, for example Europe, was much lower.

Unlike the situation among homosexual and bisexual men, in whom the prevalence of HIV infection appears to be diminishing in some areas as a result of behavioral changes,[99] there is little evidence that infection rates are decreasing among intravenous drug users in high-prevalence areas. The proportion of AIDS patients in New York City for whom intravenous drug use is the primary risk factor rose from 13% in 1982 to 36% in 1987.[96] In areas of low prevalence of HIV infection in the United States, needle sharing between homosexual and heterosexual drug users appears to be an especially important route of transmission.[2]

A nationwide compilation of local seroprevalence studies of intravenous drug users reflected widely varying prevalence of HIV infection in different geographical regions. Rates of infection were highest in the Northeast and Puerto Rico but substantially lower in many urban areas of the Midwest and far West.[41] The survey primarily encompassed studies of patients attending methadone programs and reflected seroprevalence in the mid to late 1980s. The overall prevalence rate of HIV infection was estimated to be between 5% and 33% in these pooled data, which would represent 61,000 to 398,000 individuals.

The relatively low incidence of HIV infection in many regions of the country suggested a high potential for rapid spread within intravenous drug user populations in areas of low prevalence. This is especially true because needle sharing appears to be very common among intravenous drug users in areas of low seroprevalence.[2] In various studies in the 1980s the estimated annual rate of new infections among intravenous drug users in the United States ranged from 0% to 14%, depending on the region examined.[41]

Male and female intravenous drug users appear to be at approximately equal risk of infection. Several studies have indicated higher rates of HIV seropositivity among black and Hispanic intravenous drug users than among whites.[41] It is unclear whether male intravenous drug users who are homosexual or bisexual are at greater risk of infection than those who are strictly heterosexual.

Examining HIV seroprevalence among intravenous drug users entering methadone treatment in an area of high risk (New York City), Des Jarlais and coworkers[28] found that infection rates increased rapidly in this group between 1979 (the year that AIDS was first recognized in an intravenous drug user in New York City) and 1983; however, the rate remained constant (55% to 60%) between 1984 and 1987. It was felt that at least some of this stabilization of seroprevalence reflected changes in specific drug use behavior. A survey conducted in the mid-1980s of intravenous drug users not in treatment programs had indicated that the use of unused or clean needles for injection had increased substantially, reflecting attempts to avoid risk among these active users.[27]

Hemophiliacs. Patients with hemophilia A who had received therapy with factor VIII concentrate preparations were among the first individuals recognized to be at high risk for AIDS.[31] By 1984 as many as 78% of such patients may have had evidence of HIV infection.[57] Patients treated with cryoprecipitate or fresh frozen plasma and those with hemophilia B had substantially lower rates of HIV infection.[27,56,67]

Heterosexual contacts of risk-group individuals. An understanding of the extent of heterosexual transmission of HIV infection, the specific risk factors involved, and means of prevention is vital for targeting HIV testing programs and controlling the expansion of the AIDS epidemic. Unfortunately, many important questions about this route of transmission remain unanswered.

Heterosexual transmission is an extremely important factor in the worldwide HIV/AIDS epidemic; it currently is thought to be the most common route of transmission in central Africa. In the United States and other Western countries the spread of HIV infection among male homosexuals and intravenous drug users has accounted for most cases of AIDS in the first decade of the epidemic; however, the impact of heterosexual transmission is becoming increasingly apparent. As of March 1990, 24% of all women diagnosed with AIDS in New York City appeared to have become infected by sexual contact with men at high risk for HIV infection.[71]

Rates of transmission of HIV infection by heterosexual contact appear to differ widely in various parts of the world. Epidemiological data consistently have indicated that both male-to-female and female-to-male transmission occurs, and reported AIDS cases are evenly distributed between men and women in central Africa.[76] Spread of infection from females to males, which appears to occur readily in Central Africa, has accounted for only a small minority of AIDS cases in the United States.

The reasons for these apparent differences in the nature of the HIV epidemic in different parts of the world are not completely known. It has been suggested that the AIDS epidemic spread first among homosexual and bisexual men in the United States because of the high prevalence of receptive anal intercourse and large numbers of sexual partners among subsets of this population. Anal intercourse may be a more efficient means of HIV transmission than vaginal intercourse on biological grounds.[73] Similarly, rapid spread among intravenous drug users in the United States may reflect the sharing of contaminated needles with numerous contacts. Since neither homosexual intercourse nor intravenous drug use has been found to be common in the areas of central Africa most affected by AIDS, it is possible that the epidemic in that region was established earlier, and that routes of transmission which may be less efficient (e.g., vaginal intercourse) have resulted in substantial transmission over a longer period of time.

A precise picture of the patterns of heterosexual transmission of HIV infection in the United States has not yet emerged from serological surveys. No consensus has been reached on such vital questions as the relative rate of male-to-female and female-to-male transmission or the relative risk of various types of sexual practices. Although the virus has been isolated from semen, vaginal secretions, and saliva, the relative infectivity of these fluids has not been clearly established.

Studies in which heterosexual partners of HIV-infected individuals were tested for HIV antibody have yielded divergent data. For example, 9.5% of wives of infected hemophiliac men were found to be HIV positive in one series[53]; in another study, 48% of male and female heterosexual partners of HIV-infected intravenous drug users tested positive.[42]

Use of condoms during penile-vaginal intercourse has been recommended as a means of preventing heterosexual transmission of HIV infection.[90,100] A variety of studies have been conducted to determine the degree of protection conferred by condom use. Fischl and coworkers examined rates of heterosexual transmission (male to female and female to male) over 18 months and found a transmission rate of 10% in couples using condoms and 86% in those not using condoms.[33] Some protection by condom use also has been suggested in studies of African prostitutes[62] and female partners of bisexual men.[74] It should be noted that complete prevention of HIV transmission by condom use has not been documented. In view of condoms' known failure rate in preventing pregnancy, it is likely that, used properly, they provide significant but incomplete protection against HIV infection.

Blood transfusion recipients. It has been recognized that, before screening of donated blood for HIV antibody was instituted, transfusion of contaminated blood was a likely route of infection in approximately 1% of reported AIDS cases in the United States.[25] Patients with transfusion-associated AIDS were more likely to be older and Caucasian than were AIDS patients in general.

ELISA kits for detecting HIV antibody were licensed for screening of donated blood by the FDA in March 1985. Since then, donated blood testing positive by ELISA has been discarded. Because of the possibility of false negative ELISA tests, particularly in donors who might have only recently become infected, it was subsequently recommended that individuals in certain categories be excluded as donors. These categories included men who had had homosexual intercourse after 1977, individuals who had had sex with prostitutes, and others. Despite universal screening of donated blood and exclusion of some individuals as donors, the risk of transfusion-associated HIV infection had not been entirely resolved by the late 1980s. Ward and coworkers[95] at the Centers for Disease Control reported transmission of HIV infection by seven donors who had been screened as HIV negative before donation. It was estimated that the risk of transfusion of contaminated blood remained but was extremely low, on the order of 1 in 40,000 transfusions.

It should be recognized that individuals who receive transfusions in areas of the world with significant HIV prevalence but lacking in effective HIV screening programs are at higher risk.

Because of the long asymptomatic period in most patients infected with HIV, individuals infected by blood transfusion before 1985 are expected to come to medical attention with symptomatic HIV infection well into the 1990s. It has been estimated that approximately 12,000 individuals in the United States are infected with HIV acquired through blood transfusion.[13]

Prevalence in Low-Risk Groups

Health care workers. Because HIV infection can be transmitted among intravenous drug users by shared needles and because needle-stick injuries and other forms of blood exposure are common in certain health care settings, concern about the safety of health care workers who care for HIV-infected patients has been expressed since the earliest stages of the HIV/AIDS epidemic.[101] Because HIV infection is incurable, the scientific discussion of the risk of transmission to health care workers often has been obscured by emotionalism. A wide variety of measures, some scientifically justifiable, some not, has been proposed to diminish the risk of transmission by accidental blood exposure.

Transmission of HIV infection to health care workers after puncture wounds and mucous membrane splashes of blood from infected patients has been described.[14] With needle-stick injuries, lacerations from contaminated scalpels, and other injuries in which HIV-containing blood is introduced subcutaneously, the precise risk of transmission is most likely dictated by a number of factors, such as the inoculum of viable virus in the infectious material, the amount of blood or fluid involved, the depth of the injury, and perhaps other factors such as the relative virulence of the HIV strain and unknown host factors influencing the individual's susceptibility to HIV infection. The risk in splash-type exposures, in which blood or other body fluid from an infected patient lands on unprotected skin or mucous surfaces, may be influenced by the integrity of the worker's skin at the site of the exposure.

The risk of needle-stick injury varies among different categories of health care workers. Jagger and coworkers,[49] examining patterns of such injuries in a general hospital setting, found the highest incidence reported to an employee health service to be among nurses and nursing students, followed by technicians working in laboratories, respiratory therapy, or radiology, housekeeping personnel, and, finally, physicians and medical students. Disposable syringes and intravenous equipment caused most of the injuries in this study. Since these data represented only reported injuries, the possibility of underreporting among some types of employees may have influenced the results.

Despite heightened concern about the risk of blood exposures, there is little evidence to date that educating staff members or improved methods of needle disposal have significantly diminished the incidence of needle-stick injuries.[52,82]

Following is a review of data, collected from various perspectives, that provide insight into health care workers' risk of contracting HIV infection through work-related activities. The overall risk appears to be small for workers in U.S. hospitals.

Infection following occupational exposure of health care workers. Since 1983 the Cooperative Needlestick Surveillance Group has prospectively followed health care workers who had had needle-stick, open wound, or mucous membrane exposure to blood from patients known to have AIDS or to be infected with HIV.[63] When HIV antibody tests became available in 1985, sera from exposed workers were tested at intervals for 1 year after the exposure, and attempts were made, via questionnaires, to identify other potential routes of infection. Four of the first 963 workers studied appeared to acquire HIV infection as a result of their occupational exposure, an infection rate of 0.42. All of those who seroconverted had been exposed to the virus through needle-sticks or cuts with sharp objects. None of those exposed by mucous membrane splash (103 workers) appeared to acquire infection.

Workers enrolled in this study have included nurses (63%), physicians and medical students (14%), laboratory workers (11%), and phlebotomists (7%).

Prospective evaluation of hospital workers in Zaire, which has a high prevalence of HIV infection in the general population, also has pointed to a small risk of nosocomial infection.[72]

Household contacts of HIV-infected patients. Early in the history of the HIV/AIDS epidemic, particularly before the causative agent was discovered, there was great concern that infection could be spread by casual nonsexual contact, specifically the forms of routine contact that might occur between members of the same household or between schoolchildren and their classmates.

Friedland and coworkers screened household nonsexual contacts, both adults and children, of patients with AIDS or ARC and found no evidence of such horizontal transmission of HIV infection.[36] One of 101 such household members was found to be infected: a 5-year-old child who was thought to have acquired the virus before birth.

Despite sharing of such household items as toilets, towels, and in some cases razors, nail clippers, and toothbrushes with the infected individual for a median period of 22 months, no household member acquired infection. Physical contact, including kissing, hugging, and helping to bathe and dress the HIV-positive family member, also was found to pose no risk of contagion in this study.

Although spread of HIV infection to household contacts appears to be extremely unlikely, a case of possible transmission from an infected child to a parent providing health care has been reported.[12]

Applicants for a marriage license. In 1988, a law requiring HIV testing of applicants for marriage licenses went into effect in Illinois. The results of the testing program have provided seroprevalence data on a broad-based, low-risk population of young adults. During the first 6 months of screening, only 8 of more than 70,000 applicants were found to be HIV positive, half of whom reported high-risk behavior.[93] The seroprevalence in this population was thus 0.011%.

Teenagers. Seroprevalence data gathered from applicants for military service who were under 20 years of age revealed an overall rate of HIV infection of 0.34 per 1,000.[7] As with older applicants, those from areas of the country reporting the highest incidences of AIDS were most likely to be infected, and black applicants were more likely to be infected (1.06 per 1,000) than whites (0.18 per 1,000) or Hispanics (0.31 per 1,000). The ratio of males to females among those testing HIV positive was nearly 1:1.

The extent to which these data reflect seroprevalence among U.S. teenagers in general is unclear and depends on the extent to which the applicant pool parallels the general population in risk behavior and other variables. It is clear that the risk of HIV infection varies widely among teenage military applicants, as it does among adult applicants and the adult population in general. No data are available on risk behavior of the teenagers testing positive in this study.

Prevalence in Selected Patient Groups (Table 3-3)

Pregnant women and newborns. HIV infection in pregnant women represents a doubly tragic feature of the AIDS epidemic. Most pediatric HIV infections occur in the children of infected mothers and appear to result from transmission during pregnancy or in the perinatal period. The incidence of pediatric AIDS is highest in areas where seroprevalence in adults is greatest,[92] and most infected women have a history of intravenous drug use or sexual contact with a man belonging to a high-risk group.[20] The risk of transmission to the fetus is high, and women may be asymptomatic and unaware that they are infected throughout the pregnancy.

Several large studies have been conducted to determine the prevalence of HIV infection in pregnant women. Surveys conducted in areas of high AIDS incidence have revealed alarmingly high rates of infection.

Workers at the Massachusetts Department of Public Health and the Centers for Disease Control conducted blind seroprevalence studies of HIV antibody in the blood of newborn children at 58 hospitals in Massachusetts in 1987.[46] Antibody detected in cord blood was taken to reflect the mother's antibody status. Seroprevalence rates ranged from 0.9 per 1,000 in suburban and rural hospitals to 8 per 1,000 in inner-city hospitals.

TABLE 3-3. Reported prevalence of HIV infection in the United States in selected patient categories

Patient category	Prevalence	Year
Childbearing women		
Massachusetts[46]	0.21%*	1987
New York[55,91]	2.0%,† 2.7%‡	1987-1988
Patients at a clinic for sexually transmitted diseases		
Baltimore[78]	5.2%	1987
Hospital inpatients		
Washington, D.C.[38]	3.7%	1987
Emergency room patients		
Baltimore[50]	5.2%	1988

*Range: 0.09% in suburban and rural hospitals to 0.8% in inner-city hospitals.
†Municipal hospital.
‡Voluntary hospital.

A comparable survey was carried out at Mount Sinai Medical Center in New York City in late 1987 and early 1988.[91] The overall prevalence of HIV antibody in cord blood was 2.7%, but the figure rose to 5.9% in teenage mothers.

Working in a municipal hospital in New York City serving an inner-city population, Landesman and coworkers[55] found a 2% rate of HIV seropositivity in cord blood collected from more than 600 infants. Particularly disturbing was the observation that 42% of the HIV-positive mothers denied high-risk behavior in this study. This suggests that targeting only those pregnant women who admit to high-risk behavior for HIV testing may not be an adequate screening technique.

Patients attending clinics for sexually transmitted disease. Patients seeking medical care for other sexually transmitted diseases, particularly those living in areas of high HIV prevalence, form a group for whom routine HIV testing might be appropriate. Of more than 4,000 patients attending sexually transmitted disease clinics in Baltimore, 5.2% were found to be HIV positive.[78] Men were twice as likely to be infected as women, and blacks were four times as likely to be infected as whites. As anticipated, a history of homosexuality or intravenous drug use correlated with seropositivity, but one third of the infected men and half of the infected women denied high-risk behavior on an anonymous questionnaire. Syphilis in men and genital warts in women were associated with increased risk of HIV infection.

These data suggest that patients living in areas of high HIV prevalence who manifest sexually transmitted diseases other than HIV infection should be strongly urged to undergo HIV testing, even if they deny high-risk behavior or are unaware of high-risk contacts. However, this strategy has been challenged as too costly to use in low-prevalence areas.[89] It also has been suggested that assessment of risk factors by trained interviewers might be more effective than the use of an anonymous questionnaire in identifying those at high risk.[61]

Hospitalized patients. The risk of transmission of HIV infection to health care workers by such occupational injuries as needle-sticks and scalpel cuts has led to proposals for identifying unsuspected HIV-positive hospital inpatients. Proposed strategies have included mandatory testing of all hospitalized patients, selected testing of patients undergoing surgery,[8] targeted testing of those admitting to risk behavior, and so-called universal precautions,[16] by which all patients would be regarded as potentially HIV infected. As with other populations at low risk of HIV infection, routine testing of hospitalized patients has been criticized on both scientific and ethical grounds.[40]

The prevalence of unsuspected HIV infection among hospital inpatients would be expected to vary considerably, depending on the geographical location of the hospital, the nature of the patient population served, and a host of other factors, including the specific distribution of admitting diagnoses. Seroprevalence rates for one hospital may be markedly different from those in another. Despite this obstacle, some data have been gathered on background rates of infection.

Gordin and coworkers at the Washington, D.C., Veterans Administration Medical Center found that 3.7% of 616 unselected admitted patients tested positive for HIV antibody by ELISA and the Western blot test.[38] On interviewing these patients, only two thirds of those testing positive were found to belong to high-risk groups. The authors concluded that mandatory testing could not be justified on the basis of the prevalence determined but that screening interviews were not sufficiently sensitive to identify likely HIV-positive patients. Therefore universal precautions were felt to be justified.

Emergency room patients. The prevalence of HIV infection among patients visiting an inner-city hospital emergency room was examined by Kelen and coworkers.[50] Overall, 5.2% of more than 2,000 patients had antibody to HIV. Black men between 30 and 34 years of age were found to have the highest seroprevalence, 11.4%. A statistically significant association between HIV infection and penetrating trauma was observed. Of patients denying HIV risk factors, 3.1% were seropositive. The prevalence of unrecognized HIV infection was 4%.

Hospital clinic patients. In a survey conducted at Bellevue Hospital in New York City,[64] 2.8% (3.3% of men, 2.4% of women) of more than 900 ambulatory patients who denied risk factors for HIV infection tested positive for HIV antibody by ELISA with confirmation by the Western blot test. Most of the patients attended hospital-based clinics focusing on dermatology, gynecology, prenatal care, or sexually transmitted disease. Since HIV-infected patients have a relatively high incidence of other sexually transmitted diseases, and often also have dermatological disorders, the seroprevalence in this study may have been greater than that which would be seen in a general medical clinic population. Such data most likely are not directly applicable to areas of low prevalence.

THE AVAILABILITY OF TESTING

HIV testing and counseling programs have been publicly funded through the Health Departments of all 50 states.[19] By 1989 more than 5,000 individual counseling and testing sites had been established.[19] These may be free standing, associated with appropriate ambulatory care units such as sexually transmitted disease or family planning clinics, or located in private physicians' offices or other sites. Information about these programs should be obtained from local health authorities. Testing and counseling initiatives have also been sponsored by local and state governments in some areas.[70]

Many commercial laboratories offer tests for HIV-1 infection. As discussed previously, however, quality control may vary dramatically among such laboratories.

REFERENCES

1. Anderson A: Home test kits for AIDS blocked, *Nature* 332(14):573, 1988.
2. Battjes RJ, Pickens RW, Amsel Z: Introduction of HIV infection among intravenous drug abusers in low-prevalence areas, *J Acquir Immune Defic Syndr* 2:533-539, 1989.
3. Bernard J et al: HTLV-III in cells cultured from semen of two patients with AIDS, *Science* 226:449-451, 1984.
4. Borghi V et al: Detection of serum HIV-Ag related to the major core protein (p24) in persons at risk for AIDS, *Microbiologica* 12(1):81-83, 1989.
5. Burke DS et al: Diagnosis of human immunodeficiency virus infection by immunoassay using a molecularly cloned and expressed envelope poly

peptide: comparison to Western blot on 2,707 consecutive serum samples, *Ann Intern Med* 106:671-676, 1987.
6. Burke DS et al: Human immunodeficiency virus infections among civilian applicants for United States military service, October 1985 to March 1986: demographic factors associated with seropositivity, *N Engl J Med* 317:131-136, 1987.
6a. Burke DS et al: Measurement of the false positive rate in a screening program for human immunodeficiency virus infections, *N Engl J Med* 319:961-964, 1988.
7. Burke DS et al: Human immunodeficiency virus infections in teenagers: seroprevalence among applicants for US military service, *JAMA* 263(15): 2074-2077, 1990.

8. Carey JS: Routine preoperative screening for HIV, *JAMA* 260:179, 1988.

9. Carlson JR et al: Comparison of indirect immunofluorescence and Western blot for detection of anti-human immunodeficiency virus antibodies, *J Clin Microbiol* 25:494-497, 1987.

10. *CDC AIDS Weekly*, Oct 29, 1990.

11. Centers for Disease Control: Kaposi's sarcoma and *Pneumocystis* pneumonia among homosexual men: New York City and California, *MMWR* 30:305-308, 1981.

12. Centers for Disease Control: Apparent transmission of human T-lymphotropic virus type III/lymphadenopathy–associated virus from a child to a mother providing health care, *MMWR* 35:76-79, 1986.

13. Centers for Disease Control: Human immunodeficiency virus infection in transfusion recipients and their family members, *MMWR* 36:137-140, 1987.

14. Centers for Disease Control: Update: human immunodeficiency virus infections in health care workers exposed to blood of infected patients, *MMWR* 36(19):285-289, 1987.

15. Centers for Disease Control: Public Health Service guidelines for counseling and antibody testing to prevent HIV infection and AIDS, *MMWR* 36:509-515, 1987.

16. Centers for Disease Control: Recommendations for prevention of HIV transmission in health care settings, *MMWR* 36:2S-18S, 1987.

17. Centers for Disease Control: Update: serologic testing for antibody to human immunodeficiency virus, *MMWR* 36:833-845, 1988.

18. Centers for Disease Control: Interpretation and use of the Western blot assay for serodiagnosis of human immunodeficiency virus type 1 infection, *MMWR* 38(S-7):1-7, 1989.

19. Centers for Disease Control: Publicly funded HIV counseling and testing—United States, 1985-1989, *MMWR* 39:137-152, 1990.

20. Centers for Disease Control: HIV/AIDS monthly surveillance report, August 1990.

21. Chiodi F et al: Radioimmunoprecipitation and Western blotting with sera of human immunodeficiency virus–infected patients, *AIDS Res Human Retrovirol* 3:165-176, 1987.

22. Consortium for Retrovirus Serology Standardization: Serological diagnosis of human immunodeficiency virus infection by Western blot testing, *JAMA* 260:674-679, 1988.

23. Coombs RW et al: Plasma viremia in human immunodeficiency virus infection, *N Engl J Med* 321(24):1626-1631, 1989.

24. Cooper DA, Imrie AA, Penny R: Antibody response to human immunodeficiency virus after primary infection, *J Infect Dis* 155:1113-1118, 1987.

25. Curran JW et al: Acquired immunodeficiency syndrome (AIDS) associated with transfusions, *N Engl J Med* 310:69-75, 1984.

26. Desforges JF: AIDS and preventive treatment in hemophilia, *N Engl J Med* 308:94-95, 1983.

27. Des Jarlais DC, Friedman SR, Hopkins W: Risk reduction for the acquired immunodeficiency syndrome among intravenous drug users, *Ann Intern Med* 103:755-759, 1985.

28. Des Jarlais DC et al: HIV-1 infection among intravenous drug users in Manhattan, New York City from 1977 through 1987, *JAMA* 261:1008-1012, 1989.

29. De Wolf F et al: Numbers of CD4+ cells and the levels of core antigens of and antibodies to the human immunodeficiency virus as predictors of AIDS among seropositive homosexual men, *J Infect Dis* 158:615-622, 1988.

30. Eisenstein BI: The polymerase chain reaction: a new method of using molecular genetics for medical diagnosis, *N Engl J Med* 322(3):178-183, 1990.

31. Evatt BL et al: Coincidental appearance of LAV/HTLV-III antibodies in hemophiliacs and the onset of the AIDS epidemic, *N Engl J Med* 312:483-486, 1985.

32. Eyster ME et al: Predictive markers for the acquired immunodeficiency syndrome (AIDS) in hemophiliacs: persistence of p24 antigen and low T4 cell count, *Ann Intern Med* 110:963-969, 1989.

33. Fischl MA et al: Evaluation of heterosexual partners, children, and household contacts of adults with AIDS, *JAMA* 257:640-644, 1987.

34. Fischl MA et al: The safety and efficacy of zidovudine (AZT) in the treatment of subjects with mildly symptomatic human immunodeficiency virus type 1 (HIV) infection: a double-blind, placebo-controlled trial, *Ann Intern Med* 112:727-737, 1990.

35. Forster SM et al: Decline of anti-p24 antibody precedes antigenemia as a correlate of prognosis in HIV-1 infection, *AIDS* 1(4):235-240, 1987.

36. Friedland GH et al: Lack of transmission of HTLV-III/LAV infection to household contacts of patients with AIDS or AIDS-related complex with oral candidiasis, *N Engl J Med* 314:344-349, 1986.

37. Gardner LI et al: Evidence for spread of the human immunodeficiency virus epidemic into low prevalence areas of the United States, *J Acquir Immune Defic Syndr* 2:521-532, 1989.

38. Gordin FM et al: Prevalence of human immunodeficiency virus and hepatitis B virus in unselected hospital admissions: implications for mandatory testing and universal precautions, *J Infect Dis* 161:14-17, 1990.

39. Groopman JE et al: Serological characterization of HTLV-III infection in AIDS and related disorders, *J Infect Dis* 153:736-742, 1986.

40. Hagen MD, Meyer KB, Pauker SG: Routine preoperative screening for HIV, *JAMA* 259:1357-1359, 1988.

41. Hahn RA et al: Prevalence of HIV infection among intravenous drug users in the United States, *JAMA* 261(18):2677-2684, 1989.

42. Harris CA et al: HTLV-III/LAV infection and AIDS in heterosexual partners of AIDS patients. Paper presented at the Interscience Conference on Antimicrobial Agents and Chemotherapy, Minneapolis, Minn, September 29-October 2, 1985.

43. Haseltine WA: Silent HIV infections, *N Engl J Med* 320(22):1487-1489, 1989.

44. Heyward WL, Curran JW: Rapid screening tests for HIV infection, *JAMA* 260:542-546, 1988.

45. Ho DD, Moudgil T, Alam M: Quantitation of human immunodeficiency virus type 1 in the blood of infected persons, *N Engl J Med* 321(24):1623-1625, 1989.

46. Hoff R et al: Seroprevalence of human immunodeficiency virus among childbearing women: estimation by testing samples of blood of newborns, *N Engl J Med* 318:525-530, 1988.

47. Imagawa DT et al: Human immunodeficiency virus type 1 infection in homosexual men who remain seronegative for prolonged periods, *N Engl J Med* 320:1458-1462, 1989.

48. Jackson JB et al: Absence of HIV infection in blood donors with indeterminate Western blot tests for antibody to HIV-1, *N Engl J Med* 322:217-222, 1990.

49. Jagger J et al: Rates of needle-stick injury caused by various devices in a university hospital, *N Engl J Med* 319(5):284-288, 1988.

50. Kelen GD et al: Unrecognized human immunodeficiency virus infection in

emergency department patients, *N Engl J Med* 318:1645-1650, 1988.

51. Kemp BE et al: Autologous red cell agglutination assay for HIV-1 antibodies: simplified test with whole blood, *Science* 241:1352-1354, 1988.

52. Krasinski K, LaCouture R, Holzman RS: Effect of changing needle disposal systems on needle puncture injuries, *Infect Control* 8(2):59-62, 1987.

53. Kreiss JK et al: Antibody to human T-lymphotropic virus type III in wives of hemophiliacs, *Ann Intern Med* 102:623-626, 1985.

54. Krone WJA, Sninsky JJ, Goudsmit J: Detection and characterization of HIV-1 by polymerase chain reaction, *J Acquir Immune Defic Syndr* 3:517-524, 1990.

55. Landesman S et al: Serosurvey of human immunodeficiency virus infection in parturients, *JAMA* 258:2701-2703, 1987.

56. Lederman MM et al: Impaired cell-mediated immunity in patients with classic hemophilia, *N Engl J Med* 308:79-83, 1983.

57. Lederman MM et al: Acquisition of antibody to lymphadenopathy-associated virus in patients with classic hemophilia (factor VIII deficiency), *Ann Intern Med* 102:753-757, 1985.

58. Lelie PN, Van der Poel CL, Reesink HW: Interpretation of isolated HIV anti-p24 reactivity in Western blot analysis, *Lancet* 1:632, 1987.

59. Lenette ET, Karpatkin S, Levy JA: Indirect immunofluoresence assay for antibodies to human immunodeficiency virus, *J Clin Microbiol* 25:199-202, 1987.

60. Lifson AR, Rutherford GW, Jaffe HW: The natural history of human immunodeficiency virus infection, *J Infect Dis* 158(6):1360-1367, 1988.

61. Lifson AR et al: Screening for HIV infection in sexually transmitted disease clinics, *N Engl J Med* 319:242, 1988.

62. Mann J et al: Sexual practices associated with LAV/HTLV-III seropositivity among female prostitutes in Kinshasa, Zaire. In Program and Abstracts of the Second International Conference on AIDS, Paris, June 23-25, 1986.

63. Marcus R et al: Surveillance of health care workers exposed to blood from patients infected with the human immunodeficiency virus, *N Engl J Med* 319:1118-1123, 1988.

64. Marmor M et al: Sex, drugs, and HIV infection in a New York City hospital outpatient population, J Acquir Immune Defic Syndr 3(4):307-318, 1990.

65. Mayer KH et al: Human T-lymphotropic virus type III in high-risk antibody-negative homosexual men, *Ann Intern Med* 104:194-196, 1986.

66. McDougal JS et al: Antibody response to human immunodeficiency virus in homosexual men, *J Clin Invest* 80:316-324, 1987.

67. Menitove JE et al: T-lymphocyte subpopulations in patients with classic hemophilia treated with cryoprecipitate and lyophilized concentrates, *N Engl J Med* 308:83-96, 1983.

68. Meyer KB, Pauker SG: Screening for HIV: can we afford the false positive rate? *N Engl J Med* 317:238-241, 1987.

69. National Institute of Allergy and Infectious Diseases: State-of-the-art conference on azidothymidine therapy for early HIV infection, *Am J Med* 89:335-344, 1990.

70. New York City Department of Health: Guidelines for physicians on HIV counseling and testing and related documents, July 1989.

71. New York City Department of Health: AIDS surveillance update, March 28, 1990.

72. N'Galy B et al: Human immunodeficiency virus infection among employees in an African hospital, *N Engl J Med* 319:1123-1127, 1988.

73. Padian NS: Heterosexual transmission of acquired immunodeficiency syndrome: international perspectives and national projections, *Rev Infect Dis* 9(5):947-960, 1987.

74. Padian NS et al: The heterosexual spread of AIDS virus in San Francisco: female partners of bisexual men. Program and Abstracts of the Second International Conference on AIDS, Paris, June 23-25, 1986.

75. Peterman TA, Curran JW: Sexual transmission of human immunodeficiency virus, *JAMA* 256:2222-2226, 1986.

76. Quinn TC, et al: AIDS in Africa: an epidemiologic paradigm, *Science* 234:955-963, 1986.

77. Quinn TC et al: Human immunodeficiency virus infection among patients attending clinics for sexually transmitted diseases, *N Engl J Med* 318:197-203, 1988.

78. Quinn TC et al: Rapid latex agglutination assay using recombinant envelope polypeptide for the detection of antibody to the HIV, *JAMA* 260:510-513, 1988.

79. Quinnan GV et al: *Herpesvirus* infections in the acquired immune deficiency syndrome, *JAMA* 252:72-79, 1984.

80. Ranki A et al: Long latency precedes overt seroconversion in sexually transmitted human immunodeficiency virus infection, *Lancet* 2:589-593, 1987.

81. Reddy MM et al: Tumor necrosis factor and HIV p24 antigen levels in serum of HIV-infected populations, *J Acquir Immune Defic Syndr* 1:436-440, 1988.

82. Ribner BS et al: Impact of a rigid, puncture-resistant container system upon needle-stick injuries, *Infect Control* 8(2):63-66, 1987.

83. Riggin CH et al: Detection of antibodies to human immunodeficiency virus by latex agglutination with re-combinant antigen, *J Clin Microbiol* 25:1772-1773, 1987.

84. Rinaldo C et al: Association of human immunodeficiency virus (HIV) p24 antigenemia with decrease in CD4+ lymphocytes and onset of acquired immunodeficiency syndrome during the early phase of HIV infection, *J Clin Microbiol* 27(5):880-884, 1989.

85. Ruedy J, Schecter M, Montaner JSG: Zidovudine for early human immunodeficiency virus (HIV) infection: who, when and how, *Ann Intern Med* 112(10):721-722, 1990.

86. St Louis ME et al: Seroprevalence rates of human immunodeficiency virus infection at sentinel hospitals in the United States, *N Engl J Med* 323(4):213-218, 1990.

87. Schochetman G, Ou C, Jones WK: Polymerase chain reaction, *J Infect Dis* 158(6):1154-1157, 1988.

88. Schorr JB et al: Prevalence of HTLV-III antibody in American blood donors, *N Engl J Med* 313:384-385, 1985.

89. Sienko DG et al: Screening for HIV infection in sexually transmitted disease clinics, *N Engl J Med* 319:242, 1988.

90. Solomon MZ, DeJong W: Preventing AIDS and other STDs through condom promotion: a patient education intervention, *Am J Public Health* 79(4):453-458, 1989.

91. Sperling RS et al: Umbilical cord blood serosurvey for human immunodeficiency virus in parturient women in a voluntary hospital in New York City, *Obstet Gynecol* 73(2):179-181, 1989.

92. Thomas PA et al: Unexplained immunodeficiency in children: a surveillance report, *JAMA* 252(5):639-644, 1984.

93. Turnock BJ, Kelly CJ: Mandatory premarital testing for human immunodeficiency virus: the Illinois experience, *JAMA* 261(23):3415-3418, 1989.

94. Volberding PA et al: Zidovudine in asymptomatic human immunodeficiency virus infection: a controlled trial in a person with fewer than 500 CD4-positive cells per cubic millimeter, *N Engl J Med* 322:941-949, 1990.

95. Ward JW et al: Transmission of human immunodeficiency virus (HIV) by blood transfusions screened as negative for HIV antibody, *N Engl J Med* 318:473-478, 1988.

96. Weinberg DS, Murray HW: Coping with AIDS: the special problems of New York City, *N Engl J Med* 317:1469-1472, 1987.

97. Weiss R, Thier SO: HIV testing is the answer—what's the question? *N Engl J Med* 319:1010-1012, 1988.

98. Winkelstein W et al: Sexual practices and risk of infection by the human immunodeficiency virus: the San Francisco Men's Health Study, *JAMA* 257:321-325, 1987.

99. Winkelstein W et al: The San Francisco Men's Health Study. III. Reduction in human immunodeficiency virus transmission among homosexual/bisexual men, 1982-86, *Am J Public Health* 77(6):685-689, 1987.

100. Wittkowski KM: Preventing the heterosexual spread of AIDS: what is the best advice if compliance is taken into account? *AIDS* 3(3):143-145, 1989.

101. Wormser GP, Joline C, Duncanson F: Needle-stick injuries during the care of patients with AIDS, *N Engl J Med* 310(22):1461-1462, 1984.

102. Yoshida T et al: Evaluation of passive particle agglutination test for antibody to human immunodeficiency virus, *J Clin Microbiol* 25(8):1433-1437, 1987.

CHAPTER 4

HIV Testing: Indications for Testing, Risk Assessment, and Counseling

Medical indications for HIV antibody testing
  Excluding HIV Infection in Patients at Risk with No Clinical Evidence of AIDS
  Excluding HIV Infection in Patients with Clinical Syndromes Potentially Related to HIV Infection
  Excluding HIV Infection in Patients of Unknown Risk Because of Specific Public Health Considerations
  Screening of Donated Blood
  Establishing the Diagnosis of AIDS
  Screening Programs and Seroprevalence Studies

Risk assessment
  Sexual History
  History of Drug Abuse
  Other HIV-Related History
HIV counseling
  The Role of Counseling
  Pretest Counseling
Decreasing the risk of HIV transmission
  Sexual Behavior
  Intravenous Drug Use
  Other Preventive Measures
Contact notification

The development of techniques to detect antibody to the human immunodeficiency virus type 1 (HIV or HIV-1) in the blood of infected individuals has made it possible to diagnose HIV infection before the onset of AIDS. The advantages of early detection seem obvious: both medical intervention and modification of high-risk behavior could be offered at the earliest stages of the disease. Whether such testing should be offered exclusively on a voluntary basis or made mandatory under some circumstances is a subject of controversy.[32]

Other suggested uses of HIV testing include broader public health strategies. It has been argued, for example, that identifying HIV-infected patients through testing could help reduce the risk of transmission to health care workers,[25] and that for this reason routine testing of selected patients should be undertaken.[5] Other strategies that have been proposed or established include routine screening of military recruits,[11] applicants for marriage licenses,[49,58] prison inmates,[53] and all adults under 60 years of age.[54]

Because of the low prevalence of HIV infection in the general population, however, broad-based screening of low-risk populations generally identifies few infected individuals at great financial cost. Questions about the ethics,[3] legality, utility, and scientific validity of such strategies also have been raised.[63]

Although controversy over the uses of HIV testing continues, interim strategies have been proposed to guide the practitioner. Targeted, voluntary testing of patients at increased risk of HIV infection has been recommended by the Centers for Disease Control.[7] Such a directed approach requires the practitioner to have a clear understanding of HIV transmission and to be willing and able, by means of the medical history and physical examination, to identify patients at risk. Familiarity with the medical, social, and psychological implications of HIV infection is essential for an effective and humane approach to testing and counseling.

Ever since procedures for detecting HIV infection were first developed, testing strategies have been the subject of controversy among infectious disease experts and public health authorities and within the general medical community. Surveys have indicated a significant level of dissatisfaction among some physicians over current testing procedures[24,30] and, in some cases, impatience with targeted testing.[24] The effectiveness of voluntary counseling and testing programs has not yet been established, and mandatory testing of individuals at high risk has been proposed by some[2] as a more effective strategy, although evidence for the effectiveness of this approach is also lacking. State laws currently differ on such central issues as reporting of HIV test results to public health authorities, requirements for contact tracing, and compulsory screening of selected populations.[21,29]

The indications for testing should be established individually for each patient. Except when required by law, HIV testing should be offered and strongly recommended, on a voluntary basis, to those at significant risk of infection; it should be provided for all patients who request it.

MEDICAL INDICATIONS FOR HIV ANTIBODY TESTING

The demonstrated medical benefits of early detection of HIV infection[4,12] have led to the establishment of medical indications for voluntary HIV testing.

Excluding HIV Infection in Patients at Risk with No Clinical Evidence of AIDS

HIV testing and counseling should be routinely offered to patients with a history of high-risk behavior,[1,7] including:

Men who have engaged in sexual activity with other men

Men and women with a history of intravenous drug use

Men and women who have engaged in prostitution

Women born or residing in an area with a high prevalence of infection in women

Those who received transfusions of blood or blood products between 1978 and 1985, particularly in areas with a high incidence of AIDS

Individuals who believe they are at risk of HIV infection

Heterosexual partners of individuals meeting any of these criteria

Excluding HIV Infection in Patients with Clinical Syndromes Potentially Related to HIV Infection

It has been recommended that testing and counseling also should be offered to patients with sexually transmitted diseases or medical conditions that may be related to HIV infection,[7] including:

Tuberculosis

Generalized lymphadenopathy

Unexplained dementia

Chronic, unexplained fever, diarrhea, or weight loss

Generalized herpes

Chronic candidiasis

Excluding HIV Infection in Patients of Unknown Risk Because of Specific Public Health Considerations

HIV testing should be considered for[7]:

Those considering marriage

Prison inmates

Screening of Donated Blood

Since 1985, blood donated in the United States has been screened by enzyme-linked immunosorbent assay (ELISA) for HIV antibody. Blood that tests positive is not transfused. If antibody is repeatedly detected by ELISA and confirmed by the Western blot (WB) test, the donor is informed that the test is positive.

Establishing the Diagnosis of AIDS

According to the AIDS case definition currently in use by the Centers for Disease Control, demonstration of a positive HIV antibody test is required before a diagnosis of AIDS can be made in some patients (see Chapter 1).

Screening Programs and Seroprevalence Studies

Individuals in certain groups such as active-duty military personnel, recruit applicants, and Job Corps applicants are screened for HIV infection.

Anonymous testing of certain populations such as parturient women, patients attending clinics for sexually transmitted diseases, and trauma victims has been undertaken to determine the prevalence of HIV infection (see Chapter 3).

RISK ASSESSMENT

Among adults, HIV is transmitted almost exclusively by two routes: needle sharing during intravenous drug use and sexual contact. Since HIV-infected individuals may remain asymptomatic for years after infection has occurred, the goal of risk assessment should be to identify past and present high-risk behavior. Despite the diversity of opinion on testing strategies, obtaining an accurate history of risk behavior and assessing the risk of HIV infection in patients who may not be able to provide a complete history has become an increasingly vital skill for the primary care physician, and regardless of changes in testing procedures, it is likely to remain the most important component of HIV counseling.

Sexual History

Although the sexual history is regarded as an essential element of the general medical evaluation, surveys have indicated that a large proportion of physicians do not obtain a complete history of sexual behavior from their patients.[33] The reasons for this omission vary, although embarrassment and lack of specific training in obtaining the sexual history were blamed by many physicians in one large survey.[43] Unfamiliarity with sexual practices and HIV transmission patterns may lead to improper counseling[17] and needless testing of patients at low risk of HIV infection.[65]

Discussing current and past sexual behavior at the time of initial assessment of adult and adolescent patients serves several important purposes: it allows the clinician to assess the risk of HIV infection and to make specific suggestions to the patient about necessary changes in sexual practices; it may lead to identification of sexual partners at risk for infection should the patient prove to be HIV-positive so that testing of these individuals may be explored with the patient; and it can establish an atmosphere in which the patient more freely discusses sexual behavior at subsequent visits. In addition, it should be recognized that national and international efforts to fully characterize the AIDS epidemic depend on accurate assessments of risk behavior.

All adult patients should be asked appropriate questions about past and current heterosexual behavior, including (1) number of partners, (2) frequency of anonymous encounters, (3) prostitute contact, (4) history of sexually transmitted diseases, (5) condom use, and (6) specific sexual practices.

In addition, male patients should be routinely questioned about past sexual encounters with other men. Avoiding labels by asking, "Have you ever had sex with another man?" may be more effective at eliciting accurate information than asking, "Are you homosexual?" Despite a history of homosexual activity, the patient may not describe himself as homosexual or bisexual.

Men who give a history of sexual intercourse with other men should be questioned about the number of sexual partners they have had and the circumstances (anonymous, public or private locations) in which such encounters usually occur. Information about specific sexual practices, including receptive or insertive anal intercourse, douching, and oral-anal or oral-genital contact, is important. Since receptive anal intercourse[31,56,66,67] and douching[56,66] are associated with a particularly high risk of HIV infection, such information may allow the practitioner to estimate the likelihood of HIV infection. More important, however, detailed knowledge of the patient's sexual practices may allow the physician to make specific recommendations about altering behavior.

History of Drug Abuse

Patients should be questioned carefully about previous and current drug use and needle sharing. Although HIV transmission occurs through needle sharing among parenteral drug users, the use of drugs by other routes, such as inhalation or smoking of cocaine ("crack"), may be associated with increased high-risk sexual activity.

Other HIV-Related History

Blood transfusions. The risk of HIV infection through blood transfusion was greatest between 1978 and 1985 in geographical areas, such as New York City, California, New Jersey, and the District of Columbia, where the incidence of AIDS has been highest. Patients should be questioned about all transfusions of blood or blood products. In some cases, such as major trauma, the patient may have unknowingly received a transfusion.

Artificial insemination. Transmission of HIV infection by means of artificial insemination has been reported.[15,57]

Health care employment. Although infrequent, transmission of HIV infection has occurred in health care settings. A history of health care employment, particularly exposure to blood or other body fluids from patients potentially at risk for HIV infection, may be significant.

HIV COUNSELING
The Role of Counseling

The American Medical Association,[1] the U.S. Public Health Service,[7] and local health departments[46] all have recommended that formalized counseling take place before and after HIV testing. Such an approach is advisable, because the medical and social implications of HIV testing are complex, and the individual seeking testing must deal with a large amount of information.

In pretest counseling, the likelihood of HIV infection should be discussed in light of the patient's specific history of risk behavior. Testing procedures and the meaning of a positive or negative test result must be explained (see Chapter 3). Patients testing negative must be educated about reducing risk. Those testing positive also require this information, as well as a thorough explanation of therapeutic strategies and the need to trace contacts.

The ramifications of a positive test for HIV may extend into all facets of an individual's life. Beyond the fear of suffering and death from a disease that may be both disabling and disfiguring, concern and guilt about possible exposure of loved ones, fear of disclosure of risk behavior, and fear of social abandonment may dominate an individual's reaction. The financial implications of HIV infection, including the cost of health care, potential loss of job security, and inability to purchase life insurance, may have to be confronted immediately. Because of the potentially devastating impact of a positive test result, personal contact between the practitioner and the patient, in the form of counseling before and after the test, is crucial.

There are currently no uniform national regulations governing HIV testing and counseling in the United States.[21] In some states, specific laws governing HIV counseling have been enacted.[21] Such laws may specify that certain information must be communicated to the patient during formal counseling sessions. Practitioners must consult local health authorities for requirements on counseling and testing procedures. The following are general guidelines for HIV counseling before and after testing is performed; they are not intended to take the place of local requirements.

Pretest Counseling

When the decision is made to offer HIV testing to a patient or when a patient requests such testing, counseling addressing the specific reasons for testing, as well as the test's limitations, should be offered. It is important that the patient understand the specific reasons that testing is indicated and how the test results will be used in his or her overall medical care. A judgmental attitude must be avoided, and patients should be strongly encouraged to discuss openly their feelings about the need for testing and their concerns about the testing procedure.

The practitioner should try to anticipate the reaction to a positive or negative result and explore with the patient the likely impact that a positive test would have on his or her life. Although pretest counseling cannot take the place of a thorough psychiatric evaluation, it can help identify patients who might benefit from psychiatric intervention. The reported increased risk of suicide among HIV-infected patients[38] underscores the need for a thorough exploration of the patient's feelings before testing. Asking the patient what he or she expects the test result to be may aid in anticipating the impact of a positive result.

Local regulations governing confidentiality and notification of contacts should be discussed before the test.

Objectives of pretest counseling

Pretest counseling has several objectives:
1. Establishing rapport
2. Assessing the risk of HIV infection
3. Assessing the need for testing
4. Explaining the testing procedure, including confidentiality regulations
5. Explaining the meaning of a positive or negative test result
6. Discussing possible negative consequences of testing
7. Providing information about AIDS and other HIV-related diseases
8. Reviewing means of reducing the likelihood of transmission
9. Anticipating the individual's likely reaction to a positive or negative test result
10. Obtaining informed consent according to local requirements

Establishing rapport. People undergo HIV testing for a variety of reasons. Some may realistically suspect that they are infected because of high-risk behavior, exposure to a person known to be infected, or the occurrence of symptoms. Others, such as health care workers, may fear that they may have contracted HIV infection after a single possible exposure. Occasionally people with little or no apparent risk of infection request testing because it is required for immigration, life insurance, or other purposes. In some cases, excessive fear of HIV infection may lead an individual to seek repeated testing despite assurances that infection has been excluded. The means of establishing rapport differ according to the individual's reasons for seeking testing.

Patients who believe there is a high likelihood that they are infected should be supported and encouraged in their decision to undergo testing. The patient should be questioned about past sexual behavior and drug use, both to establish the likelihood of infection on clinical grounds, and to begin the process of identifying potential contacts if the patient proves to be infected. The practitioner can offer support by acknowledging the courage the patient has shown in agreeing to be tested. It may be advisable to provide advice on safe sexual practices and other means of preventing transmission during pretest counseling.

Health care workers who request testing after a single potential exposure should be questioned carefully about the circumstances under which exposure occurred. Needle-stick injuries and splashes of blood or body fluids onto mucosal surfaces account for most such exposures. In general, individuals who have had such potential exposure can be reassured that infection is unlikely but that baseline and follow-up testing should be carried out. It has been recommended that postexposure prophylaxis with the antiviral agent zidovudine be considered,[14] although the efficacy of such prophylaxis in preventing HIV transmission is unknown. The anxiety that accompanies such incidents often is severe but usually can be lessened by clearly discussing the risk of infection (see Chapter 3).

Occasionally individuals may request repeated HIV testing despite several negative results. Such patients may be engaging in ongoing risk behavior or may be manifesting an inappropriate fear of AIDS. The practitioner should reassure such patients about the excellent reliability of current testing methods but also should probe carefully about risk behavior.

Risk assessment. See discussion earlier in this chapter.

Assessing the need for testing. Individuals requesting HIV testing, including those with a clear history of high-risk behavior, should be asked why they feel that they might be infected. A history of risk behavior or possible sexual contact with an individual at high risk of infection is the reason most commonly given. In some cases, however, additional important facts may come to light. Patients who appear to be asymptomatic on initial questioning may have sought testing after becoming aware of a subtle symptom that they suspected was HIV related. Some individuals are prompted to seek testing because they plan to begin a new sexual relationship, marry, or have children. Understanding the patient's reasons for requesting HIV testing may prove extremely helpful in directing counseling and medical management.

Explaining testing procedures, the meaning of positive and negative results, and confidentiality procedures. Two techniques are commonly used to test for HIV antibody: the enzyme-linked immunosorbent assay (ELISA) and the Western blot (WB) test. As discussed in Chapter 3, specimens testing negative by

ELISA are reported as negative for HIV antibody. Those testing repeatedly positive by ELISA are analyzed by the WB test for confirmation.

It should be explained that conventional HIV tests do not detect antibody for weeks to months after infection, and for this reason a single negative result cannot exclude HIV infection in a person actively engaged in high-risk behavior. It should be made clear during pretest counseling that repeat testing may be necessary to completely rule out the possibility of HIV infection.

Local regulations governing confidentiality of test results, as well as mechanisms by which confidentiality will be maintained, should be explained to the patient. Depending on state and local regulations, HIV test results may be disclosed under certain circumstances.[21] If anonymous testing is available, the patient should be told about this option.

Potential disadvantages of testing. Individuals who meet medical indications should be strongly urged to undergo HIV testing. Persons with no history of risk behavior who desire testing should be informed of the possibility of false positive results (see Chapter 3). Testing should take place only if confidentiality of results can be reasonably assured. Nonetheless, patients undergoing testing should be informed that discrimination on the basis of HIV infection has occurred in employment, housing, and other areas.[39]

Providing information about AIDS and other HIV-related diseases. The chronic nature of HIV infection (see Chapter 2) should be explained, and the term "AIDS" defined (see Chapter 1). Care should be taken even during pretest counseling to allow the patient to maintain a realistic level of hope. With patients who are asymptomatic, it should be pointed out that (1) AIDS most often evolves slowly, (2) therapy to delay progression to AIDS is available, and (3) additional forms of treatment are being studied extensively. Symptomatic patients can also be reassured that therapeutic options are available and likely to improve and that determining if HIV infection is present will allow for better and more appropriate medical treatment.

Reducing the risk of HIV transmission. Preventive measures are discussed later in this chapter under "Decreasing the Risk of HIV Transmission."

Anticipating the individual's reaction to the test result. Consideration should be given during pretest counseling to exploring with patients their potential reaction to a positive or negative HIV test result. Asking patients what they expect the result to be and what they would do if they learn that they are HIV infected may help identify those likely to have an extreme emotional crisis or to consider suicide or other serious acts. Such screening does not take the place of formal psychiatric evaluation, however. Individuals undergoing HIV testing had a high incidence of mood disorders in one series[48] and may be at high risk for depression. Psychiatric consultation before HIV testing and counseling should be strongly considered for patients with a history of mental illness.

Obtaining consent. Local regulations regarding procedures for obtaining informed consent vary.[21] The practitioner should be familiar with such regulations and should ensure that consent is obtained properly and in a non-coercive fashion.

Counseling after the Test

Counseling after the test should be conducted regardless of the test result. For the patient testing positive, a counseling session provides the opportunity both to review information about transmission and medical options and to assess the individual's reaction. The goals of counseling after the test should be to (1) advise the patient on ways of avoiding transmission of infection to others, (2) discuss notification of others who may have been exposed, and (3) assess the individual's emotional reaction to a positive result. For the patient testing negative, changes in behavior to eliminate the risk of HIV infection, discussed before testing, should be reinforced.

Negative test result. Individuals with a negative test result who have engaged in high-risk behavior within 6 months before testing should be advised that recent infection has not been excluded. Repeat testing after an interval of at least 3 months should be scheduled, and the patient should be advised that he or she may be capable of transmitting HIV infection to others.

Patients testing negative who remain actively engaged in high-risk behavior should be urged to change their behavior and should be informed that they remain at high risk of infection. Drug treatment options should be explored with active intravenous drug users. If high-risk behavior is to continue, HIV testing should be repeated at 3- to 6-month intervals indefinitely.

All patients testing negative should be counseled to avoid high-risk sexual practices (see below).

Positive test result. After informing the patient of the positive test result, the practitioner should allow the patient to express his or her feelings. Fears of death, abandonment by loved ones, and humiliation often are particularly acute at this time. Such patients should be assisted in identifying friends or family members with whom they might share their feelings. Establishing a plan of action for medical care, contact notification, and emotional support may lessen anxiety.

Medical treatment options should be discussed briefly during counseling after the test, although specific decisions may be postponed until an immunological evaluation has been completed (see Chapter 6).

A review of necessary changes in sexual practices and a discussion of contact notification should be included in counseling after the test.

DECREASING THE RISK OF HIV TRANSMISSION
Sexual Behavior

Sexual routes of transmission

A variety of clinical studies have attempted to stratify the risk of HIV transmission associated with various sexual practices. The high risk of receptive anal intercourse among male homosexuals has been demonstrated repeatedly, but the relative risk of other practices is less clear. It is assumed that any form of sexual contact, whether genital, oral-genital, or rectal, carries some risk of transmission.

Receptive anal intercourse. Studies of homosexual men indicate that receptive anal intercourse is an efficient means of HIV transmission.[31,66] Male-to-female transmission may also occur in this fashion.[42]

Insertive anal intercourse. Insertive anal intercourse appears to pose less of a risk of transmission than receptive anal intercourse,[31] although the risk remains significant.

Vaginal intercourse. Vaginal intercourse is clearly an important route of male-to-female HIV transmission. The importance of female-to-male transmission appears to be greater in central Africa than in Western countries.[47] Relatively few cases of AIDS in the United States have been attributed to female-to-male transmission, although patients should be informed that transmission may occur by this route.[13]

Oral-genital contact. Controversy exists over the importance of oral-genital contact in HIV transmission. Data from prospective studies of male homosexuals suggest that transmission occurs relatively rarely during fellatio,[31,34,55] although this practice was an independent risk factor for transmission in a study of heterosexual couples.[16]

Kissing. Although HIV has been isolated from saliva of infected individuals,[23] casual kissing was not found to transmit HIV infection in one large series.[18] However, it has been suggested that transmission may be possible during passionate kissing.[50]

Eliminating the risk of sexual transmission

Although specific data on the risk of HIV transmission associated with various sexual practices are available, the definition of "safe sex" is controversial.[19] Because HIV infection may occur after a single exposure and because AIDS is an incurable, fatal disease, it has been recommended that counseling be directed at eliminating, rather than simply reducing, the risk of transmission.[19] Some have suggested, however, that counseling abstinence may be unrealistic and that the use of condoms and spermicidal compounds may ultimately prove more effective in reducing HIV transmission.[68]

Abstinence. Since all forms of oral, vaginal, or rectal sexual intercourse may carry a risk of HIV transmission, it is appropriate to counsel HIV-infected individuals or those whose sexual behavior may bring them into contact with an infected person that sexual abstinence may be the only certain way to prevent transmission.

Condoms. The use of condoms has been suggested as an important strategy in limiting sexual transmission of HIV.[9] Partly as a result of such recommendations, condom sales in the United States increased substantially during the 1980s.[45] Some condom materials, particularly latex, have been shown to be impermeable to the virus.[61] Nonlatex condoms, particularly those made of sheep intestinal tissue (so-called natural condoms), may be less effective.[44] Clinical data suggest that condom use decreases HIV transmission in heterosexual couples.[16] Condoms are not uniformly protective, however, and the actual degree of protection conferred to each partner during various types of sexual activity is not known.

Reported rates of condom failure have been alarmingly high: 5% during vaginal intercourse in one study,[22] and 8% during anal intercourse in another,[60] and compliance rates may be low.[36,59] The overall efficacy of condoms in preventing HIV transmission may be less than that in preventing pregnancy.[20] Although widespread use of condoms would be likely to reduce HIV transmission within a population at risk, the level of protection provided is probably inadequate to justify their use as the sole means of preventing transmission.

Spermicides. HIV is inactivated by the spermicidal compound nonoxynol 9 in vitro.[27] It has been suggested that the use of spermicides together with condoms may further decrease the risk of transmission.[19]

Mutual masturbation. Mutual masturbation, which involves no exchange of body fluids and no deposition of semen or vaginal secretions from one partner onto mucous membrane surfaces of the other, has been suggested as a means of eliminating the risk of HIV transmission.[19] Data regarding the safety of specific practices are lacking.

Advice to the patient

All patients should be informed of the following facts about sexual behavior:

1. Mutually monogamous sexual intercourse between uninfected individuals carries no risk of HIV infection.
2. HIV-infected individuals can transmit the virus even when they appear to be completely healthy.
3. No form of oral-genital, anal, or genital sexual contact with an infected individual is known to be free of all risk of HIV transmission.

4. The use of condoms diminishes but does not eliminate the risk of sexual transmission of HIV infection.
5. If condoms are used, latex brands with spermicidal compounds are preferable and the condom should be left in place for the duration of sexual contact.

Male homosexuals. Men testing positive for HIV infection should be advised to seek forms of sexual expression other than anal or oral intercourse or oral-anal contact. All body fluids, except perhaps saliva, should be assumed to contain viable virus.

Changes in sexual behavior aimed at decreasing the risk of HIV transmission have been documented in several studies of homosexual men.[28,37,41,67] A decrease in the number of sexual partners and in receptive anal intercourse among seronegative men and a decrease in insertive anal intercourse among seropositive men was associated with a decline in transmission in one large prospective series.[67]

Men testing HIV negative on repeated determinations may remain sexually active but should be advised to avoid sexual contact with individuals who are infected or whose status is unknown. These patients also should be firmly warned about the particularly high risk of HIV infection associated with receptive anal intercourse[31] and with practices such as douching and fist insertion into the rectum ("fisting") that are associated with added trauma to the rectal mucosa.

Although condoms have been recommended as a means of preventing transmission during anal intercourse, failure rates may be high.[60]

Heterosexual females and males. The high risk of transmission associated with vaginal, oral, or anal intercourse should be stressed, and other forms of sexual contact, such as mutual masturbation, should be considered. The potential failure rate of condoms should be emphasized. Patients should be advised of the risk of fetal infection if pregnancy occurs and of the medical, financial, and emotional implications of pediatric AIDS.

Individuals testing HIV negative on repeated determinations may remain sexually active but should be advised to avoid sexual contact with persons who are known to be infected or whose HIV status is questionable.

Intravenous Drug Use

Individuals with a history of intravenous drug use should be questioned about sexual practices and counseled according to the above outline.

Needle sharing. The sharing of hypodermic needles for injecting drugs is presumed to be the primary nonsexual route of HIV transmission among intravenous drug users. Although needle sharing has become less common among intravenous drug users in some areas,[26] it remains a widespread practice, despite a rising level of awareness about AIDS.[35] Needle exchange programs, through which the drug user would be supplied with sterile injection equipment, have been proposed as a solution to this problem, but this may not be sufficient to eliminate transmission.[62] Needle sharing may be less frequent among intravenous drug users enrolled in drug abuse treatment programs.[40]

Other Preventive Measures

Nonintravenous drug use. Nonparenteral cocaine use, particularly the smoking of "crack," may be associated with an increase in unsafe sexual practices and thus an increase in the risk of HIV transmission.[64] For this reason it is important that patients are cautioned about all forms of drug use.

Alcohol. It has been suggested that alcohol consumption may exert a disinhibitory effect on high-risk sexual behavior.[51]

Protecting nonsexual household contacts. The risk of transmission of HIV infection to nonsexual household contacts appears to be extremely low. Nonetheless, HIV-infected patients should be instructed not to share toothbrushes, razors, or other items that could carry blood with household members.[6] HIV loses viability within several hours after drying on floors and other surfaces,[8] although small numbers of viable virus may persist for days. Although transmission of HIV infection has not been shown to result from this, surfaces on which blood or other body fluids from an HIV-infected person have been spilled should be cleaned thoroughly and disinfected. Household bleach (sodium hypochlorite) in a 1:10 dilution has been recommended for disinfection.[8]

Nonsexual household contacts, including friends and family members, of HIV-infected patients frequently express fear that they, too, will become infected. To prevent physical and emotional isolation of the infected person, the practitioner should allay these fears by explaining that simple precautions will eliminate any risk. A face-to-face meeting with close friends or family members may be necessary.

Informing health care workers of HIV status. Because of the small but definite risk of transmission of HIV infection in the health care setting, HIV-positive individuals should be instructed to inform physicians, dentists, or other providers that they are infected.

Blood donation. HIV-infected individuals should be instructed to refrain from donating blood, semen, plasma, body organs, or any other tissue.[6]

CONTACT NOTIFICATION

Notification of sexual contacts has been an important component of public health strategies to limit the spread of sexually transmitted diseases such as syphilis and gonorrhea. Currently there is no uniform national policy on contact notification in the United States, although this has been proposed.[52] State laws differ on tracing and notification of contacts of HIV-infected individuals.[21] However, state AIDS prevention projects funded by the Centers for Disease Control provide confidential notification of sexual and needle-sharing partners of HIV-infected individuals.[10] In these programs, contacts may be notified by the infected individual (partner referral) or by Health Department personnel (provider referral).

Practitioners should be knowledgeable about local regulations and procedures governing contact notification. HIV-infected individuals should be urged to notify sexual and needle-sharing contacts. If they refuse, confidential notification by the practitioner or other trained personnel should be offered.

REFERENCES

1. American Medical Association: HIV blood test counseling: AMA physician guidelines, Chicago, 1989, The Association.
2. Archer VE: Psychological defenses and control of AIDS, *Am J Public Health* 79(7):876-878, 1989.
3. Bayer R, Levine C, Wolf SM: HIV antibody screening: an ethical framework for evaluating proposed programs, *JAMA* 256(13):1768-1774, 1986.
4. Broder S et al: Antiretroviral therapy in AIDS, *Ann Intern Med* 113(8):604-618, 1990.
5. Carey JS: Routine preoperative screening for HIV, *JAMA* 260(2):179, 1988.
6. Centers for Disease Control: Additional recommendations to reduce sexual and drug abuse-related transmission of human T-lymphotropic virus type III/lymphadenopathy–associated virus, *JAMA* 255:1843-1844,1849, 1986.
7. Centers for Disease Control: Public Health Service guidelines for counseling and antibody testing to prevent HIV infection and AIDS, *MMWR* 36:509-515, 1987.
8. Centers for Disease Control: Recommendations for prevention of HIV transmission in health care settings, *MMWR* 36:2S-18S, 1987.
9. Centers for Disease Control: Condoms for prevention of sexually transmitted diseases, *MMWR* 37(9):133-137, 1987.
10. Centers for Disease Control: Partner notification for preventing human immunodeficiency virus (HIV) infection: Colorado, Idaho, South Carolina, Virginia, *MMWR* 37:393-402, 1988.
11. Centers for Disease Control: Trends in human immunodeficiency virus infection among civilian applicants for military service: United States, October 1985 to March 1988, *MMWR* 37:677-679, 1988.
12. Centers for Disease Control: Guidelines for prophylaxis against *Pneumocystis carinii* pneumonia for persons infected with human immunodeficiency virus, *MMWR* 38(suppl 5):1-9, 1989.
13. Centers for Disease Control: HIV/AIDS surveillance, August 1990.

14. Centers for Disease Control: Public Health Service statement on management of occupational exposure to human immunodeficiency virus, including considerations regarding zidovudine postexposure use, *MMWR* 39:1-14, 1990.
15. Chiasson MA, Stoneburner RL, Joseph SC: Human immunodeficiency virus transmission through artificial insemination, *J Acquir Immune Defic Syndr* 3:69-72, 1990.
16. Fischl MA et al: Evaluation of heterosexual partners, children, and household contacts of adults with AIDS, *JAMA* 257(5):640-644, 1987.
17. Fredman L et al: Primary care physicians' assessment and prevention of HIV infection, *Am J Prev Med* 5(4):188-195, 1989.
18. Friedland GH et al: Lack of transmission of HTLV-III/LAV infection to household contacts of patients with AIDS or AIDS-related complex with oral candidiasis, *N Engl J Med* 314:344-349, 1986.
19. Goedert JJ: What is safe sex? Suggested standards linked to testing for human immunodeficiency virus, *N Engl J Med* 316:1339-1342, 1987.
20. Gordon R: A critical review of the physics of condoms and their role in individual versus societal survival of the AIDS epidemic, *J Sex Marital Ther* 15(1):5-30, 1989.
21. Gostin LO: Public health strategies for confronting AIDS: legislative and regulatory policy in the United States, *JAMA* 261(110):1621-1630, 1989.
22. Gotzsche PC, Hording M: Condoms to prevent HIV transmission do not imply truly safe sex, *Scand J Infect Dis* 20(2):233-234, 1988.
23. Groopman JE et al: HTLV-III in saliva of people with AIDS-related complex and healthy homosexual men at risk for AIDS, *Science* 226:447-449, 1984.
24. Grove DI, Mulligan JB: Consent, compulsion, and confidentiality in relation to testing for HIV infection: the views of WA doctors, *Med J Aust* 152(4):174-178, 1990.
25. Guido LJ: Routine preoperative screening for HIV, *JAMA* 260(2):180, 1988.
26. Guydish JR et al: Changes in needle sharing behavior among intravenous drug users: San Francisco, 1986-88, *Am J Public Health* 80(8):995-997, 1990.
27. Hicks DR et al: Inactivation of HTLV-III/LAV–infected cultures of normal human lymphocytes by nonoxynol-9 in vitro, *Lancet* 2:1422-1423, 1985.
28. Joseph JG et al: Magnitude and determinants of behavior risk reduction: longitudinal analysis of a cohort at risk for AIDS, *Psychol Health* 1:73-96, 1987.
29. Judson FN: What do we really know about AIDS control? *Am J Public Health* 79(7):878-882, 1989.
30. King MB: Psychological and social problems in HIV infection: interviews with general practitioners in London, *Br Med J* 299(6701):713-717, 1989.
31. Kingsley LA et al: Risk factors for seroconversion to human immunodeficiency virus among male homosexuals, *Lancet* 1:345-348, 1987.
32. Krasinski K et al: Failure of voluntary testing for human immunodeficiency virus to identify infected parturient women in a high-risk population, *N Engl J Med* 318:185, 1988.
33. Lewis CE, Freeman HE, Corey CR: AIDS-related competence of California's primary care physicians, *Am J Public Health* 77:795-799, 1987.
34. Lyman D et al: Minimal risk of transmission of AIDS-associated retrovirus infection by oral-genital contact, *JAMA* 255(13):1703, 1986.
35. Magura S et al: Determinants of needle sharing among intravenous drug users, *Am J Public Health* 79(4):459-462, 1989.
36. Magura S et al: Variables influencing condom use among intravenous drug

users, *Am J Public Health* 80(1):82-84, 1990.

37. Martin JL: The impact of AIDS on gay male sexual behavior in New York City, *Am J Public Health* 77:578-581, 1987.
38. Marzuk PM et al: Increased risk of suicide in persons with AIDS, *JAMA* 259(9):1333-1337, 1988.
39. Matthews GW, Neslund VS: The initial impact of AIDS on public health law in the United States—1986, *JAMA* 257(3):344-352, 1987.
40. McCusker J et al: Demographic characteristics, risk behaviors, and HIV seroprevalence among intravenous drug users by site of contact: results from a community-wide HIV surveillance project, *Am J Public Health* 80(9):1062-1067, 1990.
41. McKusick L, Horstman W, Coates TJ: AIDS and sexual behavior reported by gay men in San Francisco, *Am J Public Health* 75:493-496, 1985.
42. Melbye M et al: Anal intercourse as a possible factor in heterosexual transmission of HTLV-III to spouses of hemophiliacs, *N Engl J Med* 312(13):857, 1985.
43. Merrill JM, Laux LF, Thornby JI: Why doctors have difficulty with sex histories, *South Med J* 83(6):613-617, 1990.
44. Minuk GY, Bohme CE, Bowen TJ: Condoms and hepatitis B virus infection, *Ann Intern Med* 104(4):584, 1986.
45. Moran JS et al: Increase in condom sales following AIDS education and publicity—United States, *Am J Public Health* 80(5):607-608, 1990.
46. New York City Department of Health: Guidelines for physicians on HIV counseling and testing and related documents, July 1989.
47. Padian NS: Heterosexual transmission of acquired immunodeficiency syndrome: international perspectives and national projections, *Rev Infect Dis* 9(5):947-960, 1987.
48. Perry S et al: Psychiatric diagnosis before serological testing for the human immunodeficiency virus, *Am J Psychiatry* 147(1):89-93, 1990.
49. Petersen LR et al: Premarital screening for antibodies to human immunodeficiency virus type 1 in the United States, *Am J Public Health* 80(9):1087-1090, 1990.
50. Piazza M et al: Passionate kissing and microlesions of the oral mucosa: possible role in AIDS transmission, *JAMA* 261(2):244-245, 1989.
51. Plant MA: Alcohol, sex, and AIDS, *Alcohol* 25:293-301, 1990.
52. Potterat JJ et al: Partner notification in the control of human immunodeficiency virus infection, *Am J Public Health* 79(7):874-876, 1989.
53. Quinlan JM: Mandatory testing for HIV in federal prisons, *N Engl J Med* 320:315-316, 1989.
54. Rhame FS, Maki DG: The case for wider use of testing for HIV infection, *N Engl J Med* 320(19):1248-1254, 1989.
55. Schechter MT et al: Can HTLV-III be transmitted orally? *Lancet* 1:379, 1986.
56. Stevens CE et al: Human T-cell lymphotropic virus type III infection in a cohort of homosexual men in New York City, *JAMA* 255:2167-2172, 1986.
57. Stewart GJ et al: Transmission of human T-cell lymphotropic virus type III (HTLV-III) by artificial insemination by donor, *Lancet* 2(8455):581-585, 1985.
58. Turnock BJ, Kelly CJ: Mandatory premarital testing for human immunodeficiency virus: the Illinois experience, *JAMA* 261(23):3415-3418, 1989.
59. Valdiserri RO et al: Variables influencing condom use in a cohort of gay and bisexual men, *Am J Public Health* 78(7):801-805, 1988.
60. Van Griensven GJ et al: Failure rate of condoms during anogenital intercourse in homosexual men, *Genitourin Med* 64(5):344-346, 1988.
61. Van de Perre P, Jacobs D, Sprecher-Goldberger S: The latex condom, an

efficient barrier against sexual trans-mission of AIDS-related viruses, *AIDS* 1(1):49-52, 1987.

62. Van den Hoek JAR et al: Risk reduction among intravenous drug users in Amsterdam under the influence of AIDS, *Am J Public Health* 79(10):1355-1357, 1989.

63. Weiss R, Thier SO: HIV testing is the answer—what's the question? *N Engl J Med* 319:1010-1012, 1988.

64. Weiss SH: Links between cocaine and retroviral infection, *JAMA* 261(4):607-608, 1989.

65. Williams DN et al: HIV antibody testing in a multispecialty group practice, *Minn Med* 73(7):27-29, 1990.

66. Winkelstein W et al: Sexual practices and risk of infection by the human im-munodeficiency virus: the San Fran-cisco Men's Health Study, *JAMA* 257(3):321-325, 1987.

67. Winkelstein W et al: The San Francisco Men's Health Study. III. Reduction in human immunodeficiency virus trans-mission among homosexual/bisexual men—1982-86, *Am J Public Health* 77:685-689, 1987.

68. Wittkowski KM: Preventing the het-erosexual spread of AIDS: what is the best advice if compliance is taken into account? *AIDS* 3(3):143-145, 1989.

CHAPTER 5

Overview of HIV-Related Diseases by Organ System

Dermatological disorders
   Kaposi's Sarcoma
   Infections Involving the Skin
Nervous system disorders
   HIV-1 Infection of the Central
     Nervous System
   Opportunistic Infections and
     Malignancies of the Central
     Nervous System
   Psychiatric Disturbances
   Other HIV-Related Neurological
     Disorders
Ophthalmological disorders
   Opportunistic Infections
Oral disorders
   Infections
   Malignancies
   Other Disorders
Pulmonary disorders
   HIV-Related Pulmonary Infections
   Pulmonary Involvement with HIV-
     Related Malignancies
   Other Pulmonary Conditions
     Associated with HIV Infection
Cardiovascular disorders
   Myocardial Disease
   Pericardial Disease
   Endocarditis

Gastrointestinal disorders
   Esophagitis
   Infectious Diarrhea
   Cryptosporidiosis
   Isosporiasis
   Salmonellosis
   Cytomegalovirus (CMV)
   Mycobacterium Avium-
     Intracellulare (MAI)
   Miscellaneous Enteric Infections
   Gastrointestinal Involvement with
     HIV-Related Malignancies
   HIV-Related Enteropathy
   HIV-Related Hepatic Disease
   HIV-Related Biliary Disease
Renal disorders
   HIV-Associated Nephropathy
Endocrine disorders
   Adrenal Disorders
   Gonadal Disorders
Musculoskeletal disorders
   Reiter's Syndrome
   Psoriatic Arthritis
   HIV-Associated Arthritis
   Polymyositis
   Autoimmune Phenomena
   Sjögren's Syndrome/Sicca Complex
Hematological disorders
   Cytopenias
   Autoimmune Thrombocytopenia

Infection with the human immunodeficiency virus type 1 (HIV or HIV-1) leads to a complex multisystem disease. Opportunistic infections and malignancies, resulting from the progressive immunological impairment that is central to the disorder, may involve any organ system. However, a more direct relationship between HIV-1 infection and end-organ dysfunction has been recognized in recent years. Such clinical syndromes as dementia, cardiomyopathy, enteropathy, and nephropathy, which are commonly seen in HIV-infected patients, appear to be caused by the virus itself in many cases.

Many of the clinical manifestations of HIV-1 infection may occur early in the course of the disease, before the onset of opportunistic infections and malignancies. Some infections, including pneumococcal pneumonia, oral candidiasis, and pulmonary tuberculosis, are seen more often in HIV-infected adults but are not considered AIDS-defining conditions because they are common in the general population as well. Similarly, many idiopathic disorders, including seborrheic dermatitis, autoimmune thrombocytopenia, and Reiter's syndrome, are also seen more commonly but not exclusively in patients with HIV infection and are therefore not considered diagnostic of AIDS. The term AIDS-related complex (ARC), originally coined to describe nonspecific syndromes such as chronic fever, weight loss, lymphadenopathy, and diarrhea in HIV–risk group individuals, also fails to encompass many of the currently recognized clinical disorders associated with HIV-1 infection.

The primary care physician must be able to recognize the great diversity of clinical manifestations of HIV-1 infection. Distinctions between AIDS-defining disorders and other clinical syndromes associated with HIV-1 infection, although important for surveillance purposes, often become somewhat artificial in practical management.

This chapter provides an overview of major HIV-related disorders, whether AIDS defining or not, arranged by organ system. The reader is referred to Chapter 1 for surveillance criteria for the diagnosis of AIDS and the clinical definition of ARC. The approach to diagnosis and treatment of major clinical syndromes is covered in Chapters 7 through 9.

DERMATOLOGICAL DISORDERS

Dermatological manifestations of HIV infection are seen in most patients[203] and are common at all stages of disease[29,66] (Table 5-1). Although not life threatening, seborrheic dermatitis, psoriasis, xerosis, and alopecia are often extremely disturbing to the patient. Other processes involving the skin represent serious and potentially fatal complications. These include Kaposi's sarcoma and cutaneous manifestations of opportunistic infections such as cryptococcosis, pneumocystosis, tuberculosis, histoplasmosis, and herpes simplex or herpes zoster infection.

TABLE 5-1. Major dermatological manifestations of HIV-1 infection

Disorder	Frequency
Seborrheic dermatitis	50% of AIDS and ARC patients[29]
	30% of asymptomatic HIV-positive patients[29]
Candidiasis	37% of HIV-infected patients[29]
Xerosis/ichthyosis	30% of HIV-infected patients[66]
Dermatophyte infection	21%-30% of HIV-infected patients[29,66]
Herpes simplex	22% of AIDS and ARC patients[66]
Kaposi's sarcoma	15% of U.S. AIDS cases[6]
Psoriasis	5% of HIV-infected patients[8]
Molluscum contagiosum	Frequency not reported
Varicella zoster	Frequency not reported
One or more disorders	92% of HIV-infected patients[29]

An increase in the severity of dermatological symptoms may be associated with overall clinical progression.[203]

Kaposi's Sarcoma

Kaposi's sarcoma (KS) is a cutaneous neoplasm that was among the first disorders recognized to be associated with AIDS.[20,54] Among patients with AIDS, KS is seen most frequently in individuals who acquired HIV-1 infection through sexual contact, particularly male homosexuals.[6] It has been observed that the incidence of KS among male homosexuals has declined steadily since the beginning of the AIDS epidemic, although the reasons for this decline are unclear.[80]

AIDS-related KS differs from classic KS in its tendency to produce multiple lesions and visceral involvement. In addition to the skin, frequent sites of involvement include mucous membranes, the gastrointestinal and respiratory tracts, lymph nodes, and spleen.[54,64] Involvement of the liver,[78,125] heart,[185] and several other unusual sites has also been described.

The cause of AIDS-related KS is not known. It has been suggested that infectious or chemical cofactors, particularly nitrite inhalants,[79] may be important.

KS may be associated with a variety of skin lesions. Pink or red macules ranging in size from several millimeters to over 1 cm[54] and purple plaques or nodules[54] are seen most commonly. Lesions may appear on any part of the body and commonly involve the extremities, trunk, and face.

The prognosis of AIDS-related KS correlates with the degree of immunodeficiency. Median survival has been reported to be 31 months for patients with no history of opportunistic infection and a CD4 lymphocyte count over

300/mm³, and 7 months for those with previous or concurrent opportunistic infection.[22]

Infections Involving the Skin

Viral infections

Herpes simplex. Cutaneous herpes simplex infection was found in 22% of more than 100 consecutive AIDS and ARC patients in one series.[66] Typical patterns include chronic perianal, oral,[184] or disseminated lesions.

Varicella zoster. Localized or disseminated infection with varicella zoster virus is common in HIV-infected patients and may be seen before the onset of other complications. The appearance of severe varicella zoster in risk-group patients correlates highly with the presence of HIV-1 infection and may be one of the earliest signs of the disease.[133] In one series, more than 70% of homosexual men manifesting varicella zoster developed AIDS within 6 years.[133]

Molluscum contagiosum. Molluscum contagiosum infection has been reported in association with AIDS.[99] Typical papular lesions are most commonly seen on the hands and face but may be widely disseminated.

Fungal infections

Dermatophyte. Dermatophyte infections were reported in 21%[29] and 30%[66] of HIV-infected patients in two large series.

Candida. Cutaneous candidiasis was seen in 37% of HIV-infected patients in one series[29] and was most common in patients with AIDS or ARC.

Cryptococcosis. *Cryptococcus neoformans* was recognized as a cause of nodular skin lesions with ulceration before the advent of the AIDS epidemic.[24] With HIV infection, cryptococcal infection of the skin may cause diffuse cellulitis or papular lesions resembling molluscum contagiosum.[169]

Histoplasmosis. Disseminated infection with *Histoplasma capsulatum* may produce a generalized maculopapular rash. A partial response to topical corticosteroids, as was reported in one case,[70] may lead to diagnostic confusion.

Bacterial and mycobacterial infections

Cat-scratch disease. The bacterial agent of cat-scratch disease has been reported to cause angiomatous nodules that clinically resemble Kaposi's sarcoma and respond to antimicrobial therapy in a small number of patients.[106]

Mycobacterial disorders. Abscesses, ulcers, pustules, nodules, or papules may be seen in cutaneous mycobacterial infection.[11]

Cutaneous pneumocystosis. The respiratory pathogen *Pneumocystis carinii* rarely causes skin disease but has been described in association with nodular lesions.[32] Response to therapy with trimethoprim-sulfamethoxazole has been documented.[32]

Skin disorders of unknown origin

Seborrheic dermatitis. Seborrheic dermatitis was seen in approximately 50% of AIDS and ARC patients and 30% of asymptomatic HIV-positive patients in one large series[29] and was the only consistent skin disorder seen in patients with early HIV infection in another.[7] The degree of inflammation, the tendency to progression, and overall severity appear to be greater in HIV-infected patients than in normal hosts.[131] A distinctive histopathological pattern has been described in HIV-associated cases.[192]

Although the etiology of HIV-associated seborrheic dermatitis is uncertain, the fungus *Pityrosporum orbiculare* may play a role in pathogenesis and antifungal therapy is beneficial in some cases.[73]

Xerosis/ichthyosis. In one series 30% of symptomatic HIV-infected patients were found to have xerosis or ichthyosis.[66]

Psoriasis, Reiter's syndrome. Skin lesions of psoriasis were present in 5% of HIV-infected patients in one series.[8] The association of Reiter's syndrome with HIV-1 infection is discussed in the section on musculoskeletal manifestations of HIV infection.

NERVOUS SYSTEM DISORDERS

The central nervous system (CNS) is a frequent site of involvement in HIV-related opportunistic infections and malignancies (Tables 5-2 and 5-3). In recent years there has been increasing recognition of the direct effects of HIV on the brain and spinal cord. The term "AIDS dementia complex" is used to characterize the clinical and pathological results of HIV infection.[146,147] Peripheral neuropathy is also frequently seen in these patients. Direct involvement of the nervous system appears to occur very early in the course of HIV infection in some patients.[68,84] Symptoms of AIDS dementia complex may be among the earliest recognized by physicians evaluating HIV-infected patients and by the patients themselves.[68] Pathological evidence of HIV encephalopathy is seen in most AIDS patients at autopsy,[56] often coexisting in the brain with opportunistic infections.[160]

HIV-1 Infection of the Central Nervous System

Direct infection of the central nervous system by HIV-1 may be associated with aseptic meningitis,[87] myelopathy,[65] peripheral neuropathy,[152] and AIDS dementia complex.[146,147]

Aseptic meningitis. Meningitis characterized by the presence of mononuclear cells in the cerebrospinal fluid (CSF) may occur at the time of acute HIV-1 infection or later in the illness but before the onset of AIDS symptoms.[87]

TABLE 5-2. Common AIDS-related focal neurological infections and malignancies

Disorder	Frequency	Diagnostic studies
Cerebral toxoplasmosis	Initial manifestation of AIDS in 2% of cases[91]	Computed tomography (CT) or magnetic resonance imaging (MRI) Serum antibody* Therapeutic trial Biopsy
Progressive multifocal leukoencephalopathy	2%-5% of AIDS patients[121]	CT or MRI Biopsy
CNS lymphoma	Less than 1% of AIDS patients[120]	CT or MRI Biopsy
Cerebral infarction	Not reported	CT or MRI

*High sensitivity, low specificity.

TABLE 5-3. Common AIDS-related nonfocal neurological disorders

Disorder	Frequency	Diagnostic studies
Cryptococcal meningitis	Initial manifestation of AIDS in 7% of cases[21]	Cerebrospinal fluid (CSF) examination CSF antigen Serum antigen
Tuberculous meningitis	Not reported	CSF examination CT, MRI
Cytomegalovirus (CMV) encephalitis*	Histological evidence in 24% of AIDS patients at autopsy[49]	Tissue examination

*Clinical significance is unclear.

Headache is the most common symptom, but cranial nerve palsies (V, VII, VIII) have been described. HIV-1–related aseptic meningitis appears to be self-limited and does not predict later development of AIDS dementia.

AIDS dementia complex. Dementia caused by HIV-1 infection may manifest before or after the onset of AIDS-defining opportunistic infections or malignancies and has a variable clinical course. In one series of AIDS patients, more than half developed severe dementia within 2 months of their first symptoms[146]; however, in a substantial number of cases neurological symptoms have remained stable for several months. Symptoms of dementia may suddenly worsen when the patient's general medical condition begins to deteriorate.

Early symptoms of dementia[146] may include forgetfulness, inability to concentrate, and confusion and may be accompanied by loss of balance, leg weakness or difficulty with handwriting, and pathological reflexes.[161] Patients often manifest apathy and social withdrawal or changes in mood. When mild, findings of early AIDS dementia may be misinterpreted as symptoms of depression or anxiety. Headaches or seizures occasionally are seen.

AIDS dementia typically follows a course marked by steady deterioration over a relatively short period. In advanced cases, psychomotor retardation, mutism, and incontinence may be prominent and the incidence of ataxia, motor weakness, and tremors increases.

The results of diagnostic studies are generally nonspecific in AIDS dementia. Approximately two thirds of patients are found to have a mildly elevated CSF protein, and 20% have a mononuclear pleocytosis.[146] A substantial proportion of patients has immunoglobulin IgG and oligoclonal bands in the cerebrospinal fluid.[146] Viral cultures or tests for viral antigens such as p24 may be positive. However, none of these findings, including detection of the virus, is diagnostic of AIDS dementia.

Computed tomography (CT) typically reveals findings of diffuse cerebral atrophy, including widened cortical sulci and, less commonly, enlargement of the ventricles. Atrophy may be seen without clinical findings of dementia, however; it was reported in 33% of adult AIDS patients in several recent series.[39] Diffuse white matter abnormalities with local areas of demyelination occasionally are seen.[160]

Magnetic resonance imaging (MRI) has been demonstrated to be more sensitive than CT in evaluating patients with AIDS dementia.[160] In several recent series[39] MRI detected focal lesions missed on CT in 44% of cases.

Opportunistic Infections and Malignancies of the Central Nervous System

Opportunistic infections and malignancies of the central nervous system in HIV-infected patients account for approximately 30% of neurological complications.[146] Some of these disorders typically manifest focal neurological abnormalities, and some manifest nonfocal findings.

Focal disorders. Toxoplasmosis, cerebral lymphoma, and progressive multifocal leukoencephalopathy are the most important causes of focal cerebral disorders in AIDS.

Cerebral toxoplasmosis (toxoplasmic encephalitis). Cerebral toxoplasmosis, caused by the protozoal parasite *Toxoplasma gondii*, is the initial manifestation of AIDS in approximately 2% of cases.[91] Focal neurological abnormalities, which may include hemiparesis, aphasia, ataxia, visual field deficit, cranial nerve palsies, or movement disorders, are seen in most cases. However, such nonfocal findings as lethargy, confusion, psychosis, or coma[91] are also commonly seen and may lead to diagnostic uncertainty. The incidence of seizures in cerebral toxoplasmosis has been reported to be approximately 16%,[145] comparable to that in AIDS dementia.[90]

Although only tissue examination (biopsy or autopsy) can establish a diagnosis of cerebral toxoplasmosis with certainty, imaging studies of the brain, either CT or MRI, may be suggestive enough to allow for a presumptive diagnosis. Mass lesions are almost always demonstrated by these techniques.[159] These lesions typically are located in the basal ganglia and hemispheric corticomedullary junction[45] but may be present anywhere in the brain. Lesions are most commonly multiple[45] and often bilateral. Adjacent cerebral edema with mass effect is often seen.[210] On contrast CT, toxoplasmic lesions characteristically show a peripheral pattern of contrast uptake, or ring enhancement.[45,102,210] Atypical patterns may be seen, however.

Serological studies also may aid in distinguishing between toxoplasmosis and AIDS dementia or other CNS disorders. IgG antibody to *Toxoplasma gondii* is present in the serum of 97% to 99% of AIDS patients with cerebral toxoplasmosis.[91] If the results are negative, therefore, this test may be very helpful in excluding the diagnosis of toxoplasmosis. A finding of a higher titer of antibody in the cerebrospinal fluid than in the serum is particularly suggestive of cerebral toxoplasmosis.[91] Tests for IgG antibody lack specificity, however, since most adults in the general population test positive.[112]

A therapeutic trial with the folate antagonists sulfadiazine and pyrimethamine is appropriate in cases with suggestive radiographic and clinical features. Clinical and radiographic responses often may be seen within several weeks. Such empirical therapy, if successful, provides indirect supporting evidence for the diagnosis of toxoplasmosis. The response rates of patients treated on the basis of clinical and radiographic findings are comparable to those of patients with biopsy-confirmed cerebral toxoplasmosis.[28]

Pathological examination of brain tissue currently provides the most definitive means of diagnosis.

Progressive multifocal leukoencephalopathy. Progressive multifocal leukoencephalopathy (PML), caused by the papovavirus,[150] is a progressive demyelinating disease that may be seen in association with a variety of immunodeficiency states[176] or, in rare cases, in normal hosts.[171] PML has been reported to occur in 2% to 5% of AIDS patients.[121] Symptoms include personality change, memory loss, and language disturbances. However, focal neurological abnormalities also may occur,[136] aiding in the distinction between PML and AIDS dementia complex.

Definitive diagnosis of PML requires histological confirmation by brain biopsy or autopsy. However, the diagnosis occasionally may be made presumptively on the basis of brain imaging studies. Lesions typically appear as areas of lucency within the white matter, rarely exerting mass effect.[82] Contrast enhancement tends to be absent.[113] Routine contrast CT scans may be normal in PML, however, and double-dose contrast studies have been advocated as a means of improving sensitivity.[176] Recent data suggest that PML lesions may be detected more readily by MRI than by CT.[113]

Although imaging studies may strongly suggest the diagnosis of PML, it can only be confirmed histologically.

Central nervous system lymphoma. Primary CNS lymphoma is the initial manifestation of AIDS in fewer than 1% of cases.[120] Most patients manifest clinical and radiographic findings of an intracerebral mass lesion.[57] Focal lesions with contrast enhancement are usually seen on CT.[45,58] Multiple lesions are less commonly seen than in cerebral toxoplasmosis, but distinguishing between these two disorders clinically and radiographically often is extremely difficult.

Histological examination of the brain provides conclusive evidence of lymphoma in these patients.

Miscellaneous focal cerebral disorders. Brain involvement by cryptococcosis,[55] tuberculosis,[12,77] herpes simplex,[5,212] syphilis,[9] and a variety of other disorders may be associated with clinical and radiographic signs of focal neurological disease. Cerebral infarction has been described in association with HIV-1 infection with[190] and without[46] concomitant thrombotic endocarditis.

Nonfocal disorders. In contrast to the disorders discussed previously, several AIDS-related opportunistic infections typically manifest nonfocal CNS involvement. The commonest of these is cryptococcal meningitis.

Cryptococcal meningitis. CNS infection with the yeast *Cryptococcus neoformans* is the initial manifestation of AIDS in approximately 7% of cases.[21] Fever and headache are the most common features of infection.[219] Brain imaging studies are most often normal or demonstrate only widening of the sulci and ventricular enlargement.[210] The diagnosis is confirmed by examination of the cerebrospinal fluid. India ink stain of the CSF is positive for yeast cells in more than 70% of cases,[219] and culture and cryptococcal antigen assays are positive in more than 90%.[111,219] The cellular response in the cerebrospinal fluid, when present, usually is modest, with less than 20 mononuclear cells per cubic millimeter, although higher counts may be seen.[111,219] CSF protein is elevated and glucose depressed in the minority of cases.[219]

Cytomegalovirus (CMV) encephalitis. Histological findings suggestive of CMV infection were present in the brains of 24% of AIDS patients in one study,[49] and simultaneous CMV and herpes simplex virus encephalitis has been de scribed.[116] However, the incidence and importance of CMV encephalitis are not clear.

Herpes simplex encephalitis. Herpes simplex virus (HSV) is a common cause of encephalitis in normal hosts and has been described in association with HIV-1 infection.[116] The incidence of this infection among HIV-infected individuals and its relationship to AIDS currently are unknown.

Systemic disorders. For a variety of reasons, patients infected with HIV-1, particularly those with advanced, symptomatic disease, are prone to systemic disorders that may be associated with CNS signs and symptoms. Potentially important among these are:

Hypoxemia resulting from diffuse pulmonary infections or malignancies

Anemia resulting from bone marrow effects of opportunistic infections or therapeutic agents, as well as HIV-1 infection itself

Hyponatremia[204]

Hypoglycemia, particularly in association with pentamidine isethionate therapy

Uremia resulting from HIV- or heroin-induced nephropathy or from nephrotoxic therapeutic agents such as pentamidine isethionate or amphotericin B

Vitamin B_{12} deficiency

Psychiatric Disturbances

Psychiatric disturbances, particularly depression and anxiety,[85] are common among HIV-1 infected patients. Patients with a history of risk behavior may display denial by avoiding testing. Social isolation, guilt, and uncertainty are common after a diagnosis of AIDS.[42] Stress associated with learning of a positive test for HIV-1 or being informed that an AIDS-related illness has been diagnosed may precipitate psychiatric crises and feelings of anger, fear, and confusion. It has been shown that AIDS is associated with a greatly increased risk of suicide.[129]

It may be difficult to distinguish between psychiatric symptoms and those reflecting organic disease, particularly AIDS dementia complex. Opportunistic CNS infections, including toxoplasmosis and herpes simplex encephalitis, may initially cause symptoms suggesting psychiatric disorders.[3] It has been suggested that symptoms of depression may be a harbinger of CNS infection.[41]

Other HIV-Related Neurological Disorders

Vacuolar myelopathy. Vacuolar myelopathy often accompanies AIDS dementia and is characterized by spasticity, gait disorders, and bowel and bladder dysfunction.[65]

Peripheral nervous system involvement. A variety of syndromes involving the peripheral nerves is commonly seen in association with HIV-1 infection. An acute polyneuropathy or cranial nerve palsy may occur shortly after infection.[152] Peripheral neuropathy, often in the form of a demyelinating polyneuropathy or mononeuritis multiplex, is seen in 20% of patients with ARC.[152] In more advanced cases, particularly among patients with AIDS, the most common peripheral nervous system complication is a distal, predominantly sensory neuropathy.

Myopathy. Several types of muscle disease have been described in HIV-infected patients. These are discussed in the section on musculoskeletal disorders associated with HIV-1 infection.

OPHTHALMOLOGICAL DISORDERS

The eye is a major site of involvement in HIV-related disorders (Table 5-4). Such conditions include opportunistic infections affecting the eye, Kaposi's sarcoma involving periocular structures, and AIDS-associated retinopathy. Ophthalmological consultation should be sought promptly for HIV-infected patients with visual complaints.

Opportunistic Infections

Cytomegalovirus retinitis. Cytomegalovirus (CMV), the most common opportunistic infection of the eye in AIDS, was diagnosed in 28% of patients in one large published series[92] and may be the initial manifestation of AIDS.[93] Progression to blindness is common, and vision may be threatened at the time the infection is first detected.[74] Bilateral involvement was seen in 35%[93] and 42%[74] of patients in two series. Retinal detachment is a common complication.[93] Progression of CMV retinitis despite treatment is most common in patients with severe degrees of immunodeficiency.[74] Simultaneous infection of the retina by CMV and HIV-1 has been reported.[187]

TABLE 5-4. Major ocular manifestations of HIV-1 infection

Disorder	Frequency
AIDS retinopathy	66.5% of AIDS patients[92]
	40% of ARC patients[92]
	1.3% of asymptomatic HIV-positive patients[92]
Neuroophthalmic disease	33% of AIDS patients[92]
Cytomegalovirus retinitis	28% of AIDS patients[92]
Kaposi's sarcoma (periocular)	20%[183] of KS patients

Miscellaneous opportunistic infections. A variety of other ocular infections have been reported in association with HIV-1 infection. These include syphilitic optic neuritis,[218] toxoplasmosis,[86] choroiditis[19] and optic neuropathy[123] associated with cryptococcal meningitis, endophthalmitis caused by *Mycobacterium avium-intracellulare*,[25] keratitis caused by the herpes zoster virus,[47] and choroiditis caused by *Pneumocystis carinii*.[189]

Kaposi's sarcoma. Twenty of 100 male homosexuals with Kaposi's sarcoma were found to have ocular involvement in one series.[183] Lesions were present on the eyelid in 16 patients and on the conjunctiva in seven.

AIDS-associated retinopathy. Cotton-wool spots[103,173] and retinal hemorrhages may represent the direct effects on the eye of HIV infection.[103] Although these lesions are seen most often in patients with AIDS or ARC,[53] they may be seen before the onset of other symptoms of HIV-1 infection.[52]

ORAL DISORDERS

The oral mucosa may be involved by a variety of opportunistic infections and by the AIDS-related malignancies Kaposi's sarcoma and non-Hodgkin's lymphoma. Major oral manifestations of HIV-1 infection are listed in Table 5-5.

Infections

Candidiasis. Oral candidiasis, which most often appears as white plaques on the mucosa, is common among HIV-infected patients at all stages of the disease and may be the initial clinical manifestation of immune deficiency.[104] Approximately 80% of HIV-infected homosexual men had oral colonization by *Candida albicans* in one series.[201]

Herpes simplex. In one series 10% of AIDS patients were found to have oral

TABLE 5-5. Major oral manifestations of HIV-1 infection

Disorder	Frequency
Candidiasis	91% of AIDS patients[154]
	78.8% of HIV-positive patients[201] (colonized)
	39% HIV-positive patients[201] (symptomatic)
Hairy leukoplakia	28% of homosexual men[186]
	7% of AIDS patients[154]
Periodontal disease	17% of homosexual men[186]
Herpes simplex	10% of AIDS patients[154]
Xerostomia	10% of AIDS patients[154]
Cheilitis	9% of AIDS patients[154]
Nonspecific ulcers	3% of AIDS patients[154]
Kaposi's sarcoma	Frequency not reported

herpes simplex infection.[154] Lesions are typically painful, progressive ulcerations but may appear as fissures in some cases.

Malignancies

Kaposi's sarcoma. Kaposi's sarcoma is the most common oral malignancy in AIDS.[186] Lesions typically appear on the palate, gingiva, or buccal mucosa. Oral Kaposi's sarcoma may occur in isolation or with widespread skin or visceral involvement.

Non-Hodgkin's lymphoma. AIDS-related non-Hodgkin's lymphoma may manifest nodular or ulcerating oral lesions.

Hairy leukoplakia. Hairy leukoplakia, a white lesion usually found on the sides of the tongue, has been associated with HIV-1 infection, particularly among homosexual men, and may predict progression to AIDS.[71] Evidence of an association with the Epstein-Barr virus has been reported.[72]

Other Disorders

Xerostomia, exfoliative cheilitis, and nonspecific ulcerations were seen in 10%, 9%, and 3% of patients, respectively, in one series.[154]

PULMONARY DISORDERS

Pulmonary disease is extremely common in HIV-infected patients and may be caused by virtually all of the infections and malignancies associated with AIDS. (Table 5-6 describes the radiographic patterns seen in common HIV-related pulmonary diseases). In addition, lymphocytic interstitial pneumonitis (LIP) and pulmonary lymphoid hyperplasia (PLH), disorders of uncertain origin, are common manifestations of HIV infection, particularly in children.

HIV-Related Pulmonary Infections

The lungs are a common site of involvement by opportunistic pathogens in HIV-infected patients. More than 80% of AIDS patients develop *Pneumocystis carinii* pneumonia at some point during their illness, and 25% succumb to it.[111] Other common AIDS-related pulmonary infections include tuberculosis, atypical mycobacterial infection, histoplasmosis, cryptococcosis, and cytomegalovirus infection. Both pneumococcal pneumonia and pneumonia caused by *Haemophilus* organisms appear to be more common in HIV-infected patients.

Bacterial pneumonia. HIV-1–infected patients appear to be at increased risk for pneumonia caused by *Haemophilus influenzae*[156,177] and *Streptococcus pneumoniae*.[156] Pneumonia caused by *Legionella* organisms has also been reported to occur in association with AIDS.[143]

TABLE 5-6. Radiographic patterns in common HIV-related pulmonary disease

Disorder	Radiographic patterns	
	Typical	**Atypical**
Pneumocystis pneumonia	Diffuse, bilateral infiltrates[110]; pleural involvement rare	Nodules, cavities, focal infiltrate, apical pattern[25] normal
Kaposi's sarcoma	Diffuse or nodular infiltrates; pleural involvement common[37]	
Tuberculosis	Apical infiltrates, cavities, pleural involvement, and lymphadenopathy common[155]	Diffuse infiltrates, lower lobe[155] predilection
Bacterial pneumonia	Lobar infiltrate; pleural involvement common	Diffuse infiltrates
Cryptococcosis	Nodules, pleural involvement,[98] and lymphadenopathy common[136]	Diffuse infiltrates[144]

***Pneumocystis carinii* pneumonia.** *Pneumocystis carinii* pneumonia (PCP) is the most common initial opportunistic infection in patients with AIDS in the United States and other Western countries; it is ultimately diagnosed in 80% of cases.[111] Patients with the greatest degree of immunodeficiency (i.e., those with CD4 lymphocyte counts below 200/mm³) are at substantially greater risk than other HIV-infected patients.[130]

The clinical manifestations of PCP are nonspecific. The onset of symptoms may be insidious or fulminant.[142] Most patients complain of fever, cough, and dyspnea.[110] Chills, sputum production, and chest pain are occasionally seen.[110] In rare cases fever may be the only manifestation of the disease.

Bilateral infiltrates are seen on chest roentgenograms in almost all cases,[109] although unilateral infiltrates,[110] nodules, and cavities occur occasionally. In some cases the chest roentgenogram may be completely normal.[27] Pleural effusions are rarely seen in association with PCP.

PCP is often associated with diffuse, bilateral pulmonary uptake on gallium scanning,[118,119] which may be apparent before infiltrates can be detected on a chest roentgenogram.

It should be stressed that radiographic and gallium scan findings associated with PCP are nonspecific. Other AIDS-related processes, particularly pulmonary Kaposi's sarcoma,[149] tuberculosis, histoplasmosis, and lymphocytic interstitial pneumonitis, may produce similar findings. For this reason histological confirmation of the diagnosis of PCP is necessary in most cases.[143] Bronchoscopy with bronchoalveolar lavage is particularly effective in confirming the diagnosis of PCP.[15]

It has been demonstrated that the use of prophylactic agents, particularly aerosolized pentamidine, against *Pneumocystis carinii* may alter the findings on routine roentgenograms and gallium scans.[96] Upper lobe infiltrates and cystic changes are seen more commonly in patients receiving such prophylaxis.[96]

Tuberculosis. The risk of active tuberculosis has been shown to be increased in individuals infected with HIV-1[181] who are also at high risk of tuberculosis. The clinical and radiographic presentation of tuberculosis complicating HIV-1 infection may be atypical and particularly fulminant.[195] Mediastinal lymphadenopathy and lower lobe involvement are seen particularly commonly in HIV-infected patients with tuberculosis.[155] In contrast, conventional findings of isolated apical infiltrates and pulmonary cavities are relatively unusual.[155]

Cryptococcosis. The central nervous system (CNS) is the commonest site of involvement by the yeast *Cryptococcus neoformans* in AIDS. However, respiratory involvement may occur with or without concomitant CNS disease. A variety of radiographic patterns have been associated with pulmonary cryptococcosis. Interstitial infiltrates and hilar lymphadenopathy, either alone or in combination, are the radiographic patterns most often seen in association with pulmonary cryptococcosis in AIDS.[136] Empyema[98,148,206] and the adult respiratory distress syndrome have also been described.[144]

Histoplasmosis. Disseminated infection with the fungus *Histoplasma capsulatum* is a common opportunistic infection in AIDS patients, particularly those from endemic areas. Pulmonary involvement with diffuse, bilateral infiltrates was seen in approximately 40% of cases in one series.[209]

Coccidioidomycosis. Progressive pulmonary infection caused by *Coccidioides immitis* has been reported to occur with increased frequency among AIDS patients living in endemic areas of the American Southwest.[1,16,170] Diffuse infiltrates were described in five of seven patients in one series, and dissemination to extrapulmonary sites was common.[16]

Cytomegalovirus infection. Cytomegalovirus, the most common opportunistic pathogen associated with AIDS in autopsy series,[208] frequently involves the lungs. In clinical series,[143] however, isolated CMV pneumonitis is unusual, although evidence of CMV infection is often found in lung specimens from AIDS patients with other opportunistic infections, particularly PCP.

Miscellaneous infections. Unusual causes of pulmonary infiltrates seen in association with HIV infection include strongyloidiasis,[63,127] toxoplasmosis,[134,197] nocardiosis,[172] and aspergillosis.[13]

Pulmonary Involvement with HIV-Related Malignancies

Kaposi's sarcoma and non-Hodgkin's lymphoma, the two malignancies most frequently associated with HIV infection, may both produce pulmonary disease.

Kaposi's sarcoma. Bronchopulmonary involvement with Kaposi's sarcoma has been increasingly recognized in the last several years.[57,132] Patients typically have a subacute respiratory illness characterized by dyspnea and dry cough, occasionally accompanied by hemoptysis or pleuritic chest pain. Fever may or may not be present. Airway involvement is common and may manifest as wheezing.[132] Clinical progression may be gradual or fulminant, and respiratory failure has been described as a complication.[149] Radiographic features are nonspecific, but the presence of diffuse nodular infiltrates, hilar lymphadenopathy, and pleural disease suggests the diagnosis.[37] In some patients, however, findings on the chest roentgenogram may mimic those of *Pneumocystis carinii* pneumonia (PCP) or other AIDS-related processes. In contrast to PCP, however, the gallium scan with pulmonary Kaposi's sarcoma is usually negative,[211] and serum lactate dehydrogenase levels are typically normal or only slightly elevated.[217] Cutaneous Kaposi's sarcoma lesions usually are present but may not be. The diagnosis may be confirmed by lung biopsy, although autopsy data indicate that the sensitivity of this procedure is limited.[132] Visualization of typical red-purple lesions in the large airways by bronchoscopy[132] may allow a presumptive diagnosis and therapy even without histological confirmation.

Non-Hodgkin's lymphoma. Non-Hodgkin's lymphoma (NHL) is the second most common AIDS-associated malignancy.[97] Although extranodal involvement is seen frequently in AIDS-associated NHL (occurring in 87% of cases in one large series[105]), the lungs are a relatively unusual site. The reported incidence of pulmonary involvement varies considerably, ranging from 0% to 25%.[211] Clinical features are nonspecific and respiratory symptoms are not always present. Chest roentgenograms may demonstrate abnormalities of the thoracic lymph nodes, lung parenchyma,[27] or pleura.[105] The diagnosis is confirmed histologically.

Other Pulmonary Conditions Associated with HIV Infection

Several pulmonary disorders of unknown origin characterized by diffuse infiltrates on chest roentgenogram are also associated with HIV infection. Lymphocytic interstitial pneumonitis (LIP), pulmonary lymphoid hyperplasia (PLH), and nonspecific interstitial pneumonitis are particularly common in HIV-infected children and are occasionally seen in adults. These entities may represent infection with currently unrecognized pathogens or HIV itself.[23]

CARDIOVASCULAR DISORDERS

Cardiovascular manifestations associated with HIV infection have been increasingly recognized in recent years (Table 5-7). Opportunistic infections and malignancies may involve the heart, but in many patients, perhaps most, with symptomatic cardiac disease the cause is obscure. Substantial evidence exists to indicate that HIV itself may infect heart tissue and cause clinically significant disease. In one large series, 5% of AIDS patients had symptoms of heart disease, usually caused by opportunistic infection or malignancy.[140] Homosexuals and intravenous drug users were affected equally. Echocardiographic abnormalities are commonly seen in advanced HIV-1 infection. Pericardial effusions and ventricular dysfunction were noted respectively in 29% and 29% of hospitalized AIDS patients[83] and 26% and 30% of AIDS patients overall[81] in two published series.

Myocardial Disease

Disorders of the myocardium may be related to opportunistic infections or malignancies or may appear without any definable cause in HIV-infected patients.

A large number of opportunistic pathogens have been associated with myocarditis in HIV-infected patients. These include *Pneumocystis carinii, Mycobacterium tuberculosis, Mycobacterium avium-intracellulare, Cryptococcus neoformans, Aspergillus fumigatus, Candida albicans, Histoplasma capsulatum, Coccidioides immitis, Toxoplasma gondii,* herpes simplex virus, and cytomegalovirus.[2] *T. gondii, C. neoformans, M. tuberculosis,* and cytomegalovirus have received the most attention.[2] However, myocarditis is not a common manifestation of infection with any of these organisms.[2] With some, myocardial involvement has been reported only in the setting of widespread multisystem infection and has often been first recognized at postmortem examination. The clinical significance of myocardial infection in many of these cases is unclear.

Pericardial Disease

Pericardial disease is common in AIDS patients, sometimes coexisting with cardiomyopathy. Significant but clinically silent pericardial effusions were

TABLE 5-7. Major cardiac manifestations of HIV-1 infection

Disorder	Frequency
Symptomatic heart disease	5% of AIDS patients[140]
Pericardial effusion	26%-29% of AIDS patients[81,83]
Ventricular dysfunction	29%-30% of AIDS patients[81,83]
Endocarditis	Frequency not reported

detected by echocardiography in 26% of 27 male homosexuals with AIDS in one series.[81] Pericardial involvement may complicate tuberculosis,[35] atypical mycobacterial infection,[216] cryptococcosis,[179] nocardiosis,[88] and infection with cytomegalovirus[180] or herpes simplex virus.[200] Pericardial effusions may also be seen in association with Kaposi's sarcoma.[2] In many cases the etiology of pericarditis is obscure.

Effusions may be large enough to result in hemodynamic compromise,[83,180] and both pericarditis and cardiomyopathy should be considered in the evaluation of dyspnea in patients with AIDS, AIDS-related complex, or even asymptomatic HIV infection.[83]

Endocarditis

Nonbacterial thrombotic endocarditis, a disorder of unknown etiology that has been associated with a variety of wasting diseases, has been reported in association with AIDS.[190] The condition may be associated with emboli to the brain and other sites.

HIV-infected intravenous drug users who continue to use drugs remain at high risk for infective endocarditis, which is more likely to be caused by conventional bacteria such as *Staphylococcus aureus* than by opportunistic pathogens otherwise associated with AIDS.

GASTROINTESTINAL DISORDERS

The gastrointestinal tract is a common site of disease in HIV-infected individuals. Infections involving the oral cavity, esophagus, small and large bowel, and rectum are all common in these patients. Diarrhea and other gastrointestinal complaints are extremely frequent and may occur before other manifestations of disease. In some patients, diarrhea becomes the most prominent feature of their disease, leading to progressive debilitation from dehydration and malabsorption, which may require repeated hospitalization. In many cases such AIDS-related opportunistic pathogens as *Cryptosporidium* organisms, *Isospora belli*, cytomegalovirus, *Salmonella* species, mycobacteria, and others account for these symptoms by infection of the small or large bowel or biliary system. Kaposi's sarcoma and lymphoma may also involve the gastrointestinal tract. In many patients, however, no specific infection or malignancy can be identified. This fact has given rise to the concept of an HIV-related enteropathy that may cause chronic diarrhea and malabsorption and may be associated with histological abnormalities of the bowel mucosa.[59]

Esophagitis

Candidiasis is the most common cause of esophagitis in AIDS[166] and is usually but not always seen in association with oral candidiasis. In one series 48% of

AIDS patients undergoing routine upper endoscopy were found to have candidal esophagitis, although only 60% of those with documented esophagitis had symptoms of dysphagia or odynophagia.[158] Other AIDS-related infections and malignancies that may cause esophagitis include herpes simplex virus, cytomegalovirus,[198] Kaposi's sarcoma,[153] lymphoma, and occasionally other opportunistic infections.[67] HIV-1 itself may be the cause of esophageal ulcerations, particularly before the onset of AIDS.[164]

A specific etiologic diagnosis usually requires upper endoscopy, since barium studies lack sensitivity.[30] Empiric antifungal therapy may be appropriate for patients with symptoms of esophagitis who have oral candidiasis.

Infectious Diarrhea

Pathogenic organisms were isolated in 85% of AIDS patients with diarrhea in one series.[188] Although the microbiological yield may not be as high in patients with diarrhea at earlier stages of their HIV infection, a thorough search often yields a specific, potentially treatable infectious cause.

Cryptosporidiosis

The parasite *Cryptosporidium* was not recognized as a significant human pathogen before the AIDS epidemic. The organism is now known to cause intestinal infection in both normal[214] and immunocompromised hosts. In the setting of HIV-1 infection, *Cryptosporidium* organisms are a frequent and largely untreatable cause of chronic, watery diarrhea[191] and biliary disease.[178]

The diagnosis of cryptosporidiosis is usually made by microscopic examination of stool stained by the modified Kinyoun acid-fast technique.[126] Occasionally the organism is detected only in small bowel specimens or on endoscopic small bowel biopsy. Since the organism is not generally detected by routine stool examination, laboratory personnel should be notified when *Cryptosporidium* infection is suspected.

Isosporiasis

The parasite *Isospora belli* is a frequent cause of a syndrome of watery diarrhea generally indistinguishable from that caused by *Cryptosporidium*. The diagnosis is confirmed by direct stool examination. In contrast to cryptosporidiosis, isosporiasis typically responds to treatment with a variety of agents, including sulfonamide antibiotics and pyrimethamine.[207]

Salmonellosis

Nontyphi *Salmonella* species were identified by stool culture in 25% of AIDS patients with diarrhea in one series.[188] Disseminated, bacteremic salmonella infections may be seen in AIDS as well as in HIV-infected patients before the onset of AIDS.[60,94] Fever, diarrhea, and abdominal cramps are common in patients with salmonellosis,[60] although bacteremia may occur without intestinal complaints.[60]

Cytomegalovirus (CMV) Infections

Cytomegalovirus, a particularly common cause of infection in homosexual men,[138] has been shown to cause esophagitis, gastritis, colitis,[95] and appendicitis[122] in the setting of AIDS. The symptoms of esophagitis and gastritis are nonspecific,[95] consisting of odynophagia and epigastric pain. In one series 45% of AIDS patients with diarrhea had evidence of CMV enteritis.[188] Symptoms of CMV colitis are nonspecific and include diarrhea and cramping or continuous abdominal pain.[95] Hemorrhage and mucosal ulcerations are seen in virtually all patients on colonoscopy,[50] although specific diagnosis requires biopsy of colonic mucosa and demonstration of viral inclusions.

It has been suggested that HIV-1 itself, rather than CMV, may be the primary cause of colitis and other infections commonly attributed to CMV,[141] and that CMV may produce secondary infection.

Mycobacterium avium-intracellulare

Mycobacterium avium-intracellulare is frequently identified in bowel tissue specimens from patients with AIDS[36] and has been associated with colitis.[215]

Miscellaneous Enteric Infections

A variety of organisms has been associated with intestinal infections in homosexual men. *Neisseria gonorrhoeae, Chlamydia trachomatis*, and herpes simplex virus are frequent causes of proctitis,[162] whereas infectious diarrhea may be seen in association with *Entamoeba histolytica, Giardia lamblia, Clostridium difficile*, and *Campylobacter* species.[162,163] With the exception of progressive, chronic herpes simplex infection, the relationship of infection with these agents to HIV-1 infection is not clear.

Gastrointestinal Involvement with HIV-Related Malignancies

Kaposi's sarcoma. Autopsy studies indicate that Kaposi's sarcoma involves the gastrointestinal tract in approximately 30% of cases.[167,208] Although gastrointestinal involvement is most common in patients with widespread cutaneous lesions, it may also occur without such lesions. There may be few or no symptoms, although bleeding from eroding lesions occurs occasionally.

Lymphoma. The gastrointestinal tract was the commonest (24%) extranodal site of involvement by non-Hodgkin's lymphoma in AIDS patients in one large series.[105] Any segment of the bowel may be involved. Symptoms are typically nonspecific.

Anorectal neoplasia. Dysplasia[51] and carcinoma in situ[33,151] have been reported within anal warts in HIV-infected homosexual men.

HIV-Related Enteropathy

In some HIV-1 infected patients with chronic diarrhea, no bowel pathogen is identified by routine studies. Malabsorption and mucosal abnormalities have been described in some of these patients[108]; such abnormalities included villous atrophy and lymphocytic infiltration in the small bowel, and viral inclusions and mast cell infiltration in the large bowel.[108] In some patients with similar clinical syndromes, acid-fast organisms of uncertain identity have been seen on duodenal biopsy.[59] A gastropathy of unclear origin associated with achlorhydria,[114] which may become clinically significant,[115] has also been described.

HIV-Related Hepatic Disease

HIV-1 itself has not been shown to have a direct effect on the liver[117]; however, hepatic involvement by opportunistic infections and malignancies, hepatic toxicity by drugs used in therapy, and possible interactions between HIV-1 infection and hepatitis viruses may cause liver dysfunction in AIDS patients.

A high incidence of hepatomegaly has been reported in autopsy[208] and clinical[76] series. Histological abnormalities commonly seen in association with AIDS include steatosis, sinusoidal dilation, and atrophy of hepatic parenchymal cells.[208] AIDS-related disorders commonly involving the liver include mycobacteriosis,[17] CMV infection,[208] Kaposi's sarcoma,[208] and lymphoma.[105]

Although evidence of prior hepatitis B infection is common among HIV-infected male homosexuals and intravenous drug users, severe chronic or progressive hepatitis is rare,[174] for reasons that are unclear. Evidence exists that hepatitis D may be activated by HIV infection.[182]

HIV-Related Biliary Disease

Several AIDS-related disorders may be associated with biliary obstruction. Both cryptosporidiosis and cytomegaloviral infection may be associated with stenosis of the common bile duct,[128,178] sclerosing cholangitis,[178] or both. Cytomegalovirus has also been reported in association with acalculous cholecystitis.[100] Biliary involvement in AIDS produces typical symptoms of abdominal pain, nausea, and vomiting,[178] and obstruction may predispose to secondary bacterial infection.

RENAL DISORDERS

HIV-infected patients are susceptible to a variety of renal disorders. Opportunistic pathogens, particularly cytomegalovirus and mycobacteria,[208] as well as *Cryptococcus* and *Histoplasma* organisms,[62] may cause infection of the kidneys, and Kaposi's sarcoma[208] and non-Hodgkin's lymphoma[62] have been reported to involve the renal parenchyma. A number of medications commonly used to treat HIV-infected patients, most notably pentamidine isethionate, amphotericin B, and trimethoprim-sulfamethoxazole, are associated with renal toxicity. Heroin nephropathy may be difficult to distinguish from renal disease of other causes in active intravenous drug users, and renal manifestations of intercurrent infections such as infective endocarditis may arise.

HIV-Associated Nephropathy

As with several other end-organ diseases seen in HIV-infected patients (e.g., dementia, enteropathy, cardiomyopathy, and neuropathy), evidence has accumulated that HIV itself may cause renal parenchymal disease that may progress to renal failure. This so-called HIV nephropathy has been described in all HIV high-risk groups and at all stages of HIV infection, including asymptomatic, ARC, and AIDS.[18] It is seen most commonly in blacks and intravenous drug users.[18] HIV nephropathy appears to be more prevalent among patients in New York and Miami than in San Francisco.[62]

HIV nephropathy appears to be a direct effect of HIV-1 on the kidneys[26] and is associated with characteristic pathological changes. Typical findings include focal and segmental glomerulosclerosis, tubular necrosis, and microcystic tubular dilation.[62]

HIV nephropathy is typically characterized by proteinuria, hypertension, normal-size or slightly enlarged kidneys, and rapidly progressive renal failure[62] leading to end-stage disease within 1 year. No intervention is known to be beneficial, although the effect of antiviral therapy has not been determined. Hemodialysis extends life by only a few months in most cases.

A variety of other conditions have been described in association with HIV infection,[62] including mesangial proliferative glomerulonephritis, minimal-change disease, membranoproliferative glomerulonephritis, membranous glomerulonephritis, postinfectious glomerulonephritis, and hemolytic-uremic syndrome.

ENDOCRINE DISORDERS

Although several AIDS-related opportunistic infections may involve the adrenal gland and some commonly used medications may interfere with endocrine functions, clinically significant abnormalities of the endocrine system are rare in HIV-infected patients.[4]

Adrenal Disorders

Cytomegalovirus infection of the adrenal glands was found in 40% of AIDS patients in one autopsy series.[208] Adrenal involvement in cryptococcosis, disseminated mycobacterial infection,[61,196] and Kaposi's sarcoma has also been described.[61] Functional hypoadrenalism was found in 20% of patients in an early clinical study,[69] although the overall incidence of clinically significant adrenal dysfunction is not known. Ketoconazole, an imidazole compound commonly used to treat HIV-associated fungal infections, inhibits adrenal steroid synthesis.[157]

Gonadal Disorders

In one autopsy series,[40] 39% of AIDS patients were found to have testicular involvement by opportunistic infections. The most common pathogens are cytomegalovirus, mycobacteria, and toxoplasma organisms. Functional hypogonadism was documented in 50% of male AIDS patients in one series,[43] and significant depression of circulating testerone levels was seen in both AIDS and ARC patients, with the degree of depression correlating with overall clinical status. Ketoconazole inhibits testosterone secretion and may be associated with gynecomastia.[75]

MUSCULOSKELETAL DISORDERS

Musculoskeletal complaints are common during the course of HIV infection and may arise at any stage of the disease (Table 5-8). In some cases these symptoms are among the first experienced by the HIV-infected patient. It has been pointed out that the initial manifestations of disease in some cases are reminiscent of those of systemic lupus erythematosus[107] and may include arthralgias, cytopenias, butterfly rash, proteinuria, and abnormal urinary sediment.

In one recent survey 72% of HIV-positive patients were found to have rheumatological manifestations,[8] including arthralgias (34.7%), arthritis (11.9%), Reiter's syndrome (9.9%), painful articular syndrome (9.9%), psoriatic arthritis

TABLE 5-8. Major musculoskeletal manifestations of HIV-1 infection

Disorder	Frequency among HIV-positive patients
Arthralgia	34.7%
Arthritis	11.9%
Reiter's syndrome	9.9%
Painful articular syndrome	9.9%
Psoriatic arthritis	1.9%
Polymyositis	1.9%

Modified from Berman A et al: Rheumatic manifestations of human immunodeficiency virus infection, *Am J Med* 85:59-64, 1988.

(1.9%), and polymyositis (1.9%). Arthralgias most typically involve the knees, shoulders, elbows, or ankles, although the spine or small joints of the feet or hands may also be involved.[8] The arthralgia may range from mild to severe and debilitating.[8] Features suggestive of sicca complex[31] syndrome or Sjögren's syndrome[38] have also been described in some cases. The causes of these various conditions are unknown. HIV-1 may play a direct role in the pathogenesis of some of these disorders, whereas others, such as Reiter's syndrome, may represent reactive states reflecting infection with other organisms commonly seen in HIV-infected patients.

Myalgias and arthralgias are often a feature of the acute syndrome associated with seroconversion[199] and may also occur later. Reiter's syndrome, psoriatic arthritis, and nonspecific reactive arthritis are all commonly seen in HIV-infected patients and may be more common than in the general population.[44,48] Polymyositis has also been associated with HIV infection, as have a variety of autoimmune phenomena, including autoimmune thrombocytopenia[205]; rheumatoid factor and anticardiolipin antibodies[193]; and antinuclear, antilymphocyte, antigranulocyte, and other autoantibodies.[101]

Further complicating the interpretation of musculoskeletal complaints is the fact that opportunistic infections, including cryptococcosis,[168] sporotrichosis,[124] and mycobacteriosis,[14] and therapy with the antiretroviral agent zidovudine have been associated with myositis.[10]

Because the causes of most HIV-related bone and joint diseases are not known, the classification of specific clinical syndromes is not well established. Following are some of the specific patterns that have been recognized.

Reiter's Syndrome

Reiter's syndrome typically affects young men and appears to be more common in HIV-infected individuals than in the general population. Nearly 10% of patients in various stages of HIV infection had findings consistent with Reiter's syndrome in one prospective series.[8] In contrast, the annual incidence of Reiter's syndrome was only 0.0035% among a general population of men under 50 years of age.[135]

Several possible reasons for the association between Reiter's syndrome and HIV infection have been proposed.[101] Coinfection with organisms such as *Chlamydia*, which are known to precipitate Reiter's syndrome, may account for some cases, particularly among patients positive for the HLA-B27 antigen. Bowel infections caused by organisms commonly seen in HIV-infected patients but not previously linked to Reiter's syndrome, such as *Cryptosporidium* or other pathogens not yet characterized, may prove to be important. The stimulation of the immune response seen with the onset of Reiter's syndrome may trigger the progression of a preexisting HIV infection. Conversely, the immunodeficiency produced by HIV infection may lead to the development of Reiter's syndrome by unknown mechanisms.

Winchester and coworkers[213] described 13 HIV-infected patients with complete or incomplete Reiter's syndrome, manifested by arthritis in all cases and by urethritis and conjunctivitis in the majority. Several patients in this series, as well as in a comparable series by Berman and coworkers,[8] had such typical features as keratosis blennorrhagia, stomatitis, or balanitis. Nine of 12 patients tested positive for HLA-B27 antigen.

The arthritis in these patients tended to be severe, most often involving the knees and shoulders. Bone erosions were documented in seven cases. Three patients in the series by Winchester and colleagues were found to be infected with organisms known to precipitate Reiter's syndrome (*Shigella flexneri:* 2; *Campylobacter fetus:* 1), and several other patients had concomitant culture-negative diarrhea or urethritis.

Treating HIV-related Reiter's syndrome with nonsteroidal antiinflammatory agents or corticosteroids is often unsuccessful.[213] Progressive Kaposi's sarcoma and overall clinical deterioration occurred in two patients following treatment for Reiter's syndrome with methotrexate.[213]

Psoriatic Arthritis

Papulosquamous skin rashes such as seborrheic dermatitis and psoriasis appear to occur more often in HIV-infected patients. In one series,[8] 5% of patients manifested psoriasis and 2% had findings compatible with psoriatic arthritis. Duvic and coworkers[44] described 13 HIV-infected patients with psoriasis, including nine in whom skin lesions developed after the onset of HIV-related symptoms. Three of these patients had coexistent Reiter's-like symptoms with arthritis, urethritis, and conjunctivitis. Psoriasis-associated arthritis in some reported cases has been severe and deforming.[8]

As with Reiter's syndrome, the relationship between HIV and psoriasis and its associated arthritis currently is not well understood. No definite association has been established in these patients between HLA-B27 antigen expression and psoriasis-associated arthritis. In fact, two patients with severe, deforming arthritis were HLA-B27 negative.[8]

HIV-Associated Arthritis

A form of seronegative arthritis not associated with Reiter's syndrome or psoriasis has also been described in some HIV-infected patients.[101] Rynes and coworkers[175] described four patients with oligoarticular arthritis involving the lower extremities. Three of these patients met criteria for the diagnosis of AIDS. In all four cases the arthritis was severe and debilitating, although synovial fluid examinations demonstrated little or no inflammation. No infections known to precipitate reactive arthritis were documented in any of the patients. Three of the four were HLA-B27 positive.

Polymyositis

Polymyositis is the most frequent muscle disorder seen in association with HIV infection.[34] In one large, prospective series[8] 2% of the patients were found to have polymyositis on initial evaluation. As with other HIV-related musculoskeletal syndromes, it may manifest at various stages of HIV infection and may in fact be the initial manifestation.[34]

Polymyositis typically manifests proximal muscle weakness, muscle wasting, and elevated creatine kinase levels, often to more than five times normal.[101] Electromyographic studies demonstrate abnormalities characteristic of myopathy. In reported cases in which histological information is available, inflammatory infiltrates of the involved muscles have usually been demonstrated.[101]

Autoimmune Phenomena

A variety of autoantibodies has been reported in HIV-infected patients. Clinical similarities between the manifestations of HIV infection in some individuals and those of systemic lupus erythematosus have been pointed out.[107] These similarities include arthralgias, lymphadenopathy, butterfly rash, and other skin disorders, as well as frequent involvement of the kidneys and central nervous system. The similarities led to initial diagnostic confusion in some reported cases of HIV infection.[107] Antinuclear antibody can be detected in some HIV-positive patients.[107]

Sjögren's Syndrome/Sicca Complex

Sicca complex (xerostomia, xerophthalmia) has been described in a small number of HIV-infected patients[31] with and without typical features of Sjögren's syndrome.[31] Couderc and coworkers[31] described five HIV-positive patients with progressive generalized lymphadenopathy and sicca complex with lymphocytic infiltration of salivary glands. Lymphocytic infiltration of one or more extrasalivary sites, including the lungs, liver, kidneys, or bone marrow, was also demonstrated in each of these patients, all of whom had serological evidence of infection with the Epstein-Barr virus. In contrast to most cases of classic Sjögren's syndrome, none of these patients were found to have antinuclear antibodies, rheumatoid factor, or other autoantibodies. The relationship between sicca complex, Sjögren's syndrome, and HIV infection is uncertain.

HEMATOLOGICAL DISORDERS

A remarkable array of hematological disorders has been described in HIV-infected patients. These disorders include anemia, leukopenia, thrombocytopenia, coagulopathy, myelofibrosis, hemophagocytosis, plasma cell hyperplasia, and lymphoma.

The causes of these disorders vary. Some represent the direct effects of HIV infection on hematopoietic precursor cells; other reflect the production of autoantibodies and perhaps other autoimmune mechanisms. Depletion of helper/inducer (CD4) lymphocytes is, of course, characteristic of HIV infection and at the heart of the immunological disorders associated with AIDS. Other cells, however, including red blood cells, granulocytes, and monocytes, may also be directly or indirectly affected by HIV. Abnormalities of the peripheral blood smear may include anisocytosis, poikilocytosis, and rouleau formation.[202] Bone marrow examination may reveal dyserythropoiesis, erythroid hypoplasia, megaloblastosis, reticuloendothelial iron block, and a variety of other abnormalities.[202]

Several of the opportunistic infections associated with AIDS, most notably mycobacteriosis, may involve the bone marrow and lymphoid tissue. A number of therapeutic agents commonly used to treat AIDS-related complications (e.g., pentamidine, amphotericin B, trimethoprim-sulfamethoxazole, gancyclovir, and acyclovir) may be associated with clinically significant hematological toxicity. Finally, hematological side effects of antiretroviral agents such as zidovudine may predominate in some patients.

In rare cases patients may have hematological abnormalities as their first manifestation of HIV infection. For example, autoimmune thrombocytopenia, perhaps detected on a routine blood test, may be seen long before other HIV-related disorders. In some patients, particularly those with advanced AIDS, it may be difficult to distinguish among the various possible causes of hematological abnormalities.

AIDS-Related Cytopenias

Among HIV-infected patients, depletion of red cells, white cells, and platelets is seen most commonly in those with advanced disease. Mir and coworkers[139] found anemia in 92%, neutropenia in 85%, monocytopenia in 75%, and thrombocytopenia in 61% of patients with full-blown AIDS. The abnormalities in these patients were felt to be caused by a number of factors representing the effects of therapy, opportunistic infections, or HIV infection itself. Bone marrow biopsy typically revealed erythroid hypoplasia.

Autoimmune Thrombocytopenia

Thrombocytopenia is common in HIV-infected individuals. It may be seen at all stages of the disease[165] and does not have clear prognostic significance.[90] Proposed mechanisms include the elaboration of antiplatelet antibodies[194] and the deposition of immune complexes on the platelet surface.

The diagnosis of autoimmune thrombocytopenia should be made only after bone marrow examination confirms that platelet production is not depressed. Involvement of the marrow by opportunistic infections such as histoplasmosis or disseminated mycobacterial infection or by lymphoma may result in thrombocytopenia, although typically these patients have other evidence of bone marrow depression. Several medications commonly prescribed for HIV-infected patients may interfere with platelet production. The most common of these are zidovudine, sulfonamides, pyrimethamine, and acyclovir. Other causes of peripheral consumption of platelets must also be excluded; this can occur through sequestration in the spleen in patients with portal hypertension, through disseminated intravascular coagulation, or through autoimmune destruction associated with drug therapy.[165]

REFERENCES

1. Abrahms DI et al: Disseminated coccidioidomycosis in AIDS, *N Engl J Med* 310(15):986-987, 1984.
2. Acierno LJ: Cardiac complications in acquired immunodeficiency syndrome (AIDS): a review, *J Am Coll Cardiol* 13(5):1144-1154, 1989.
3. Adams F: The "sheet sign," *JAMA* 251:342, 1984.
4. Aron DC: Endocrine complications of the acquired immunodeficiency syndrome, *Arch Intern Med* 149:330-333, 1989.
5. Barza M, Pauker SG: The decision to biopsy, treat, or wait in suspected herpes encephalitis, *Ann Intern Med* 92:641-649, 1980.
6. Beral V et al: Kaposi's sarcoma among persons with AIDS: a sexually transmitted infection? *Lancet* 335(8682):123-128, 1990.
7. Berger RS et al: Cutaneous manifestations of early human immunodeficiency virus exposure, *J Am Acad Dermatol* 19:298-303, 1988.
8. Berman A et al: Rheumatic manifestations of human immunodeficiency virus infection, *Am J Med* 85:59-64, 1988.
9. Berry CD et al: Neurologic relapse after benzathine penicillin therapy for secondary syphilis in a patient with HIV infection, *N Engl J Med* 316(25):1587-1589, 1987.
10. Bessen LJ et al: Severe polymyositis-like syndrome associated with zidovudine therapy of AIDS and ARC, *N Engl J Med* 318:708, 1988.
11. Beyt BE et al: Cutaneous mycobacteriosis: analysis of 34 cases with a new classification of the disease, *Medicine* 60(2):95-109, 1980.
12. Bishburg E et al: Central nervous sys-

tem tuberculosis with the acquired immunodeficiency syndrome and its related complex, *Ann Intern Med* 105:210-213, 1986.

13. Blaser MJ, Cohn DL: Opportunistic infections in patients with AIDS: clues to the epidemiology of AIDS and relative virulence of pathogens, *Rev Infect Dis* 8(1):21-30, 1986.

14. Blumenthal DR, Zucker JR, Hawkins CC: *Mycobacterium avium* complex–induced septic arthritis and osteomyelitis in a patient with the acquired immunodeficiency syndrome, *Arthritis Rheum* 33(5):757-758, 1990.

15. Broaddus C et al: Bronchoalveolar lavage and transbronchial biopsy for the diagnosis of pulmonary infections in the acquired immunodeficiency syndrome, *Ann Intern Med* 102:747-752, 1985.

16. Bronnimann DA et al: Coccidioidomycosis in the acquired immunodeficiency syndrome, *Ann Intern Med* 106:372-379, 1987.

17. Cappell MS et al: Clinical utility of liver biopsy in patients with serum antibodies to the human immunodeficiency virus, *Am J Med* 88:123-130, 1990.

18. Carbone L et al: Course and prognosis of human immunodeficiency virus–associated nephropathy, *Am J Med* 87:389-395, 1989.

19. Carney MD, Combs JL, Waschler W: Cryptococcal choroiditis, *Retina* 10(1):27-32, 1990.

20. Centers for Disease Control: Kaposi's sarcoma and *Pneumocystis* pneumonia among homosexual men—New York and California, *MMWR* 30:305-308, 1981.

21. Centers for Disease Control: Update: acquired immunodeficiency syndrome—United States, *MMWR* 35:17-20, 1986.

22. Chachoua A et al: Prognostic factors and staging classification of patients with epidemic Kaposi's sarcoma, *J Clin Oncol* 7(6):774-780, 1989.

23. Chayt KJ et al: Detection of HTLV-III RNA in lungs of patients with AIDS and pulmonary involvement, *JAMA* 256(17):2356-2359, 1986.

24. Chu AC, Hay RJ, MacDonald DM: Cutaneous cryptococcosis, *Br J Dermatol* 103:95-100, 1980.

25. Cohen JI, Saragas SJ: Endophthalmitis due to *Mycobacterium avium* in a patient with AIDS, *Ann Ophthalmol* 22(2):47-51, 1990.

26. Cohen AH et al: Demonstration of human immunodeficiency virus in renal epithelium in HIV-associated nephropathy, *Mod Pathol* 2:125-128, 1989.

27. Cohen BA et al: Pulmonary complications of AIDS: radiologic features, *Am J Radiol* 143:115-122, 1984.

28. Cohn JA et al: Evaluation of the policy of empiric treatment of suspected *Toxoplasma* encephalitis in patients with the acquired immunodeficiency syndrome, *Am J Med* 86(5):521-527, 1989.

29. Coldiron BM, Bergstresser PR: Prevalence and clinical spectrum of skin disease in patients infected with human immunodeficiency virus, *Arch Dermatol* 125:357-361, 1989.

30. Connolly GM et al: Investigation of upper gastrointestinal symptoms in patients with AIDS, *AIDS* 3(7):453-456, 1989.

31. Couderc L et al: Sicca complex and infection with human immunodeficiency virus, *Arch Intern Med* 147:898-901, 1987.

32. Coulman CU, Greene I, Archibald RWR: Cutaneous pneumocystosis, *Ann Intern Med* 106:396-398, 1987.

33. Croxson T et al: Intraepithelial carcinoma of the anus in homosexual men, *Dis Colon Rectum* 27(5):325-330, 1984.

34. Dalakas MC, Pezeshkpour GH: Neuromuscular diseases associated with human immunodeficiency virus in-

fection, *Ann Neurol* 23(suppl):S38-S48, 1988.

35. Dalli E et al: Tuberculous pericarditis as the first manifestation of acquired immunodeficiency syndrome, *Am Heart J* 114(4 part 1):905-906, 1987.

36. Damsker B, Bottone EJ: *Mycobacterium avium–Mycobacterium intracellulare* from the intestinal tracts of patients with the acquired immunodeficiency syndrome: concepts regarding acquisition and pathogenesis, *J Infect Dis* 151(1):179-181, 1985.

37. Davis SD et al: Intrathoracic Kaposi sarcoma in AIDS patients: radiographic-pathologic correlation, *Radiology* 163:495-500, 1987.

38. De Clerck LS et al: Acquired immunodeficiency syndrome mimicking Sjögren's syndrome and systemic lupus erythematosus, *Arthritis Rheum* 31(2):272-275, 1988.

39. De La Paz R, Enzmann D: Neuroradiology of acquired immunodeficiency syndrome. In Rosenblum ML, Levy RM, Bredesen DE, editors: *AIDS and the nervous system*, New York, 1988, Raven Press.

40. De Paepe ME, Guerrieri C, Waxman M: Opportunistic infections of the testis in the acquired immunodeficiency syndrome, *Mt Sinai J Med* 57(1):25-29, 1990.

41. Dilley JW, Macks J: Secondary depression in patients with AIDS. Paper presented at the International Conference on Acquired Immunodeficiency Syndrome, Paris, June 23-25, 1986 (abstract).

42. Dilley JW et al: Findings in psychiatric consultations with patients with acquired immune deficiency syndrome, *Am J Psychiatry* 142:82-85, 1985.

43. Dobs AS et al: Endocrine disorders in men infected with human immunodeficiency virus, *Am J Med* 84:611-616, 1988.

44. Duvic M et al: Acquired immunodeficiency syndrome–associated psoriasis and Reiter's syndrome, *Arch Dermatol* 123:1622-1632, 1987.

45. Elkin CM et al: Intracranial lesions in the acquired immunodeficiency syndrome: radiological (computed tomographic) features, *JAMA* 253(3):393-396, 1985.

46. Engstrom JW, Lowenstein DH, Bredesen DE: Cerebral infarctions and transient neurologic deficits associated with acquired immunodeficiency syndrome, *Am J Med* 86(5):528-532, 1989.

47. Engstrom RE, Holland GN: Chronic herpes zoster virus keratitis associated with the acquired immunodeficiency syndrome, *Am J Ophthalmol* 105(5):556-558, 1988.

48. Espinoza LR et al: Psoriatic arthritis and acquired immunodeficiency syndrome, *Arthritis Rheum* 31(8):1034-1040, 1988.

49. Fiala M et al: Responses of neurologic complications of AIDS to 3'-azido-3' deoxythymidine and 9-(1,3-dihydroxy-2-propoxymethyl) guanine. I. Clinical features, *Rev Infect Dis* 10:250-256, 1988.

50. Frager HH et al: Cytomegalovirus colitis in acquired immune deficiency syndrome: radiologic spectrum, *Gastrointest Radiol* 11:241-246, 1986.

51. Frazer IH et al: Association between anorectal dysplasia, human papillomavirus, and human immunodeficiency virus infection in homosexual men, *Lancet* 2(8508):657-660, 1986.

52. Freeman WR et al: Retinopathy before the diagnosis of AIDS, *Ann Ophthalmol* 21(12):468-474, 1989.

53. Freeman WR et al: Prevalence and significance of acquired immunodeficiency syndrome–related retinal microvasculopathy, *Am J Ophthalmol* 107(3):229-235, 1989.

54. Friedman-Kien AE et al: Disseminated Kaposi's sarcoma in homosexual men, *Ann Intern Med* 96:693-700, 1982.

55. Fujita NK et al: Cryptococcal intracerebral mass lesions: the role of computed tomography and nonsurgical management, *Ann Intern Med* 94:382-388, 1981.

56. Gabuzda DH, Hirsch MS: Neurologic manifestations of infection with human immunodeficiency virus: clinical features and pathogenesis, *Ann Intern Med* 107:383-391, 1987.

57. Gill PS et al: Pulmonary Kaposi's sarcoma: clinical findings and results of therapy, *Am J Med* 87:57-61, 1989.

58. Gill PS et al: Primary central nervous system lymphoma in homosexual men: clinical, immunologic, and pathologic features, *Am J Med* 78:742-748, 1985.

59. Gillin JS et al: Malabsorption and mucosal abnormalities of the small intestine in the acquired immunodeficiency syndrome, *Ann Intern Med* 102:619-622, 1985.

60. Glaser JB et al: Recurrent *Salmonella typhimurium* bacteremia associated with the acquired immunodeficiency syndrome, *Ann Intern Med* 102:189-193, 1985.

61. Glasgow BJ et al: Adrenal pathology in the acquired immune deficiency syndrome, *Am J Clin Pathol* 84:594-597, 1985.

62. Glassock RJ et al: Human immunodeficiency virus (HIV) infection and the kidney, *Ann Intern Med* 112:35-49, 1990.

63. Glezerov V, Masci JR: Disseminated strongyloidiasis and other selected unusual infections in patients with the acquired immunodeficiency syndrome. In Rotterdam H, editor: *Progress in AIDS pathology*, Philadelphia, 1990, Field & Wood.

64. Gnepp DR et al: Primary Kaposi's sarcoma of the head and neck, *Ann Intern Med* 100:107-114, 1984.

65. Goldstick L, Mandybur TI, Bode R: Spinal cord degeneration in AIDS, *Neurology* 35:103-106, 1985.

66. Goodman DS et al: Prevalence of cutaneous disease in patients with acquired immunodeficiency syndrome (AIDS) or AIDS-related complex, *J Am Acad Dermatol* 17:210-220, 1987.

67. Goodman P et al: Mycobacterial esophagitis in AIDS, *Gastrointest Radiol* 14(2):103-105, 1989.

68. Grant I et al: Evidence for early central nervous system involvement in the acquired immunodeficiency syndrome (AIDS) and other human immunodeficiency virus infections: studies with neuropsychologic testing and magnetic resonance imaging, *Ann Intern Med* 107:828-836, 1987.

69. Green LW et al: Adrenal insufficiency as a complication of the acquired immunodeficiency syndrome, *Ann Intern Med* 101:497-498, 1984.

70. Greenberg RG, Berger TG: Progressive disseminated histoplasmosis in acquired immune deficiency syndrome: presentation as a steroid-responsive dermatosis, *Cutis* 43(6):535-538, 1989.

71. Greenspan D et al: Relation of oral hairy leukoplakia to infection with the human immunodeficiency virus and the risk of developing AIDS, *J Infect Dis* 155(3):475-481, 1987.

72. Greenspan JS et al: Replication of Epstein-Barr virus within the epithelial cells of oral "hairy" leukoplakia, an AIDS-associated lesion, *N Engl J Med* 313(25):1564-1571, 1985.

73. Groisser D, Bottone EJ, Lebwohl M: Association of *Pityrosporum orbiculare (Malassezia furfur)* with seborrheic dermatitis in patients with the acquired immunodeficiency syndrome (AIDS), *J Am Acad Dermatol* 20:770-773, 1989.

74. Gross JG et al: Longitudinal study of cytomegalovirus retinitis in acquired immune deficiency syndrome, *Ophthalmology* 97(5):681-686, 1990.

75. Grosso DS et al: Ketoconazole inhibition of testicular secretion and dis-

placement of steroid hormones from serum proteins, *Antimicrob Agents Chemother* 23(2):207-211, 1983.

76. Grumbach K et al: Hepatic and biliary tract abnormalities in patients with AIDS: sonographic-pathologic correlation, *J Ultrasound Med* 8(5): 247-254, 1989.

77. Harder E, Al-Kawi MZ, Carney P: Intracranial tuberculoma: conservative management, *Am J Med* 74:570-576, 1983.

78. Hasan FA et al: Hepatic involvement as the primary manifestation of Kaposi's sarcoma in the acquired immunodeficiency syndrome, *Am Gastroenterol* 84(11):1449-1451, 1989.

79. Haverkos HW: The search for cofactors in AIDS, including an analysis of the association of nitrite inhalant abuse and Kaposi's sarcoma, *Prog Clin Biol Res* 325:93-102, 1990.

80. Haverkos HW et al: The changing incidence of Kaposi's sarcoma among patients with AIDS, *J Am Acad Dermatol* 22(6 part 2):1250-1253, 1990.

81. Hecht SR et al: Unsuspected cardiac abnormalities in the acquired immune deficiency syndrome: an echocardiographic study, *Chest* 96:805-808, 1989.

82. Heinz ER et al: Computed tomography in white-matter disease, *Radiology* 130:371-378, 1979.

83. Himelman RB et al: Cardiac manifestations of human immunodeficiency virus infection: a two-dimensional echocardiographic study, *J Am Coll Cardiol* 13(5):1030-1036, 1989.

84. Ho DD et al: Isolation of HTLV-III from cerebrospinal fluid and neural tissues of patients with neurologic syndromes related to the acquired immunodeficiency syndrome, *N Engl J Med* 313:1493-1497, 1985.

85. Holland JC, Tross S: The psychosocial and neuropsychiatric sequelae of the acquired immunodeficiency syndrome and related disorders, *Ann Intern Med* 103:760-764, 1985.

86. Holland GN et al: Ocular toxoplasmosis in patients with acquired immunodeficiency syndrome, *Am J Ophthalmol* 106(6):653-657, 1988.

87. Hollander H, Stringari S: Human immunodeficiency virus–associated meningitis: clinical course and correlations, *Am J Med* 83:813-816, 1987.

88. Holtz HA, Lavery DP, Kapila R: Actinomycetales infection in the acquired immunodeficiency syndrome, *Ann Intern Med* 102(2):203-205, 1985.

89. Holtzman DM et al: New-onset seizures associated with human immunodeficiency virus infection: causation and clinical features in 100 cases, *Am J Med* 87:173-177, 1989.

90. Holzman RS, Walsh CM, Karpatkin S: Risk for the acquired immunodeficiency syndrome among thrombocytopenic and nonthrombocytopenic homosexual men seropositive for the human immunodeficiency virus, *Ann Intern Med* 106:383-386, 1987.

91. Israelski DM, Remington JS: Toxoplasmic encephalitis in patients with AIDS, *Infect Dis Clin North Am* 2:429-445, 1988.

92. Jabs DA et al: Ocular manifestations of acquired immunodeficiency syndrome, *Ophthalmology* 96(7):1092-1099, 1989.

93. Jabs DA, Enger C, Bartlett JG.: Cytomegalovirus retinitis and acquired immunodeficiency syndrome, *Arch Ophthalmol* 107(1):75-80, 1989.

94. Jacobs JL et al: Salmonella infections in patients with the acquired immunodeficiency syndrome, *Ann Intern Med* 102:186-188, 1985.

95. Jacobson MA, Mills J: Serious cytomegalovirus disease in the acquired immunodeficiency syndrome (AIDS): clinical findings, diagnosis, and treatment, *Ann Intern Med* 108:585-594, 1988.

96. Jules-Elysee KM et al: Aerosolized pentamidine: effect on diagnosis and presentation of *Pneumocystis carinii* pneumonia, *Ann Intern Med* 112:750-757, 1990.

97. Kaplan MH et al: Neoplastic complications of HTLV-III infection: lymphomas and solid tumors, *Am J Med* 82:389-396, 1987.

98. Katz AS, Niesenbaum L, Mass B: Pleural effusion as the initial manifestation of disseminated cryptococcosis in acquired immune deficiency syndrome: diagnosis by pleural biopsy, *Chest* 96(2):440-441, 1989.

99. Katzman M et al: Molluscum contagiosum and the acquired immunodeficiency syndrome: clinical and immunological details of two cases, *Br J Dermatol* 116(1):131-138, 1987.

100. Kavin H et al: Acalculous cholecystitis and cytomegalovirus infection in the acquired immunodeficiency syndrome, *Ann Intern Med* 104:53-54, 1986.

101. Kaye BR: Rheumatologic manifestations of infection with human immunodeficiency virus (HIV), *Ann Intern Med* 111:158-167, 1989.

102. Kelly WM, Brant-Zawadzki M: Acquired immunodeficiency syndrome: neuroradiologic findings, *Radiology* 149:485-491, 1983.

103. Khadem M et al: Ophthalmologic findings in acquired immune deficiency syndrome (AIDS), *Arch Ophthalmol* 102(2):201-206, 1984.

104. Klein RS et al: Oral candidiasis in high-risk patients as the initial manifestation of the acquired immunodeficiency syndrome, *N Engl J Med* 311:354-358, 1984.

105. Knowles DM et al: Lymphoid neoplasia associated with the acquired immunodeficiency syndrome (AIDS): the New York University Medical Center experience with 105 patients (1981-1986), *Ann Intern Med* 108:744-753, 1988.

106. Koehler JE et al: Cutaneous vascular lesions and disseminated cat-scratch disease in patients with the acquired immunodeficiency syndrome (AIDS) and AIDS-related complex, *Ann Intern Med* 109:449-455, 1988.

107. Kopelman RG, Zolla-Pazner S: Association of human immunodeficiency virus infection and autoimmune phenomena, *Am J Med* 84:82-88, 1988.

108. Kotler DP et al: Enteropathy associated with the acquired immunodeficiency syndrome, *Ann Intern Med* 101:421-428, 1984.

109. Kovacs JA, Masur H: *Pneumocystis carinii* pneumonia: therapy and prophylaxis, *J Infect Dis* 158(1):254-259, 1988.

110. Kovacs JA et al: *Pneumocystis carinii* pneumonia: a comparison between patients with the acquired immunodeficiency syndrome and patients with other immunodeficiencies, *Ann Intern Med* 100:663-671, 1984.

111. Kovacs JA et al: Cryptococcosis in the acquired immunodeficiency syndrome, *Ann Intern Med* 103:533-538, 1985.

112. Krick JA, Remington JS: Toxoplasmosis in the adult: an overview, *N Engl J Med* 298(10):550-553, 1978.

113. Krupp LB et al: Progressive multifocal leukoencephalopathy in AIDS. In Wormser GP, Stahl RE, Bottone EJ, editors: *Acquired immune deficiency and other manifestations of HIV infection*, Park Ridge, NJ, 1987, Noyles Publications.

114. Lake-Bakaar G et al: Gastric secretory failure in patients with the acquired immunodeficiency syndrome (AIDS), *Ann Intern Med* 109:502-504, 1988.

115. Lake-Bakaar G et al: Gastropathy and ketoconazole malabsorption in the acquired immunodeficiency syndrome (AIDS), *Ann Intern Med* 109:471-473, 1988.

116. Laskin OL, Stahl-Bayliss CM, Morgello S: Concomitant herpes simplex virus type 1 and cytomegalovirus ventriculoencephalitis in acquired immunodeficiency syndrome, *Arch Neurol* 44(8):843-847, 1987.

117. Lebovics E et al: The hepatobiliary manifestations of human immunodeficiency virus infection, *Am J Gastroenterol* 83:1-7, 1988.

118. Levenson SM et al: Abnormal pulmonary gallium accumulation in *P. carinii* pneumonia, *Radiology* 119:395-398, 1976.

119. Levin M et al: *Pneumocystis* pneumonia: importance of gallium scan for early diagnosis and description of a new immunoperoxidase technique to demonstrate *Pneumocystis carinii*, *Am Rev Respir Dis* 128:182-185, 1983.

120. Levy RM, Bredesen DE: Central nervous system dysfunction in acquired immunodeficency syndrome. In Rosenblum ML, Levy RM, Bredesen DE, editors: *AIDS and the nervous system*, New York, 1988, Raven Press.

121. Levy RM et al: Neurological manifestations of the acquired immunodeficiency syndrome (AIDS): experience at UCSF and review of the literature, *J Neurosurg* 62:475-495, 1985.

122. Lin J et al: Cytomegalovirus-associated appendicitis in a patient with the acquired immunodeficiency syndrome, *Am J Med* 89:377-379, 1990.

123. Lipson BK et al: Optic neuropathy associated with cryptococcal arachnoiditis in AIDS patients, *Am J Ophthalmol* 107(5):523-527, 1989.

124. Lipstein-Kresch E et al: Disseminated *Sporothrix schenckii* infection with arthritis in a patient with acquired immunodeficiency syndrome, *J Rheumatol* 12(4):805-808, 1985.

125. Luburich P et al: Hepatic Kaposi sarcoma in AIDS: US and CT findings, *Radiology* 175(1):172-174, 1990.

126. Ma P, Soave R: Three-step stool examination for cryptosporidiosis in 10 homosexual men with protracted watery diarrhea, *J Infect Dis* 147:824-828, 1983.

127. Maayan S et al: *Strongyloides stercoralis* hyperinfection in a patient with the acquired immune deficiency syndrome, *Am J Med* 83:945-948, 1987.

128. Margulis SJ et al: Biliary tract obstruction in the acquired immunodeficiency syndrome, *Ann Intern Med* 105:207-210, 1986.

129. Marzuk PM et al: Increased risk of suicide in persons with AIDS, *JAMA* 259(9):1333-1337, 1988.

130. Masur H et al: CD4 counts as predictors of opportunistic pneumonias in human immunodeficiency virus (HIV) infection, *Ann Intern Med* 111(3):223-231, 1989.

131. Mathes BM, Douglass MC: Seborrheic dermatitis in patients with acquired immunodeficiency syndrome, *J Am Acad Dermatol* 13:947-951, 1985.

132. Meduri GU et al: Pulmonary Kaposi's sarcoma in the acquired immune syndrome: clinical, radiographic, and pathologic manifestations, *Am J Med* 81:11-18, 1988.

133. Melbye M et al: Risk of AIDS after herpes zoster, *Lancet* 1(8535):728-731, 1987.

134. Mendelson M et al: Pulmonary toxoplasmosis in AIDS, *Scand J Infect Dis* 19:703-706, 1987.

135. Michet CJ et al: Epidemiology of Reiter's syndrome in Rochester, Minnesota: 1950-1980, *Arthritis Rheum* 31(3):428-431, 1988.

136. Miller WT, Edelman JM, Miller WT: Cryptococcal pulmonary infection in patients with AIDS: radiographic appearance, *Radiology* 175(3):725-728, 1990.

137. Miller JR et al: Progressive multifocal leukoencephalopathy in a male homosexual with T-cell immune deficiency, *N Engl J Med* 307(23):1436-1438, 1982.

138. Mintz L et al: Cytomegalovirus infections in homosexual men: an epidemiological study, *Ann Intern Med* 99:326-329, 1983.

139. Mir N et al: HIV disease and bone marrow changes: a study of 60 cases, *Eur J Haematol* 42(4):339-343, 1989.

140. Monsuez J et al: Comparison among acquired immune deficiency syndrome patients with and without clinical evidence of cardiac disease, *Am J Cardiol* 62:1311-1313, 1988.

141. Morris DJ: Is human immunodeficiency virus (HIV) rather than cytomegalovirus the cause of retinitis and colitis in HIV-infected patients? *J Infect Dis* 12(3):557-559, 1990.

142. Murray JF, Mills J: Pulmonary infectious complications of human immunodeficiency virus infection, *Am Rev Respir Dis* 141:1582-1598, 1990.

143. Murray JF et al: Pulmonary complications of the acquired immunodeficiency syndrome: report of a National Heart, Lung and Blood Institute workshop, *N Engl J Med* 310(25):1682-1688, 1984.

144. Murray RJ et al: Recovery from cryptococcemia and the adult respiratory distress syndrome in the acquired immunodeficiency syndrome, *Chest* 93:1304-1306, 1988.

145. Navia BA et al: Cerebral toxoplasmosis complicating the acquired immune deficiency syndrome: clinical and neuropathological findings in 27 patients, *Ann Neurol* 19:224-238, 1986.

146. Navia BA et al: The AIDS dementia complex. I. Clinical features, *Ann Neurol* 19:517-524, 1986.

147. Navia BA et al: The AIDS dementia complex. II. Neuropathology, *Ann Neurol* 19:525-535, 1986.

148. Newman TG et al: Pleural cryptococcosis in the acquired immunodeficiency syndrome, *Chest* 91:459-461, 1988.

149. Ognibene FP et al: Kaposi's sarcoma causing pulmonary infiltrates and respiratory failure in the acquired immunodeficiency syndrome, *Ann Intern Med* 102:471-475, 1985.

150. Padgett BL et al: JC papovavirus in progressive multifocal leukoencephalopathy, *J Infect Dis* 133(6):686-690, 1976.

151. Palefsky JM et al: Anal intraepithelial neoplasia and anal papillomavirus infection among homosexual males with group IV HIV disease, *JAMA* 263(21):2911-2916, 1990.

152. Parry GJ: Peripheral neuropathies associated with human immunodeficiency virus infection, *Ann Neurol* 23(suppl):S49-S53, 1988.

153. Patow CA et al: Pharyngeal obstruction by Kaposi's sarcoma in a homosexual male with acquired immune deficiency syndrome, *Otolaryngol Head Neck Surg* 92(6):713-716, 1984.

154. Phelan JA et al: Oral findings in patients with acquired immunodeficiency syndrome, *Oral Surg Oral Med Oral Pathol* 64(1):50-56, 1987.

155. Pitchenik AE, Rubinson HA: The radiographic appearance of tuberculosis in patients with the acquired immune deficiency syndrome (AIDS) and pre-AIDS, *Am Rev Respir Dis* 131:393-396, 1985.

156. Polsky B et al: Bacterial pneumonia in patients with the acquired immunodeficiency syndrome, *Ann Intern Med* 104:38-41, 1986.

157. Pont A et al: Ketoconazole blocks adrenal steroid synthesis, *Ann Intern Med* 97:370-372, 1982.

158. Porro GB, Parente F, Cernuschi M: The diagnosis of esophageal candidiasis in patients with acquired immune deficiency syndrome: is endoscopy always necessary? *Am J Gastroenterol* 84(2):143-146, 1989.

159. Post MJD et al: Cranial CT in ac-

quired immunodeficiency syndrome: spectrum of diseases and optimal contrast enhancement technique, *Am J Radiol* 145:929-940, 1985.

160. Post MJD et al: CT, MR, and pathology in HIV encephalitis and meningitis, *Am J Radiol* 151(2):373-380, 1988.

161. Price RW et al: AIDS encephalopathy, *Neurol Clin* 4(1):285-301, 1986.

162. Quinn TC et al: The polymicrobial origin of intestinal infections in homosexual men, *N Engl J Med* 309(10):576-582, 1983.

163. Quinn TC et al: Infections with *Campylobacter jejuni* and *Campylobacter*-like organisms in homosexual men, *Ann Intern Med* 101:187-192, 1984.

164. Rabeneck L et al: Acute HIV infection presenting with painful swallowing and esophageal ulcers, *JAMA* 263(17):2318-2322, 1990.

165. Ratner L: Human immunodeficiency virus–associated autoimmune thrombocytopenic purpura: a review, *Am J Med* 86:194-198, 1989.

166. Raufman JP: Odynophagia/dysphagia in AIDS, *Gastroenterol Clin North Am* 17(3):599-614, 1988.

167. Reichert CM et al: Autopsy pathology in the acquired immune deficiency syndrome, *Am J Pathol* 112:357-382, 1983.

168. Ricciardi DD et al: Cryptococcal arthritis in a patient with acquired immune deficiency syndrome: case report and review of the literature, *J Rheumatol* 13(2):455-458, 1986.

169. Rico MJ, Penneys NS: Cutaneous cryptococcosis resembling molluscum contagiosum in a patient with AIDS, *Arch Dermatol* 121:901-902, 1985.

170. Roberts CJ: Coccidioidomycosis in the acquired immune deficiency syndrome: depressed humoral as well as cellular immunity, *Am J Med* 76:734-736, 1984.

171. Rockwell D et al: Absence of immune deficiencies in a case of progressive multifocal leukoencephalopathy, *Am J Med* 61:433-436, 1976.

172. Rodriguez JL et al: Pulmonary nocardiosis in the acquired immunodeficiency syndrome: diagnosis with bronchoalveolar lavage and treatment with non-sulphur-containing drugs, *Chest* 90(6):912-914, 1986.

173. Rosenberg PR et al: Acquired immunodeficiency syndrome: ophthalmic manifestations in ambulatory patients, *Ophthalmology* 90(8):874-878, 1983.

174. Rustgi VK et al: Hepatitis B virus infection in the acquired immunodeficiency syndrome, *Ann Intern Med* 101:795-797, 1984.

175. Rynes RI et al: Acquired immunodeficiency syndrome–associated arthritis, *Am J Med* 84:810-816, 1988.

176. Saxton CR et al: Progressive multifocal leukoencephalopathy in a renal transplant recipient: increased diagnostic sensitivity of computed tomographic scanning by double-dose contrast with delayed films, *Am J Med* 77:333-337, 1984.

177. Schlamm HT, Yancovitz SR: *Haemophilus influenzae* pneumonia in young adults with AIDS, ARC, or risk of AIDS, *Am J Med* 86:11-14, 1989.

178. Schneiderman DJ, Cello JP, Laing FC: Papillary stenosis and sclerosing cholangitis in the acquired immunodeficiency syndrome, *Ann Intern Med* 106:546-549, 1987.

179. Schuster M, Valentine F, Holzman R: Cryptococcal pericarditis in an intravenous drug abuser, *J Infect Dis* 152(4):842, 1985.

180. Scott PJ, Conway SP, Da Costa P: Cardiac tamponade complicating cytomegalovirus pericarditis in a patient with AIDS, *J Infect Dis* 20(1):92-93, 1990.

181. Selwyn PA et al: A prospective study

of the risk of tuberculosis among intravenous drug users with human immunodeficiency virus infection, *N Engl J Med* 320(9):545-550, 1989.

182. Shattock AG, Finlay H, Hillary IB: Possible reactivation of hepatitis D with chronic delta antigenaemia by human immunodeficiency virus, *Br Med J* 294:1656-1657, 1987.

183. Shuler JD et al: Kaposi sarcoma of the conjunctiva and eyelids associated with the acquired immunodeficiency syndrome, *Arch Ophthalmol* 107(6):858-862, 1989.

184. Siegal FP et al: Severe acquired immunodeficiency in male homosexuals, manifested by chronic perianal ulcerative herpes simplex lesions, *N Engl J Med* 305:1439-1444, 1981.

185. Silver MA et al: Cardiac involvement by Kaposi's sarcoma in acquired immune deficiency syndrome (AIDS), *Am J Cardiol* 53(7):983-985, 1984.

186. Silverman S et al: Oral findings in people with or at high risk for AIDS: a study of 375 homosexual males, *J Am Dent Assoc* 112(2):187-192, 1986.

187. Skolnik PR et al: Dual infection of retina with human immunodeficiency virus type 1 and cytomegalovirus, *Am J Ophthalmol* 107(4):361-372, 1989.

188. Smith PD et al: Intestinal infections in patients with acquired immunodeficiency syndrome (AIDS): etiology and response to therapy, *Ann Intern Med* 108:328-333, 1988.

189. Sneed SR et al: *Pneumocystis carinii* choroiditis in patients receiving inhaled pentamidine, *N Engl J Med* 322(13):936-937, 1990.

190. Snider WD et al: Neurological complications of acquired immune deficiency syndrome: analysis of 50 patients, *Ann Neurol* 14:403-418, 1983.

191. Soave R et al: Cryptosporidiosis in homosexual men, *Ann Intern Med* 100:504-511, 1984.

192. Soeprono FF et al: Seborrheic-like dermatitis of acquired immunodefi-

ciency syndrome: a clinicopathologic study, *J Am Acad Dermatol* 14:242-248, 1986.

193. Stimmler MM et al: Anticardiolipin antibodies in acquired immunodeficiency syndrome, *Arch Intern Med* 149:1833-1836, 1989.

194. Stricker RB et al: Target platelet antigen in homosexual men with immune thrombocytopenia, *N Engl J Med* 313:1375-1380, 1985.

195. Sunderam G et al: Tuberculosis as a manifestation of the acquired immunodeficiency syndrome (AIDS), *JAMA* 256(3):362-366, 1986.

196. Tapper ML et al: Adrenal necrosis in the acquired immunodeficiency syndrome, *Ann Intern Med* 100(2):239-241, 1984.

197. Tawney S et al: Pulmonary toxoplasmosis: an unusual nodular radiographic pattern in a patient with the acquired immunodeficiency syndrome, *Mt Sinai J Med* 53:683-685, 1986.

198. Teixidor HS et al: Cytomegalovirus infection of the alimentary canal: radiologic findings with pathologic correlation, *Radiology* 163(2):317-323, 1987.

199. Tindall B et al: Characterization of the acute clinical illness associated with human immunodeficiency virus infection, *Arch Intern Med* 148:945-948, 1988.

200. Toma E et al: Herpes simplex type 2 pericarditis and bilateral facial palsy in a patient with AIDS, *J Infect Dis* 160(3):553-554, 1989.

201. Torssander J et al: Oral *Candida albicans* in HIV infection, *Scand J Infect Dis* 19(3):291-295, 1987.

202. Treacy M et al: Peripheral blood and bone marrow abnormalities in patients with HIV related disease, *Br J Haematol* 65:289-294, 1987.

203. Valle SL: Dermatologic findings related to human immunodeficiency virus infection in high-risk individuals,

J Am Acad Dermatol 17:951-961, 1987.

204. Vitting KE et al: Frequency of hyponatremia and nonosmolar vasopressin release in the acquired immunodeficiency syndrome, *JAMA* 263(7):973-978, 1990.

205. Walsh C et al: Thrombocytopenia in homosexual patients: prognosis, response to therapy, and prevalence of antibody to the retrovirus associated with the acquired immunodeficiency syndrome, *Ann Intern Med* 103:542-545, 1985.

206. Wasser L, Talavera W: Pulmonary cryptococcosis in AIDS, *Chest* 92:692-695, 1987.

207. Weiss LM et al: *Isospora belli* infection: treatment with pyrimethamine, *Ann Intern Med* 109:474-475, 1988.

208. Welch K et al: Autopsy findings in the acquired immune deficiency syndrome, *JAMA* 252(9):1152-1159, 1984.

209. Wheat LJ et al: Histoplasmosis in the acquired immune deficiency syndrome, *Am J Med* 78:203-210, 1985.

210. Whelan MA et al: Acquired immunodeficiency syndrome: cerebral computed tomographic manifestations, *Radiology* 149:477-484, 1983.

211. White DA, Matthay RA: Noninfectious pulmonary complications of infection with the human immunodeficiency virus, *Am Rev Respir Dis* 140:1763-1787, 1989.

212. Whitley RJ et al: Diseases that mimic herpes simplex encephalitis: diagnosis, presentation, and outcome, *JAMA* 262(2):234-239, 1989.

213. Winchester R et al: The co-occurrence of Reiter's syndrome and acquired immunodeficiency, *Ann Intern Med* 106:19-26, 1987.

214. Wolfson JS et al: Cryptosporidiosis in immunocompetent patients, *N Engl J Med* 312:1278-1282, 1985.

215. Wolke A et al: *Mycobacterium avium-intracellulare*–associated colitis in a patient with the acquired immunodeficiency syndrome, *J Clin Gastroenterol* 6:225-229, 1984.

216. Woods GL, Goldsmith JC: Fatal pericarditis due to *Mycobacterium avium-intracellulare* in acquired immunodeficiency syndrome, *Chest* 95(6):1355-1357, 1989.

217. Zaman MK, White DA: Serum lactate dehydrogenase levels and *Pneumocystis carinii* pneumonia, *Am Rev Respir Dis* 137:796-800, 1988.

218. Zambrano W, Perez GM, Smith JL: Acute syphilitic blindness in AIDS, *J Clin Neuro Ophthalmol* 7(1):1-5, 1987.

219. Zuger A et al: Cryptococcal disease in patients with the acquired immunodeficiency syndrome: diagnostic features and outcome of treatment, *Ann Intern Med* 104:234-240, 1986.

CHAPTER **6**

General Medical Evaluation of the Asymptomatic HIV-Infected Patient

Early in the AIDS epidemic, many medical practitioners, as well as individuals at high risk, felt that there was little reason to test for the presence of HIV-1 infection before the onset of symptoms because no therapy was available to alter the course of the disease. Beginning in the late 1980s, however, testing of asymptomatic individuals became increasingly widespread. Many who believed that they were at risk sought testing or were offered testing by their physicians.

Several developments accounted for this change in approach, including aggressive public information campaigns and easier access to testing; most important, however, was the fact that therapies had become available that could benefit HIV-infected patients before symptoms appeared.

The development of life-prolonging antiretroviral therapy and effective prophylaxis of *Pneumocystis carinii* pneumonia, the most common initial opportunistic infection in AIDS, has provided a strong medical indication for HIV-1 testing. Increasingly attention has focused on the appropriate role of the primary care physician in carrying out screening of patients with a history of risk behavior for infection with HIV-1.[35]

Unfortunately, primary care physicians, including those practicing in areas where HIV-1 infection is common, may lack familiarity with HIV-related diseases[31,56] and with relevant laboratory diagnostic tests.[16] Sexual counseling of patients at risk for HIV infection varies greatly from practitioner to practitioner.[16] Nonetheless, as the HIV-1 epidemic expands, increasing numbers of infected patients in an asymptomatic stage of disease will see primary care physicians for comprehensive care. Such care should include a thorough evaluation for evidence of HIV-related disorders, immunological staging, appropriate use of prophylactic and antiretroviral therapy when indicated, counseling about the risk of spreading infection to others, and support for the patient in coping with the disease.

The medical assessment of asymptomatic HIV-infected patients should be directed toward several goals. Most important among these is determining the clinical and immunological stage of disease. As was discussed in Chapter 2, accurate staging is essential for selecting initial diagnostic screening tests and for identifying patients for whom therapy or prophylaxis is indicated. Medical conditions not related to HIV-1 infection must also be identified, characterized, and treated, if necessary. An understanding of the individual's personal life and, particularly, HIV-related risk behavior is essential for effective counseling and support.

OBTAINING THE MEDICAL HISTORY FROM AN HIV-INFECTED PATIENT: SPECIAL CONSIDERATIONS

A carefully obtained medical history of a patient with HIV-1 infection can provide the clinician with many important insights (see the box below). Because HIV-1 infection is largely a disease of young adults, patients in an early, asymptomatic stage most commonly feel quite well and have no significant chronic illnesses. Many patients doubt that they are infected at all, particularly those referred for medical assessment simply because of a positive screening test. This attitude stems in part from the popular conception that HIV-1 infection and AIDS are synonymous and represent a rapidly progressive, debilitating disease. In later stages of the disease, some patients may be inclined either to deny or exaggerate somatic complaints. Cognitive defects, perhaps reflecting the AIDS dementia complex, may interfere with patients' ability to relate their medical history or current complaints.

HIV-infected patients are regarded as asymptomatic only if there is no history of AIDS-related opportunistic infections or malignancies and no symptoms compatible with AIDS-related complex. (These diagnostic categories are discussed in detail in Chapter 1; the differential diagnosis and recommended diagnostic workup for HIV-related symptoms is discussed in detail in Chapter 7.) Following are several goals that should be kept in mind when obtaining the medical history of an HIV-infected patient.

Evaluating the Patient's Reaction to the Diagnosis of HIV Infection

HIV-infected patients who have received appropriate counseling should be questioned about their understanding of the disease, routes of transmission, and recommended changes in their sexual practices and life-style. If counseling has not taken place, it should be approached as outlined in Chapter 4.

When informed of a positive HIV test result, patients may react with a range of feelings, including denial, anger, guilt, depression, or apparent in-

---

Major Elements of Medical History

Current symptoms
General past medical history
History of potentially HIV-related complaints (see box on p. 125)
Place of birth, travel history
Immunization history
Risk behavior history
Employment history

difference. Although individual practitioners' styles may differ, questions designed to explore such reactions should be asked in an understanding, accepting way and, in general, patients should be encouraged to discuss their feelings (see Chapter 4).

Many asymptomatic patients do not initially believe that they are infected and question the validity of positive test results. In such cases the meaning of the test result should be reviewed and discussed (see Chapter 4) and, if doubt remains, repeat testing should be considered.

Most asymptomatic HIV-infected patients are young adults with little or no history of significant health problems. It is important for the primary care physician to determine the impact of HIV infection on the patient's daily life. Disruption of family support systems or, for some patients, further alienation from family and friends is common. Employment, housing, and financial concerns may become paramount for some individuals. Appropriate questioning about these areas may lead the physician to arrange family counseling or social service intervention and demonstrates to the patient that there is an interest in providing assistance and support.

Asymptomatic patients frequently are confused about the distinction between HIV-1 infection and AIDS. The relatively long natural history that HIV-related disease usually pursues (see Chapter 2) should be carefully explained. Questions about the prognosis are almost always asked by the patient at the first encounter (see box on p. 124). Although specific predictions are unwise and in fact likely to be inaccurate, an atmosphere of both realism and hope should be established. After immunological staging has been completed, the short-term risk of AIDS-related complications should be easier to assess (see Chapter 2).

Evaluating for Symptoms of HIV-1 Infection

The patient may ignore or minimize important symptoms of HIV-1 infection. For this reason patients should be systematically questioned about nonspecific symptoms associated with HIV-1 infection (see the box on p. 125), and AIDS-associated opportunistic infections and malignancies (see the box on p. 126). It should be noted that there is substantial overlap between nonspecific signs of HIV-1 infection and early signs and symptoms of potentially life-threatening opportunistic infections and malignancies.

Evaluating for Current or Previous Evidence of Immunodeficiency

Several infections, although not considered diagnostic of AIDS, are common among HIV-1 infected patients and may indicate the duration of infection and the rate at which immunodeficiency is progressing (see Chapter 2).

Questions Frequently Asked by HIV-Infected Patients

1. DO I HAVE AIDS? (Chapter 1)
   AIDS is the culmination of HIV infection, marked by the onset of opportunistic infections and malignancies. Most HIV-infected patients do not currently have AIDS.
2. WILL I DEVELOP AIDS? (Chapter 1)
   It appears that all or virtually all HIV-infected patients will develop AIDS, barring
   major advances in therapy.
3. HOW LONG WILL I LIVE? (Chapters 1 and 2)
   The prognosis of HIV infection for an individual depends to a large extent on the
   degree of immunodeficiency at the time of diagnosis. Survival can range from
   months to years.
4. CAN THE PEOPLE I LIVE WITH CATCH HIV INFECTION FROM ME? (Chapters 1
   and 4)
   Studies indicate that nonsexual household contacts are not at risk of contagion;
   however, precautions should be taken with body fluids.
5. SHOULD I TELL ANYONE THAT I AM INFECTED? (Chapter 4)
   Patients should be urged to tell sexual or blood contacts. The need to inform others
   of the diagnosis should be individualized.
6. CAN ANYONE FIND OUT THAT I AM INFECTED? (Chapter 4)
   Confidentiality laws regarding HIV test results vary by state.
7. SHOULD I CONTINUE TO WORK?
   The patient should be encouraged to avoid dramatic changes in life-style unless
   these are dictated by physical limitations. Specific job-related activities should be
   assessed for risk of HIV transmission to others.
8. WHAT SHOULD I EAT?
   The patient should be encouraged to eat a balanced diet. Fad diets should be dis-
   couraged.
9. SHOULD I EXERCISE?
   Exercise to tolerance is of no proven risk or benefit.
10. WILL THERE BE A CURE? (Chapter 10)
    The answer to this question is currently unknown. Current therapeutic strategies
    have been shown to be partially effective and new, more effective therapies can be
    anticipated.

Assessing the Risk of Specific HIV-Related Disorders

A history of previous tuberculin skin test results, as well as serological tests
for syphilis, should be obtained, since these tests may lose diagnostic sensitivity as immunodeficiency progresses,[23] and both tuberculosis[51] and syphilis[1]
may progress with HIV-1 infection.[1]

A thorough travel history, including country of birth, areas of residence
during childhood and adolescence, and military history, can aid in evaluating
subsequent AIDS-related illnesses. Tuberculosis, histoplasmosis, strongyloi-

---

Common Nonspecific Signs and Symptoms of HIV-1 Infection

General

Fever
Weight loss
Generalized lymphadenopathy

Dermatological

Seborrheic dermatitis
Xerosis/ichthyosis
Dermatophyte infection
Candidiasis
Molluscum contagiosum
Herpes zoster
Herpes simplex

Ocular

Retinal hemorrhages, exudates
Dry eyes

Oral

Ulcerations
Angular cheilitis
Thrush

Parotid gland enlargement
Dry mouth
Hairy leukoplakia

Cardiovascular

Pericardial rub
S3 gallop

Gastrointestinal

Diarrhea
Splenomegaly

Musculoskeletal

Arthralgias
Arthritis
Reiter's syndrome

Neurological

Peripheral neuropathy
Cognitive defects: difficulty concentrating, decreased short-term memory

---

diasis, and other opportunistic infections are more likely in patients who lived under conditions of high prevalence early in life.

Immunization status. Information about immunizations against polio, measles, mumps, rubella, pneumococcal infection, and hepatitis B should be obtained.

General medical history. Because of the multisystem nature of HIV-1 infection and its complications (see Chapter 5), it may be difficult to interpret physical complaints, and clues to the presence of non-HIV–related disorders may be overlooked. For this reason it is important that a thorough history of previously diagnosed medical conditions be elicited and recorded and that a risk-factor assessment for cardiovascular and neoplastic disease be made.

Assessing past and current risk behaviors. Details of risk behavior should be discussed, and misconceptions about contagion corrected. A discussion of post-test counseling for HIV-infected patients at all stages of disease is presented in Chapter 4.

Selected Signs and Symptoms of AIDS-Related Opportunistic Infections and Malignancies*

General

Fever, weight loss
Generalized or localized lymphadenopathy

Dermatological

Ulcerations (herpes simplex)
Pustules (herpes simplex, disseminated mycobacterial or fungal infection)
Nodules (Kaposi's sarcoma, lymphoma, disseminated mycobacterial, or fungal infection)

Ocular

Decreased visual acuity (infectious retinitis)
Visual field deficit (cerebral toxoplasmosis, lymphoma)
Periocular skin lesions (Kaposi's sarcoma)

Oral

Painful ulcerations (herpes simplex)
Nodules (Kaposi's sarcoma, lymphoma)

Respiratory

Persistent cough (*Pneumocystis carinii* pneumonia or other opportunistic infection, Kaposi's sarcoma)
Dyspnea (*P. carinii* pneumonia or other opportunistic infection, Kaposi's sarcoma)

Gastrointestinal

Dysphagia/odynophagia (infectious esophagitis, Kaposi's sarcoma)
Diarrhea
Hepatomegaly (mycobacterial or other opportunistic infection involving the liver, lymphoma, Kaposi's sarcoma)
Jaundice (biliary tract involvement with cytomegalovirus infection, cryptosporidiosis)

Neurological

Cognitive dysfunction (AIDS dementia)
Focal deficit (cerebral toxoplasmosis, lymphoma, or other space-occupying lesion; cerebral infarction)
Headache (cryptococcal meningitis; cerebral toxoplasmosis, lymphoma, or other space-occupying lesion)

*Common AIDS-related disorders are in parentheses; for a more extensive discussion of clinical syndromes, see Chapters 5 and 7.

PHYSICAL EXAMINATION

The physical examination of HIV-infected patients should be thorough and appropriate for the patient's age and past medical history. In addition, it should be specifically directed toward identifying HIV-related abnormalities. The differential diagnosis and recommended diagnostic workup of abnormal physical findings at all stages of HIV infection is discussed in Chapter 7.

General Condition and Nutritional Status

The patient's height and body weight should be recorded at the first visit, and his or her weight should be noted at each subsequent visit. The patient's usual weight, as well as recent changes in weight, should be ascertained.

Standardized measurements of the triceps skinfold or arm anthropometry may be helpful in following the nutritional status over time.

Skin

HIV-infected patients frequently have abnormalities of the skin, hair, and nails. Common mucocutaneous disorders such as seborrheic dermatitis, xerosis, psoriasis, and folliculitis are generally easily recognized. Herpes simplex oral or genital infections are often present as ulcerating lesions on the lips, the anterior oral cavity, the perineum, penis, or perirectal region. Occasionally the herpes simplex virus may produce more disseminated infection, with ulcerating lesions on the trunk, face, and extremities. Persistent herpes simplex infection is regarded as an AIDS-defining condition.

Varicella zoster virus may produce any of its typical manifestations, including primary varicella (chickenpox), dermatomal zoster (shingles), or disseminated zoster. Dermatomal zoster may manifest as a severe infection years before the onset of AIDS-defining opportunistic infections.[36]

Several AIDS-related opportunistic infections may cause papular or pustular lesions. These disorders include cryptococcosis,[49] histoplasmosis, tuberculosis, and pneumocystosis.[13]

Molluscum contagiosum is seen frequently in HIV-infected patients at all stages of immunodeficiency and may appear on the face, neck, trunk, or extremities. The lesions are smooth, dome-shaped papules often having an umbilicated center containing a waxy plug.

The lesions of Kaposi's sarcoma may be seen on any part of the body but most commonly appear on the face, particularly the tip of the nose and the ears; they are also found on the trunk and extremities. Mucous membrane involvement is particularly common in patients with Kaposi's sarcoma, and lesions are often seen on the gingival surfaces, palate, and peritonsillar areas.

Lymphatics

A careful assessment for lymph node enlargement should be made each time an HIV-infected patient is examined. Although generalized lymphadenopathy is a common finding, particularly in patients who have not yet become profoundly immunodepressed, asymmetrical lymphadenopathy or rapidly enlarging nodes in one or more areas may be a clue to the presence of a lymphadenopathic opportunistic infection or malignancy. The cervical (anterior and posterior), supraclavicular, axillary, epitrochlear, inguinal, and femoral areas should be systematically palpated and the size and character of any palpable nodes carefully documented.

Eyes

The conjunctival sacs should be carefully examined. Petechiae detected here may be a clue to the presence of systemic emboli, as may be seen in infective or thrombotic endocarditis. The fundoscopic examination is extremely important. Detecting fundal hemorrhages or exudates may provide evidence of retinitis, caused by cytomegalovirus, *Toxoplasma* organisms, or other pathogens, and should prompt a thorough examination by an ophthalmologist. Visual field deficits suggest focal neurological disorders such as toxoplasmosis or lymphoma, and if confirmed justify neurological referral and appropriate brain imaging studies.

Oropharynx

The examination of the oropharynx in HIV-infected patients must be particularly thorough. Common lesions include thrush (a cheesy exudate that typically appears on the dorsum of the tongue, buccal mucosa, and palate), hairy leukoplakia, herpes simplex infection, Kaposi's sarcoma, and nonspecific ulcerations (see Chapter 5).

Chest

Breathlessness, tachypnea, and a dry cough exacerbated by deep inspiration often signal the presence of HIV-related pulmonary disorders. However, the chest examination may be normal in patients with early respiratory infections or malignancies.[40]

Bronchial breath sounds, dullness to percussion, or other signs of consolidation suggest an alveolar process, such as bacterial pneumonia. Localized wheezing may indicate compression of the airway by a tumor or an endobronchial obstructing lesion, such as Kaposi's sarcoma.

Pleural disease is commonly associated with tuberculosis, pulmonary Kaposi's sarcoma, and bacterial pneumonia and may also complicate other AIDS-related pulmonary disorders. However, pleural effusions are rarely seen in infection caused by *Pneumocystis carinii*.

Cardiovascular Examination

Patients should be evaluated for evidence of orthostatic hypotension, reflecting intravascular volume depletion or autonomic neuropathy.

Because of the high incidence of HIV-related myocardial and pericardial disease, evidence of left ventricular dysfunction (e.g., S3 gallop) or pericardial sounds should be carefully sought.

Valvular disease is particularly common in patients with a history of intravenous drug use and previous endocarditis, but noninfectious, thrombotic endocarditis may also occur in patients in other high-risk groups.

Abdomen

Because of the variety of disorders that may involve abdominal organs, examination of the abdomen is particularly important in HIV-infected patients. Enlargement of the liver or spleen or ascites should be noted and documented. Splenomegaly, in particular, is common at all stages of HIV infection, and the approach to diagnostic evaluation may be dictated by the duration of this finding.

Genitals

Because of the frequency of associated sexually transmitted disease, a thorough genital examination, including a pelvic examination in women, is essential in the initial evaluation of the HIV-infected patient and in follow-up. The possible association between HIV-1 infection and cervical neoplasia[21] necessitates that Papanicolaou's test (Pap smear) be performed initially. The optimum frequency of repeat Pap smears in this population has not been determined.

Rectal Examination

Sexually transmitted diseases, particularly genital herpes and genital warts, frequently manifest in the perianal area, particularly in homosexual men. Rectal fissures are also commonly seen. A digital rectal examination and test of the stool for occult blood should be performed routinely at initial assessment, particularly because of the association between rectal malignancies and HIV infection.[14]

Neurological Examination

A thorough neurological assessment directed toward detecting evidence of peripheral neuropathy (motor and sensory examination, deep tendon reflexes), focal neurological deficits, and evidence of myelopathy, as well as a careful evaluation of mental status, is important at any stage of HIV infection. Subtle cognitive deficits can be detected in a large proportion of patients, including many in the early, asymptomatic phase of disease,[18] with the so-called AIDS dementia complex.[41] An attempt should be made to identify and characterize such problems as memory loss and difficulty concentrating.

INITIAL LABORATORY SCREENING
Complete Blood Count

Because of the high incidence of anemia, thrombocytopenia, and white blood cell abnormalities (see Chapter 5), a complete blood count should be part of the initial evaluation and routine follow-up screening in all patients (see the box below).

Biochemical Profile

A number of abnormalities may be detected in asymptomatic patients at various stages of HIV infection on routine biochemical tests. Common among these disorders are hyponatremia,[60] liver function abnormalities, elevation of bilirubin, and abnormalities of creatinine and urea nitrogen.

Urinalysis

The presence of red blood cells or excess protein in the urine may be an early indication of HIV nephropathy or, less likely, involvement of the kidneys by opportunistic infection or malignancy.

Screening Chest Roentgenogram

In HIV-infected patients with respiratory symptoms, the value of the chest roentgenogram is clear.[40] The yield of screening roentgenograms performed

---

Recommended Initial Screening Blood Tests

Complete blood count	Hepatitis B surface antigen, antibody
Electrolytes	Lymphocyte subset analysis
Liver function tests	*Toxoplasma* antibody*
Creatinine	Cryptococcal antigen*
VDRL	

*Value as a screening test has not been established.

in cases of asymptomatic HIV infection has not yet been established. Nonetheless, even in asymptomatic patients evidence of healed or active tuberculosis, enlargement of thoracic lymph nodes, pleural disease, and interstitial lung disease may be detected by routine chest roentgenograms and may require further diagnostic evaluation.

Other Screening Blood Tests of Potential Value

HIV-infected patients should have serological tests for syphilis. Patients testing positive by VDRL and a confirmatory treponemal test should be treated according to the stage of syphilis.[4] Because of the risk of relapse after adequate therapy,[1] it has been suggested that such patients should be followed with monthly VDRL tests for at least 6 months[24] to determine if therapy has been curative.[3]

Hepatitis B surface antigen assay may also be an appropriate routine screening test because of the parallel epidemiology of hepatitis B and HIV infection. Sexual partners and household contacts of patients with hepatitis B antigenemia should be immunized.[5]

Routine antibody assays for *Toxoplasma gondii* are recommended by some. Patients testing positive for such antibody are at risk of subsequent cerebral toxoplasmosis, whereas this infection has rarely been described in patients without detectable antibody.

Such testing of all patients on initial assessment and, perhaps, at intervals during follow-up could provide important diagnostic information in patients who subsequently manifest intracerebral mass lesions. The implications for prophylaxis are not clear as yet.[44]

Cryptococcal antigen assays may detect cryptococcal infection in a pre-symptomatic state,[34] although the value of this as a routine screening test has been challenged[43] and apparent false positives have been reported.[19]

THE ROLE OF IMMUNOLOGICAL TESTING
Immunological Parameters in Disease Staging

Immunological staging by means of lymphocyte subset analysis is essential for adequate evaluation and management of HIV-infected patients. Although this type of testing was not available in clinical laboratories until recently, it now is commonly performed by many hospital and commercial laboratories, particularly in areas of the country with high HIV prevalence.

As was discussed in Chapter 2, the CD4 lymphocyte count provides invaluable guidance to the clinician and to a large extent dictates the approach to therapy and the follow-up strategy, as well as the overall prognosis.

PREVENTING SECONDARY INFECTIONS

In recent years, strategies aimed at reducing the incidence of some major HIV-related infectious diseases by appropriate use of vaccines and antibiotic prophylaxis have emerged. The most encouraging development so far is the effectiveness of a number of drugs in preventing *Pneumocystis carinii* pneumonia, the most frequent initial opportunistic infection in AIDS. In addition, isoniazid appears to be effective in preventing active tuberculosis in some HIV-infected patients, and preliminary data suggest that the incidence of other important infections might be lessened by appropriate use of prophylactic antimicrobial agents. Increasing attention has been focused on vaccination against pneumococcal infection, hepatitis B, and certain other infections that often occur concomitantly with HIV infection.

Routine administration of prophylaxis against *Pneumocystis carinii* and use of selected vaccines are vital parts of the comprehensive care of HIV-infected patients.

IMMUNIZATIONS

Vaccines are available against several of the infectious diseases for which HIV-infected individuals are at increased risk (see the box below). However, concerns have been expressed about the effectiveness of the commonly used vaccines in patients with HIV-related immunodeficiency.[29] It has been demonstrated in serological studies that patients with advanced HIV infection frequently have little or no measurable immunological response to vaccination. Patients with asymptomatic or early symptomatic HIV infection often mount impaired but adequate responses. Clinical studies confirming the efficacy of vaccines in patients with HIV infection are not yet available.

Recommended Immunizations for HIV-Infected Patients

Pneumococcal vaccine*[9]
Haemophilus influenzae vaccine (HbCV)[6]
Influenza vaccine†[6]
Hepatitis B vaccine (if nonimmune)[22]
Measles, mumps, and rubella (MMR)‡[6]
Diphtheria, pertussis, and tetanus (DPT)‡[6]
Inactivated polio vaccine (not oral vaccine)‡[6]

*23-Valent vaccine should be administered to patients who previously received only 14-valent vaccine or who were vaccinated more than 6 years previously.
†HIV-symptomatic patients only.
‡ If nonimmune.

Recommendations on routine vaccination of HIV-infected patients have largely been made on the basis of previous experience in other types of patients, both immunocompromised and immunocompetent. The need for readministering vaccines given in childhood to HIV-infected adults has also not been clearly demonstrated. Following is a brief discussion of available data and current recommendations about the use of currently available vaccines in the context of HIV infection.

Pneumococcal Vaccine

HIV-infected patients are at increased risk of pneumococcal infection.[48] Immunization against pneumococcal infection with a polysaccharide vaccine is generally recommended for patients with chronic cardiopulmonary disease or certain other chronic medical problems.[8] Studies of antibody response to pneumococcal vaccine in HIV-infected patients have indicated that most asymptomatic patients mount an impaired but significant response.[25,27] IgM antibody response appears to be particularly impaired in symptomatic patients,[26] and frank vaccine failure has been reported.[54]

Despite these potential limitations, routine vaccination of all HIV-infected patients has been recommended.[9] Revaccination with the current 23-valent vaccine is recommended for patients at high risk who previously received only the 14-valent vaccine or who received the 23-valent vaccine more than 6 years previously.

Haemophilus Influenzae Vaccine

Patients infected with HIV may be at increased risk for invasive infection caused by *Haemophilus influenzae* type b.[50] For this reason, vaccination with *Haemophilus influenzae* type b conjugate vaccine (HbCV) has been encouraged.[6] However, data on the use of this vaccine in the presence of HIV infection currently are limited.

Influenza Vaccine

It has been recommended that influenza vaccine be administered annually during the influenza season to symptomatic HIV-infected patients.[6] Although influenza A pneumonia has been described in association with HIV infection,[58] it is not known if the incidence or severity of influenza and its complications are greater with HIV infection. It is possible that vaccination of HIV-infected patients against influenza may lessen the risk of infection with *Streptococcus pneumoniae* and *Haemophilus influenzae*, bacteria that often cause superinfection with influenza.

Unfortunately the influenza vaccine may not be very effective, especially in patients with symptomatic HIV infection. The standard one-dose vaccine fails to elicit protective levels of antibody in more than half of patients with AIDS or AIDS-related complex and a significant proportion of asymptomatic HIV-infected patients.[42] Even a two-dose vaccine regimen may be inadequate for most symptomatic patients.[38]

Despite these limitations, vaccination of HIV-infected patients may be prudent until further data become available on the clinical efficacy of such vaccinations in preventing bacterial superinfection. The option of chemoprophylaxis with amantadine has been proposed for patients with advanced HIV infection,[22] although the effectiveness of this approach has not been established.

Hepatitis B Vaccine

Behaviors associated with HIV infection (i.e., intravenous drug use and male homosexuality) are also associated with hepatitis B infection. In addition, evidence has accumulated to suggest that the course of hepatitis B may be affected by concomitant HIV infection. The duration of viral replication may be prolonged,[28] and superimposed hepatitis D may be reactivated.[53] For these reasons, vaccination against hepatitis B has been recommended for nonimmune HIV-infected patients.[22] As with other vaccines, however, the immunological response of HIV-infected patients to the hepatitis B vaccine is often inadequate. More than 40% of homosexual men at various stages of HIV infection failed to respond adequately to a standard three-dose vaccine regimen in one study.[12]

Measles Immunization

In recent years several large outbreaks of measles have occurred among young children in the United States. Measles has been reported in association with HIV infection in both children and adults, and fatal childhood cases have occurred.[7]

It has been recommended that symptomatic HIV-infected adults who are exposed to measles receive immune globulin (0.5 ml/kg, maximum dose 15 ml) regardless of their vaccination status.[6]

Other Immunizations

Other immunizations that have been recommended for nonimmune patients include the routine childhood vaccinations: measles, mumps, and rubella (MMR) and diphtheria, pertussis, and tetanus (DPT), but not the oral polio vaccine.[6] Because of the risk of vaccine-induced polio, it is recommended that only the inactivated polio vaccine be administered to HIV-infected patients, regardless of age.[6] Antibody responses to the bacterial toxoid vaccines against diphtheria, pertussis, and tetanus may be impaired.[2]

PROPHYLAXIS AGAINST OPPORTUNISTIC INFECTIONS

In recent years increasing emphasis has been placed on the use of antimicrobial agents to prevent opportunistic infections in HIV-infected patients. This strategy has been most thoroughly studied and most successful in preventing *Pneumocystis carinii* pneumonia (PCP). Following is an overview of recent data regarding prophylaxis against PCP and tuberculosis. These recommendations apply to symptomatic and asymptomatic HIV-infected patients.

Pneumocystis Carinii Pneumonia

Patients with a previous history of AIDS-related opportunistic infection or malignancy and those with a CD4 lymphocyte count below 200/mm^3 or less than 20% of the total lymphocyte count are at high risk for developing PCP.[8] At particularly high risk are patients with a previous episode of PCP or other AIDS-defining conditions. Sixteen of 30 patients with Kaposi's sarcoma who received no prophylaxis developed PCP within approximately 2 years in one prospective series.[15] One third of the patients with an initial CD4 lymphocyte count of 200/mm^3 or less developed PCP by 36 months in the Multicenter AIDS Cohort Study,[8] and approximately 80% of patients receiving zidovudine (AZT) but no specific PCP prophylactic drug had recurrences within 24 months.[8] On the basis of these and other data, routine administration of prophylactic therapy to prevent PCP has been recommended for high-risk patients, including those receiving antiretroviral drugs.[8]

Although a number of agents, including trimethoprim-sulfamethoxazole, pyrimethamine-sulfadoxine, pentamidine isethionate, and dapsone, have been shown to be effective in preventing PCP in HIV-infected patients, little controlled data comparing these drugs have yet been published. It currently is unclear which agent confers the greatest degree of protection, and what dose and route of administration are best. Despite the fact that prophylaxis to prevent PCP has justifiably become standard practice, much of the clinical data supporting various strategies has appeared so far only in the form of preliminary reports.

The following specific agents are effective in preventing PCP.

Trimethoprim-sulfamethoxazole. Trimethoprim-sulfamethoxazole in a variety of dosing regimens has been shown to be highly effective in the primary prophylaxis and secondary prevention of PCP. In a randomized, prospective study of patients with Kaposi's sarcoma and no previous opportunistic infection, Fischl and coworkers demonstrated that trimethoprim-sulfamethoxazole, in a double-strength dose given twice daily, completely protected patients from developing PCP.[15] During a 3-year follow-up, 53% of patients receiving no prophylaxis developed PCP. Secondary prevention of PCP in patients recovering from a first episode has also been demonstrated with this regimen.[46]

Unfortunately, 50% of patients may have adverse reactions to trimethoprim-sulfamethoxazole, particularly rash and fever.[15] It should be noted that many patients who have these side effects can continue therapy[15] and that patients manifesting hypersensitivity reactions may tolerate the drug upon rechallenge.[52] However, because many patients cannot take trimethoprim-sulfamethoxazole, other effective prophylactic agents have been sought.

Pentamidine isethionate (aerosol). Pentamidine, when administered in periodic aerosol treatments, may be effective in primary and secondary prevention of PCP.[39] In a large prospective study, aerosolized pentamidine administered monthly was shown to reduce the relapse rate of PCP by 50% in patients treated after an initial episode.[17] On the basis of several preliminary studies, the Food and Drug Administration approved the use of aerosolized pentamidine to prevent PCP in patients with a history of PCP or a CD4 lymphocyte count below 200/mm^3. The recommended dose is 300 mg once a month diluted in 6 ml of sterile water and administered at 6 liters per minute from a 50-psi compressed air source by Respirgard II nebulizer.[8,61] As other types of nebulizers are more carefully evaluated and the results of large-scale prospective trials are analyzed, specific recommendations for administering aerosolized pentamidine may be revised.

Patients receiving aerosolized pentamidine prophylaxis who develop PCP may manifest predominant upper lobe disease,[11] an otherwise unusual radiographic pattern. It has been suggested that keeping the patient in a supine position during the aerosol treatment might improve distribution of the drug to the lung apices.[45] Spontaneous pneumothoraces[33] and extrapulmonary *Pneumocystis carinii* infections at a variety of sites[20,55] have been described in HIV-infected patients receiving aerosolized pentamidine prophylaxis.

Dapsone. Dapsone is a sulfone antibiotic long used in the treatment of leprosy. In preliminary studies, dapsone has been shown to confer varying degrees of protection against the development of PCP in high-risk, HIV-infected patients. In one published study of primary prophylaxis with dapsone,[32] the drug was given to patients who had a CD4 lymphocyte count below 200/mm^3 but no history of a previous PCP episode; these patients showed significantly lower rates of PCP. In another study only two episodes of PCP occurred in 173 high-risk patients receiving dapsone (25 mg four times daily), whereas 26 episodes occurred in 23 patients who refused prophylaxis over a mean follow-

---

Recommended Regimens for Prophylaxis against Pneumocystis Carinii Pneumonia*[8]

1. Trimethoprim-sulfamethoxazole (double-strength), twice daily and leucovorin, 5 mg once daily†

or

2. Aerosolized pentamidine, 300 mg every 4 weeks by nebulizer (see text)

*Prophylaxis is recommended for HIV-infected patients with a CD4 lymphocyte count below $200/mm^3$ or that is less than 20% of the total lymphocyte count, or for any patient with a history of *Pneumocystis carinii* infection.[8]
†Should not be given if patient has known severe hypersensitivity.
Note: Neither regimen has been established as safe for use during pregnancy.

---

up period of approximately 9 months.[37] Protection may also be conferred at lower doses, including 50 mg daily[30] and 100 mg twice weekly.[59]

Pyrimethamine-sulfadiazine. It has been suggested that combination therapy with pyrimethamine and sulfadiazine for cerebral toxoplasmosis may also confer partial or complete protection against PCP.[47] This observation has not yet been confirmed in prospective studies.

In summary, several agents are effective in preventing PCP (see the box above). Comparative studies will determine which agent is superior, although preliminary data suggest that trimethoprim-sulfamethoxazole may be the best first-line drug in patients who can tolerate it.

Tuberculosis

HIV-infected patients, particularly intravenous drug abusers and those from tropical or subtropical countries, are at high risk for tuberculosis.[57] A large prospective study of HIV-infected intravenous drug users in New York City demonstrated that skin testing with purified protein derivative (PPD) was an effective means of identifying those at highest risk of developing active tuberculosis.[51]

Preventive therapy for tuberculosis is currently recommended for all HIV-infected patients with tuberculin skin test reactions of 5 mm or more and no evidence of active tuberculosis,[10] regardless of age. The recommended regimen is isoniazid, 300 mg daily for adults and 10 mg/kg to a maximum daily dose of 300 mg for children, continued for 12 months.

THE ROLE OF ANTIRETROVIRAL THERAPY

The use of antiretroviral therapy in all stages of HIV-1 infection is discussed in Chapter 10.

Common Indications for Urgent Intervention*

New fever   Focal neurological deficit
Dyspnea   Decreased visual acuity
Persistent cough   Severe diarrhea
Persistent headache   Persistent nausea and vomiting
Seizure   Jaundice
Loss of consciousness

*See Chapter 7 for recommended diagnostic evaluation.

FOLLOW-UP CARE OF THE ASYMPTOMATIC PATIENT
Frequency of Visits

Routine follow-up every 3 to 6 months is appropriate for the asymptomatic patient with a normal CD4 lymphocyte count who is not receiving antiviral therapy. Recommended follow-up strategies for patients receiving antiviral therapy are discussed in Chapter 10.

Access to Emergency Care

HIV-infected patients, particularly those with CD4 lymphocyte counts below 200/mm^3, may develop serious infectious or neoplastic complications suddenly. Such patients should be carefully instructed on when to seek emergency care (see the box above) and advised to reveal their HIV status to any health care provider involved in their care. Patients should also be encouraged to contact the primary care provider if questions arise about the significance of symptoms or if emergency care has been obtained. Ideally, a system for non-emergency walk-in visits should be established. Symptom-oriented approaches to diagnosis and management are discussed in Chapter 7.

REFERENCES

1. Berry CD et al: Neurologic relapse after benzathine penicillin therapy for secondary syphilis in a patient with HIV infection, *N Engl J Med* 316(25): 1587-1589, 1987.

2. Borkowsky W et al: Antibody responses to bacterial toxoids in children infected with human immunodeficiency virus, *J Pediatr* 110(4):563-566, 1987.

3. Brown ST et al: Serological response to syphilis treatment: a new analysis of old data, *JAMA* 253(9):1296-1299, 1985.

4. Brown ST: Update on recommendations for the treatment of syphilis, *Rev Infect Dis* 4:S837-S841, 1982.

5. Centers for Disease Control: Recommendations for protection against viral hepatitis, *MMWR* 34(22):313-335, 1985.

6. Centers for Disease Control: Recommendations of the Advisory Commit-

tee on Immunization Practices (ACIP): immunization of children with human immunodeficiency virus–supplementary ACIP statement, *MMWR* 37(12):181-183, 1988.

7. Centers for Disease Control: Measles in HIV-infected children—United States, *MMWR* 37(12):183-186, 1988.

8. Centers for Disease Control: Guidelines for prophylaxis against *Pneumocystis carinii* pneumonia for persons infected with human immunodeficiency virus, *MMWR* 38(S-5):1-9, 1989.

9. Centers for Disease Control: Recommendations of the immunization practices advisory committee: pneumococcal polysaccharide vaccine, *JAMA* 261(9):1265-1267, 1989.

10. Centers for Disease Control: Screening for tuberculosis and tuberculous infection in high-risk populations and the use of preventive therapy for tuberculous infection in the United States: recommendations of the Advisory Committee for Elimination of Tuberculosis, *MMWR* 39(RR-8):1-12, 1990.

11. Chaffey MH et al: Radiographic distribution of *Pneumocystis carinii* pneumonia in patients with AIDS treated with prophylactic inhaled pentamidine, *Radiology* 175(3):715-719, 1990.

12. Collier AC et al: Antibody to human immunodeficiency virus (HIV) and suboptimal response to hepatitis B vaccination, *Ann Intern Med* 109:101-105, 1988.

13. Coulman CU, Greene I, Archibald RWR: Cutaneous pneumocystosis, *Ann Intern Med* 106:396-398, 1987.

14. Croxson T et al: Intraepithelial carcinoma of the anus in homosexual men, *Dis Colon Rectum* 27(5):325-330, 1984.

15. Fischl MA, Dickinson GM, LaVoie L: Safety and efficacy of sulfamethoxazole and trimethoprim chemoprophylaxis for *Pneumocystis carinii* pneumonia in AIDS, *JAMA* 259(8):1185-1189, 1988.

16. Fredman L et al: Primary care physi-

cians' assessment and prevention of HIV infection, *Am J Prev Med* 5(4):188-195, 1989.

17. Golden JA et al: Prevention of *Pneumocystis carinii* pneumonia by inhaled pentamidine, *Lancet* 1(8639):654-657, 1989.

18. Grant I et al: Evidence for early central nervous system involvement in the acquired immunodeficiency syndrome (AIDS) and other human immunodeficiency virus (HIV) infections, *Ann Intern Med* 107:828-836, 1987.

19. Gurtman A et al: The significance of isolated positive cerebrospinal fluid cryptococcal antigen in HIV-infected patients. Paper presented at the Sixth International Conference on AIDS, San Francisco, June 21, 1990 (abstract).

20. Hardy WD, Northfelt DW, Drake TA: Fatal, disseminated pneumocystosis in a patient with acquired immunodeficiency syndrome receiving prophylactic aerosolized pentamidine, *Am J Med* 87(3):329-331, 1989.

21. Henry MJ et al: Association of human immunodeficiency virus–induced immunosuppression with human papillomavirus infection and cervical intraepithelial neoplasia, *Am J Obstet Gynecol* 160(2):352-353, 1989.

22. Hibberd PL, Rubin RH: Approach to immunization in the immunosuppressed host, *Infect Dis Clin North Am* 4(1):123-142, 1990.

23. Hicks CB et al: Seronegative secondary syphilis in a patient infected with the human immunodeficiency virus (HIV) with Kaposi's sarcoma: a diagnostic dilemma, *Ann Intern Med* 107:492-495, 1987.

24. Hook EW: Syphilis and HIV infection, *J Infect Dis* 160(3):530-534, 1989.

25. Huang S et al: Antibody responses after influenza and pneumococcal immunization in HIV-infected homosexual men, *JAMA* 257(15):2047-2050, 1987.

26. Janoff EN et al: Class-specific antibody

response to pneumococcal capsular polysaccharides in men infected with human immunodeficiency virus type 1, *J Infect Dis* 158(5):983-990, 1988.

27. Klein RS et al: Response to pneumococcal vaccine among asymptomatic heterosexual partners of persons with AIDS and intravenous drug users infected with human immunodeficiency virus, *J Infect Dis* 160(5):826-831, 1989.

28. Krogsgaard K et al: The influence of HTLV-III infection on the natural history of hepatitis B virus infection in male homosexual HBsAg carriers, *Hepatology* 7(1):37-41, 1987.

29. La Montagne JR: Immunization programs and human immunodeficiency virus, *Rev Infect Dis* 11(suppl 3):S639-S643, 1989.

30. Lang OS et al: Low-dose dapsone prophylaxis of *Pneumocystis carinii* pneumonia. Paper presented at the Fifth International Conference on AIDS, Montreal, June 6, 1989 (abstract).

31. Lewis CE, Freeman HE, Corey CR: AIDS-related competence of California's primary care physicians, *Am J Public Health* 77:795-799, 1987.

32. Lucas CR et al: Primary dapsone chemoprophylaxis for *Pneumocystis carinii* pneumonia in immunocompromised patients with the human immunodeficiency virus, *Med J Aust* 151(1):30-33, 1989.

33. Martinez CM et al: Spontaneous pneumothoraces in AIDS patients receiving aerosolized pentamidine, *Chest* 94(6):1317-1318, 1988.

34. Masci J, Pierone G, Nicholas P: Serum cryptococcal antigen screening in the early diagnosis of cryptococcal infection in patients with HIV infection. Paper presented at the Fifth International Conference on AIDS, Montreal, June 7, 1989 (abstract).

35. Mathews WC, Linn LS: AIDS prevention in primary care clinics: testing the market, *J Gen Intern Med* 4:34-38, 1989.

36. Melbye M et al: Risk of AIDS after herpes zoster, *Lancet* 1(8535):728-731, 1987.

37. Metroka CE, Jacobus D, Lewis N: Successful chemoprophylaxis for *Pneumocystis* with dapsone or Bactrim. Paper presented at the Fifth International Conference on AIDS, Montreal, June 6, 1989 (abstract).

38. Miotti PG et al: The influence of HIV infection on antibody responses to a two-dose regimen of influenza vaccine, *JAMA* 262(6):779-784, 1989.

39. Montgomery AB: Prophylaxis of *Pneumocystis carinii* pneumonia in patients infected with the human immunodeficiency virus type 1, *Semin Respir Infect* 4(4):311-317, 1989.

40. Murray JF, Mills J: State of the art: pulmonary infectious complications of human immunodeficiency virus infection, *Am Rev Respir Dis* 141:1356-1372, 1990.

41. Navia BA, Jordan BD, Price RW: The AIDS dementia complex. I. Clinical features, *Ann Neurol* 19:517-524, 1986.

42. Nelson KE et al: The influence of human immunodeficiency virus (HIV) infection on antibody responses to influenza vaccines, *Ann Intern Med* 109:383-388, 1988.

43. Nelson MR et al: The limited value of routine serum antigen screening for cryptococcal infection. Paper presented at the Fifth International Conference on AIDS, Montreal, June 7, 1989 (abstract).

44. Nicholas P et al: Trimethoprim-sulfamethoxazole in the prevention of cerebral toxoplasmosis. Paper presented at the Sixth International Conference on AIDS, San Francisco, June 21, 1990 (abstract).

45. O'Doherty MJ et al: Does inhalation of pentamidine in the supine position increase deposition in the upper part of the lung? *Chest* 97(6):1343-1348, 1990.

46. Pierone G, Masci J, Nicholas P: Trimethoprim-sulfamethoxazole for secondary prophylaxis of *Pneumocystis*

carinii pneumonia in AIDS. Paper presented at the Fifth International Conference on AIDS, Montreal, June 6, 1989 (abstract).

47. Pierone G et al: Pyrimethamine-sulfadiazine in the prophylaxis of *Pneumocystis carinii* pneumonia in AIDS patients with cerebral toxoplasmosis. Paper presented at the Fifth International Conference on AIDS, Montreal, June 6, 1989 (abstract).

48. Polsky B et al: Bacterial pneumonia in patients with the acquired immunodeficiency syndrome, *Ann Intern Med* 104:38-41, 1986.

49. Rico MJ, Penneys NS: Cutaneous cryptococcosis resembling molluscum contagiosum in a patient with AIDS, *Arch Dermatol* 121:901-902, 1985.

50. Schlamm HT, Yancovitz SR: *Haemophilus influenzae* pneumonia in young adults with AIDS, ARC or risk of AIDS, *Am J Med* 86:11-14, 1989.

51. Selwyn PA et al: A prospective study of the risk of tuberculosis among intravenous drug users with human immunodeficiency virus infection, *N Engl J Med* 320(9):545-550, 1989.

52. Shafer RW, Seitzman PA, Tapper ML: Successful prophylaxis of *Pneumocystis carinii* pneumonia with trimethoprim-sulfamethoxazole in AIDS patients with previous allergic reactions, *J Acquir Immune Defic Syndr* 2:389-393, 1989.

53. Shattock AG, Finlay H, Hillary IB: Possible reactivation of hepatitis D with chronic delta antigenemia by human immunodeficiency virus, *Br Med J* 294(6588):1656-1657, 1987.

54. Simberkoff MS et al: *Streptococcus pneumoniae* infections and bacteremia in patients with acquired immune deficiency syndrome, with report of a pneumococcal vaccine failure, *Am Rev Respir Dis* 130(6):1174-1176, 1984.

55. Sneed SR et al: *Pneumocystis carinii* choroiditis in patients receiving inhaled pentamidine, *N Engl J Med* 322(13):936-937, 1990.

56. Somogyi AA et al: Attitudes toward the care of patients with acquired immunodeficiency syndrome: a survey of community internists, *Arch Intern Med* 150:50-53, 1990.

57. Sunderam G et al: Tuberculosis as a manifestation of the acquired immunodeficiency syndrome (AIDS), *JAMA* 256(3):362-366, 1986.

58. Thurn JR, Henry K: Influenza A pneumonitis in a patient infected with the human immunodeficiency virus (HIV), *Chest* 95(4):807-810, 1989.

59. Torres R et al: Randomized trial of intermittent dapsone versus aerosolized pentamidine for primary and secondary prophylaxis of *Pneumocystis carinii* pneumonia. Paper presented at the Sixth International Conference on AIDS, San Francisco, June 21, 1990 (abstract).

60. Vitting KE et al: Frequency of hyponatremia and nonosmolar vasopressin release in the acquired immunodeficiency syndrome, *JAMA* 263(7):973-978, 1990.

61. Young FE et al: Aerosolized pentamidine: approved for HIV-infected individuals at high risk for *Pneumocystis carinii* pneumonia, *Arch Intern Med* 149(11):2412-2413, 1989.

CHAPTER 7

Symptom-Oriented Evaluation and Management of HIV-Infected Patients

Recognizing the clinical signs of HIV
 infection
Evaluation of specific complaints
 General Signs
 Cardiopulmonary Signs

Gastrointestinal/Intraabdominal
 Signs
Musculoskeletal Signs
Neurological Signs

Infection with the human immunodeficiency virus type 1 (HIV or HIV-1), may dramatically alter the meaning of clinical signs and symptoms. Among patients with significant HIV-related immunodeficiency, relatively minor complaints such as a headache or cough may signify life-threatening opportunistic infections or malignancies. Even at earlier stages of the natural history of HIV infection, such common problems as diarrhea, chest pain, or fatigue must be viewed from the unique perspective of the complex, multisystem disorder that the virus causes.

This chapter presents an approach to the differential diagnosis and diagnostic evaluation of symptoms commonly encountered with HIV infection. Although minor complaints, particularly related to skin and mucous membrane disorders, are common among HIV-infected patients, this chapter emphasizes the presenting manifestations of serious, debilitating, and life-threatening complications of HIV infection.

RECOGNIZING THE CLINICAL SIGNS OF HIV INFECTION

After an asymptomatic phase that typically lasts for several years, HIV-infected patients may come to medical attention with signs of disease long before the appearance of the more dramatic and recognizable opportunistic infections or malignancies associated with acquired immunodeficiency syndrome (AIDS) (Chapter 2).

Because of the multisystem nature of HIV infection and the remarkable variety of associated clinical disorders (Chapter 5), recognizing early signs of HIV infection may be quite difficult, even in patients who are known to be infected. When there is no clinical suspicion of HIV infection, this task may be impossible. The true significance of such nonspecific HIV-related symptoms as lymph node enlargement, diarrhea, or weight loss may not be initially recognized. Diagnostic confusion is particularly likely when the patient is not known to be at high risk for HIV infection and in geographical areas where prevalence rates are low. Even disorders associated with advanced stages of HIV infection, such as invasive herpes simplex infection or non-Hodgkin's lymphoma, may not initially be appreciated as being related to HIV infection.

Diagnosing disorders that result from HIV infection, therefore, requires familiarity with the commonly seen syndromes, an ability to assess the likelihood of HIV infection, and a high "index of suspicion."

As discussed in Chapter 4, the likelihood that HIV-related signs or symptoms will be recognized as such can be increased by routinely and systematically questioning all patients about risk behavior during the course of the initial medical evaluation. Routinely asking all male patients if they have ever had sex with other men, asking female patients about the sexual patterns of current and former male sexual partners, and asking patients of both sexes if they have used intravenous drugs or received blood transfusions before 1985 should be regarded as appropriate and medically important.

Patients giving a history of risk behavior should be offered counseling and testing for HIV infection (Chapter 4). Such patients who initially test negative and who have engaged in risk behavior within the preceding 3 to 6 months should be retested subsequently (e.g., at 3 and 6 months) to rule out early infection. Those who continue to engage in high-risk behavior despite counseling should be retested at intervals of 3 to 6 months indefinitely. If HIV infection is confirmed, staging by immunological testing, including measuring of the absolute CD4 lymphocyte count and the CD4/CD8 ratio, should be conducted, since the interpretation of symptoms may vary according to the stage of HIV infection at which the patient is seen (Chapter 2). As will be seen, immunological staging often provides invaluable insight into the differential diagnosis of specific complaints.

Such a program of risk factor assessment, directed testing, and immunological staging of those who are infected may nonetheless fail to identify some HIV-infected patients.

Although some disorders, such as Kaposi's sarcoma, may be virtually diagnostic of HIV infection, all the symptoms and many of the specific disorders discussed in this chapter are encountered frequently in patients not infected with HIV. The new appearance of certain signs or symptoms (such as severe seborrheic dermatitis or persistent diarrhea) in a patient not known to be HIV positive should prompt careful assessment or reassessment of potential HIV risk factors. Under some circumstances (e.g., the appearance of several nonspecific signs simultaneously), it may be appropriate to recommend HIV testing to patients who have these disorders, even if they deny or are unaware of potential exposure to the virus. It should be kept in mind that many patients first come to medical attention with manifestations of advanced HIV infection, including AIDS, without any history of earlier HIV-related complaints.

Following is an overview of the differential diagnosis and suggested diagnostic evaluation of common presenting symptoms and signs in HIV-infected patients. Of course, disorders unrelated to HIV infection may occur in HIV-infected individuals. The purpose of this discussion is not to provide a comprehensive approach to all disorders that may produce these clinical manifestations, but rather to highlight HIV-related signs and symptoms and the unique aspects of the pathogenesis and management of these problems in patients with HIV infection. As with all patients, the evaluation of symptoms and signs of disease in HIV-infected patients must be individualized. The morbidity and cost of diagnostic studies must be taken into account, and the extent of the diagnostic workup should reflect the likelihood that a treatable cause of the disorder can be identified.

EVALUATION OF SPECIFIC COMPLAINTS
General Signs

Fever of unknown origin
Incidence. Unexplained persistent fever (i.e., fever of several weeks' duration for which no cause can be identified after a routine diagnostic evaluation) is a common phenomenon in HIV-infected patients and may be encountered at any stage of the disease.

Differential diagnosis. The differential diagnosis of persistent fever varies, depending on the stage of the disease (Figure 7-1). Self-limited fever is a common feature of acute HIV infection,[38] but it usually is accompanied by other clinical signs, including a rash, headache, or oral ulcerations.[38] Persistent fever is often seen in early symptomatic patients, often in association with generalized lymphadenopathy; along with other constitutional signs, it may be associated with earlier progression to AIDS.[57]

In patients with advanced HIV infection, particularly those with CD4 lym-

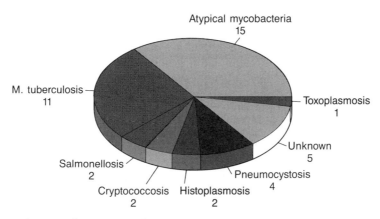

FIGURE 7-1. Causes of persistent fever in 42 AIDS patients.

Data from Pierone G et al: Fever of unknown origin in AIDS. Paper presented at the Sixth International Conference on AIDS, San Francisco, California, June 21, 1990.

phocyte counts under 200/mm³ or with a previous diagnosis of AIDS, opportunistic infections may give rise to fever before the onset of more specific symptoms. Disseminated mycobacterial infection is probably the most common specific cause of fever of obscure origin in AIDS patients. Early *Pneumocystis carinii* pneumonia and disseminated cryptococcosis, histoplasmosis, and cytomegalovirus infection may become apparent in this fashion. Visceral Kaposi's sarcoma and lymphoma may also cause nonspecific fever.

Diagnostic evaluation. The approach to a patient with HIV infection who has a fever of unknown origin should be directed at identifying treatable infections (Figure 7-2). If a thorough history and physical examination, routine laboratory and radiographic studies, and cultures of blood, urine, and stool fail to provide a clue to the source of the fever, radionuclide scans, a biopsy of the liver and/or bone marrow, or special culture techniques may lead to a diagnosis.

Radionuclide studies. Gallium-67 and indium-111 scanning may identify localized infections in some patients. In a study by Fineman and colleagues of 36 AIDS patients with unexplained fever, 21 (78%) and 12 (44%) of 27 documented localized infections were identified by indium scanning and gallium scanning, respectively.[34] Although less sensitive overall, gallium studies were particularly effective in detecting early *P. carinii* pneumonia and infections involving the lymph nodes.

Liver biopsy. Because of the high incidence of liver involvement by opportunistic infections in AIDS, the efficacy of liver biopsy in evaluating unexplained fever in HIV-infected patients (particularly those with a history of

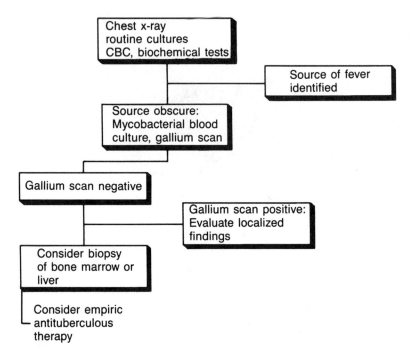

FIGURE 7-2. Evaluation of persistent fever without localizing findings.

AIDS-related infections) appears to be substantially higher than in non-HIV–infected patients.[14] In one series, liver biopsy provided a specific diagnosis in most patients at various stages of HIV infection referred for evaluation of fever, but the diagnostic yield was more than twice as high in patients with a history of AIDS-defining infections than in those with no history of AIDS.[14] In this series, liver biopsy was substantially more effective than bone marrow biopsy in detecting mycobacterial infection. The serum alkaline phosphatase was significantly higher (mean, 774 IU/L) in cases where the liver biopsy yielded a specific diagnosis. The role of liver biopsy remains controversial, however. Advocates point to the high diagnostic accuracy for mycobacterial infection,[66] whereas others believe that most treatable infections diagnosed by liver biopsy may be identified by less invasive means.[97]

Bone marrow biopsy. Examination and culture of bone marrow may identify the cause of unexplained fever in as many as 25% of patients with AIDS.[43] Disseminated infection with mycobacteria[39] and *Histoplasma capsulatum*[29,61] is commonly identified in this way, particularly among patients with a previous diagnosis of AIDS-defining opportunistic infection or malignancy. *Mycobacterium avium-intracellulare* was isolated from 20% of bone marrow biopsies performed on AIDS patients for a variety of indications in one series,[16] although no granulomas were seen on histological examination in most of the culture-positive specimens. Bone marrow lymphoma was also found in several patients.

In the evaluation of unexplained fever in HIV-infected patients, bone marrow biopsy is probably most helpful in patients with CD4 lymphocyte counts below 200/mm³ or with previous opportunistic infections or malignancies. Hematological indications for bone marrow examination, such as thrombocytopenia or anemia, may arise at earlier stages of HIV infection.

Special culture techniques. Blood and tissue specimens, particularly of bone marrow and the liver, should be stained specifically for mycobacteria[18] and fungi. Since mycobacteria do not grow on routine culture media, pathology and microbiology laboratories should be informed when these organisms are suspected so that the specimen can be preserved properly and specific culture media can be used. A variety of culture systems are available for this purpose.[84,112]

Disseminated histoplasmosis may be diagnosed by appropriate culture of blood or tissue specimens,[108] although these tests are often negative or require as long as 4 weeks for identification.[106] Serological studies for histoplasmosis are relatively insensitive in immunocompromised patients,[58] although antigen tests may be of value.[107]

Weight loss and malnutrition

Incidence. Weight loss and malnutrition are common features of HIV infection, particularly among patients at advanced stages of disease. However, significant weight loss may occur before the onset of AIDS, either in isolation or accompanied by other nonspecific manifestations of HIV infection such as diarrhea, fever, or lymphadenopathy.

A variety of nutritional deficiencies have been described in association with HIV infection. The most important of these is protein-calorie malnutrition. Protein-calorie intake may be normal[98] or abnormal[21] in malnourished patients. Triglyceride levels tend to rise as the disease progresses,[48] whereas total cholesterol remains normal or falls.[11]

Preliminary data suggest that significant deficiencies of vitamins B_6 and B_{12},[8] as well as copper, selenium,[35] and zinc,[103] may be seen even in patients with early, asymptomatic disease. Although the significance of these observations is not yet clear, copper and zinc deficiencies may be associated with progression to more symptomatic disease and AIDS.[103] It has been suggested that correcting such nutritional deficiencies may be beneficial.[6,74] However, current data are insufficient to determine the value of this approach.

Differential diagnosis. Patients with AIDS or other forms of symptomatic

HIV infection may lose weight and become malnourished for various reasons (Table 7-1). In many patients with advanced disease, gastrointestinal disorders, systemic infections, depression, and dementia may all play important roles.

Gastrointestinal causes of weight loss may be apparent in some cases. Oral disease in the form of gingivitis, herpes simplex infection, candidiasis, or other disorders may make chewing painful or alter the sense of taste. In some cases dysphagia resulting from esophagitis may significantly interfere with eating. Patients with small bowel involvement by cryptosporidiosis, isosporiasis, cytomegalovirus, or other pathogens may suffer from recurrent abdominal pain, nausea, or vomiting, with or without malabsorption. HIV enteropathy may result in decreased gastric acid production,[63] as well as frank malabsorption.[41,60] Hepatitis or biliary disease related to HIV infection may also cause anorexia, nausea, or vomiting.

Other causes of malnutrition may be prominent in some individuals. Advanced AIDS encephalopathy or opportunistic infections or malignancies involving the brain may interfere with the patient's ability to feed himself or herself. Depression, which is common at all stages of HIV infection, may lead to anorexia and a lack of will to eat. Many of the medications commonly prescribed for HIV infection and its related disorders may cause nausea or anorexia. Some of these drugs (e.g., isoniazid and ketoconazole) may cause hepatitis, whereas others (e.g., dideoxyinosine and pentamidine) may be associated with pancreatitis.

A wasting syndrome marked by dramatic loss of lean body mass is a common feature of AIDS and may also be seen at earlier stages of HIV infection.

TABLE 7-1. Reasons for weight loss in HIV-infected patients

Decreased intake	Poor dentition
	Oral lesions
	Esophageal lesions
	Anorexia
	Dementia
	Depression
	Unavailability of food
Malabsorption	Intestinal infections
	Intestinal lymphoma
	HIV enteropathy
Systemic disorders	HIV wasting syndrome
	Opportunistic infections
	HIV-related malignancies

Evidence has emerged that tumor necrosis factor, a protein derived from macrophages that is associated with cachexia in a number of diseases, may have an important role in this syndrome.[62] Patients with advanced AIDS complicated by acute infections may become markedly hypermetabolic.

The patient's dietary habits and home situation may also have a negative impact on nutrition. Some HIV-infected individuals are attracted to fad diets which may be nutritionally inadequate.[75] Fear of contagion may make family and household members, as well as health care workers, reluctant to help debilitated HIV-infected patients feed themselves.

Although malnutrition may be difficult or impossible to correct in many patients, identifying specific causes may permit effective nutritional support. The means of providing adequate nutrition may range from simple steps, such as encouraging the patient to eat despite a poor appetite or arranging for dental care, to progressively more complex measures, such as treating depression, providing adequate home care, supplementing the diet with standard oral preparations, or using specialized diets or, in patients with advanced disease, enteral tube feedings, peripheral hyperalimentation, or total parenteral nutrition.

Diagnostic evaluation. A nutritional assessment is considered an important part of the general medical evaluation. Because malnutrition is so common in HIV-infected individuals and because many HIV-related disorders may interfere with nutrition, a detailed assessment of these patients may be particularly valuable.

Complete medical history. Patients should be asked their usual weight and questioned about recent weight changes and changes in activity level. When reviewing systems, particular attention should be paid to complaints about oral disease, swallowing difficulties, nausea, vomiting, diarrhea, and symptoms suggesting depression or dementia. Patients should be questioned specifically about relevant aspects of their home situation (i.e., how they obtain and pay for food and whether they need assistance in feeding themselves). The specifics of their usual diet should be ascertained, and they should be questioned about fad diets.

Physical examination. The height and body weight should be recorded at the first visit, and the weight should be noted at each subsequent visit. Standardized measurements of the triceps skin fold or arm anthropometry may be helpful in following the nutritional status serially. The mouth should be examined thoroughly for lesions of Kaposi's sarcoma and infections such as thrush, herpes simplex, and hairy leukoplakia. The teeth and gums should be evaluated because of the high incidence of gingivitis and tooth decay seen in association with HIV infection.

Laboratory assessment. An elevated prothrombin time, macrocytic anemia, hypoalbuminemia, or hypocholesterolemia may indicate significant malnutrition.

Lymphadenopathy

Incidence. Nonspecific lymph node enlargement was recognized as a common finding in HIV-infected patients early in the history of the AIDS epidemic,[79] and it may arise at any time in the course of HIV infection. In one large study, 71% of HIV-infected homosexual men at various stages of disease were found to have significant lymphadenopathy.[64]

The syndrome of persistent generalized lymphadenopathy, defined as unexplained palpable lymph node enlargement of more than 1 cm in two or more extrainguinal sites for at least 3 months,[17] may be a direct effect of HIV infection. This syndrome, which may occur early in the course of the disease, is seen in the minority of patients, and its prognostic significance is not clear.

Nonspecific lymphadenopathy in early HIV infection often regresses over time,[37] although the incidence of lymph node enlargement in AIDS and other advanced stages of HIV infection is less clear. Because hyperplastic lymph nodes tend to involute with progression to AIDS, autopsy series have shown low rates of significant lymphadenopathy.[105] However, involvement of the lymph nodes by opportunistic infections or AIDS-related malignancies becomes increasingly common as HIV infection progresses.

Differential diagnosis. The diagnostic significance of lymph node enlargement varies with the stage of HIV infection. As noted previously, a nonspecific generalized lymphadenopathy may be seen at any point in the disease but is most common before the onset of profound immunodeficiency and AIDS-related infections or malignancies. Histological examination of lymph nodes from patients with persistent generalized lymphadenopathy typically reveals nonspecific hyperplasia.[79] The challenge to the clinician is to distinguish persistent generalized lymphadenopathy, which requires no specific therapy, from opportunistic infection or malignancy involving the lymph nodes. Among the HIV-related infections that manifest lymph node enlargement, mycobacteriosis, particularly tuberculosis, has been the most common in a number of clinical series. Infection with *Mycobacterium tuberculosis* was found on lymph node biopsy in 12 of 21 intravenous drug users referred for evaluation of generalized lymphadenopathy in one series from New York City.[50] Infection with *Cryptococcus neoformans, Histoplasma capsulatum,*[105] *Toxoplasma gondii,*[30] and other organisms may also involve the lymph nodes. Lymphoma may manifest generalized or localized lymph node enlargement. Metastatic involvement of the lymph nodes was found in 44% of patients with cutaneous Kaposi's sarcoma in one autopsy series[105] and has also been reported in clinical series.[20]

Diagnostic evaluation. No general guidelines have been agreed on for evaluating lymph node enlargement in HIV-infected patients. Until such guidelines are devised, a cautious approach to the diagnostic workup is appropriate. Lymph node biopsy should be performed in all cases in which a reasonable working diagnosis cannot be established on other grounds. Nonetheless, the decision to biopsy must be individualized. Patients with CD4 lymphocyte counts in the normal range (over 500/mm³) who have symmetrical lymph node enlargement may not require immediate biopsy (Figure 7-3) because of the relatively small chance of opportunistic infection. It should be noted, however, that HIV-related lymphoma or lymphadenopathic Kaposi's sarcoma may occur before the onset of severe immunodeficiency. Patients with more advanced HIV infection, particularly those with a history of AIDS or with a CD4 lymphocyte count below 200/mm³, who present with new lymph node enlargement generally should undergo biopsy. Patients at any stage of the disease with asymmetrical lymphadenopathy at one or more noninguinal sites should also be evaluated with biopsy. Those with inguinal lymphadenopathy should

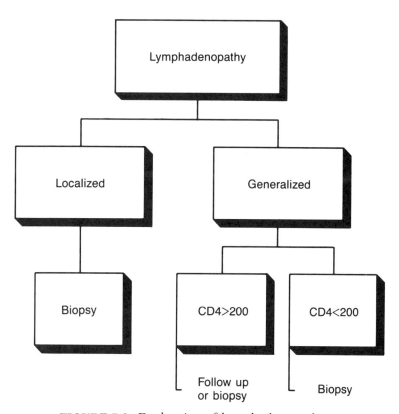

FIGURE 7-3. Evaluation of lymphadenopathy.

have a rapid but thorough evaluation for syphilis and other sexually transmitted diseases (e.g., chancroid, lymphogranuloma venereum) before being considered for biopsy.

If lymph node tissue is obtained, specific stains and cultures for mycobacteria and fungi should be performed on all specimens, since the histopathology may be misleading (e.g., granulomas may be absent in cases of disseminated mycobacterial infection). With possible cryptococcal or *Toxoplasma* infection of the lymph nodes, serological studies may be helpful in confirming the diagnosis.

Preliminary reports indicate that radionuclide scanning with either gallium[85] or rhenium sulfide colloid[81] may aid in distinguishing between reactive lymph nodes and those involved by opportunistic infection or malignancy.

Cardiopulmonary Signs

Persistent cough/dyspnea

Incidence. Respiratory complaints are very common, particularly at advanced stages of HIV infection.

Differential diagnosis. The differential diagnosis of persistent cough or dyspnea in HIV-infected patients varies greatly with the stage of disease (Table 7-2). In patients with absolute CD4 lymphocyte counts under $200/mm^3$ or with a history of AIDS, opportunistic respiratory infections such as *Pneumocystis carinii* pneumonia (PCP) must be excluded,[77] particularly in those with fever or other systemic signs of infection.

Bacterial pneumonia is common among HIV-infected patients, including those with CD4 lymphocyte counts over $200/mm^3$. Patients who have recovered from diffuse pneumonias such as PCP may complain of a persistent, dry cough for months afterward.

TABLE 7-2. Common causes of respiratory complaints in HIV-infected patients

CD4 lymphocyte count	Respiratory disorders
$>200/mm^3$	Bacterial pneumonia
	Tuberculosis
$<200/mm^3$	*Pneumocystis carinii* pneumonia
	Other opportunistic infection
	Tuberculosis
	Bacterial pneumonia
	Congestive heart failure
	Kaposi's sarcoma

Diagnostic evaluation. The evaluation of HIV-infected patients with a new or persistent cough should be guided, if time and the clinical situation permit, by the results of immunological staging (Figure 7-4). New respiratory complaints in patients with a CD4 lymphocyte count under 200/mm^3 should be promptly evaluated with a chest roentgenogram and sputum Gram and acid-fast stain. Blood cultures should be done in febrile patients. The patient should be quickly assessed for evidence of disseminated opportunistic infection or malignancy, particularly Kaposi's sarcoma. Determination of arterial blood gases and immediate hospitalization may be necessary, particularly for patients with progressive dyspnea accompanying a cough. If the chest roentgenogram is normal and there is no evidence of systemic bacterial infection, pulmonary gallium scanning may be useful in detecting early *P. carinii* pneumonia.[69,70]

If radiographic and radionuclide studies provide no insight into the cause of the cough, echocardiography may identify patients with occult cardiomyopathy or pericardial disease (Figure 7-5).[49,51]

Evaluation of a cough in patients with a CD4 lymphocyte count over 200/mm^3 also should include an early chest roentgenogram and assessment for systemic infection, caused particularly by *Streptococcus pneumoniae* or *Haemophilus influenzae*. However, in these patients, particularly those with a CD4 lymphocyte count over 500/mm^3, the diagnostic workup should also be directed at respiratory disorders unrelated to HIV infection.

Chest pain

Incidence. Chest pain is an uncommon symptom in HIV-infected patients, although the exact incidence is not known.

Differential diagnosis. Because most HIV-infected patients are young, coronary artery disease is unusual. However, esophagitis, pleural disease, myocarditis, or pericarditis may have chest pain as a prominent feature, and a detailed history should be directed at distinguishing among these disorders.

Diagnostic evaluation. All HIV-infected patients with chest pain should be evaluated by chest roentgenogram and electrocardiography. If the pain is substernal in location, esophageal (Figure 7-6) and cardiac causes are most likely. Patients with esophagitis usually notice pain on swallowing (the evaluation of such patients is outlined in the discussion of dysphagia).

Gastrointestinal/Intraabdominal Signs

Dysphagia and odynophagia

Incidence. Difficulty swallowing (dysphagia) and pain on swallowing (odynophagia) are common complaints in HIV-infected patients, particularly among those at advanced stages of immunodeficiency. The frequency of these com-

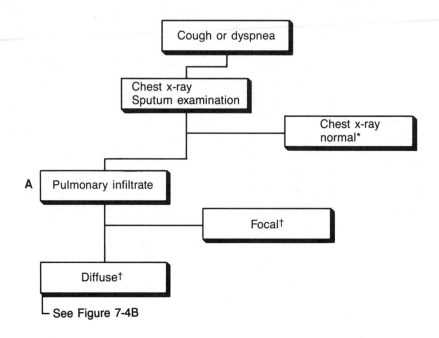

A

Cough or dyspnea

Chest x-ray
Sputum examination

Chest x-ray
normal*

Pulmonary infiltrate

Focal†

Diffuse†

└ See Figure 7-4B

*Consider gallium scanning, pulmonary function tests, and echocardiography.
†Bronchoscopy if no specific diagnosis on routine evaluation and sputum examination.

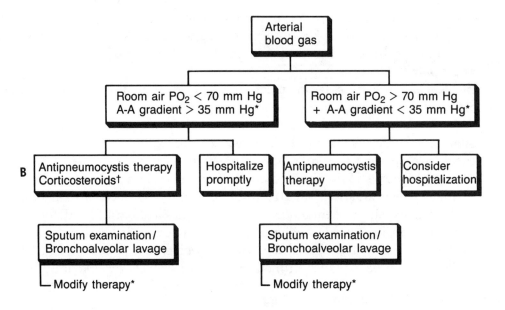

B

Arterial
blood gas

Room air PO_2 < 70 mm Hg
A-A gradient > 35 mm Hg*

Room air PO_2 > 70 mm Hg
+ A-A gradient < 35 mm Hg*

Antipneumocystis therapy
Corticosteroids†

Hospitalize
promptly

Antipneumocystis
therapy

Consider
hospitalization

Sputum examination/
Bronchoalveolar lavage

Sputum examination/
Bronchoalveolar lavage

└ Modify therapy*

└ Modify therapy*

*See Chapter 9.
†Unless diagnosis other than pneumocystosis likely.

FIGURE 7-4. A, Evaluation of respiratory complaints. **B,** Management of diffuse pulmonary infiltrates.

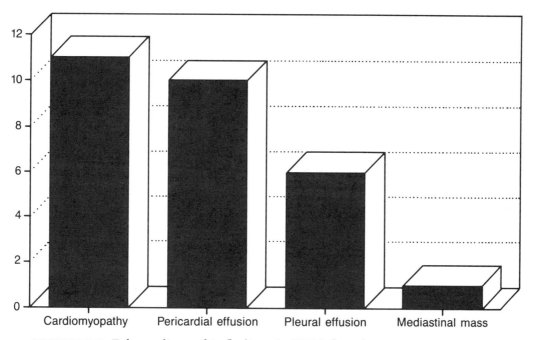

FIGURE 7-5. Echocardiographic findings in HIV-infected patients.

Data from Himelman RB, et al: Cardiac manifestations of human immunodeficiency virus infection: a two-dimensional echocardiographic study, *J Am Coll Cardiol* 13:1030-1036, 1989.

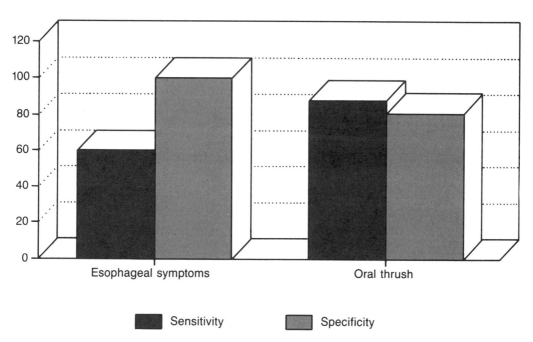

■ Sensitivity   ■ Specificity

FIGURE 7-6. Value of clinical parameters in diagnosing candidal esophagitis.

Data from Porro GB, Parente F, Cernuschi M: The diagnosis of esophageal candidiasis in patients with acquired immune deficiency syndrome: is endoscopy always necessary? *Am J Gastroenterol* 84(2):143-146, 1989.

plaints reflects the high incidence of esophagitis caused by opportunistic infections and involvement of the esophagus by AIDS-related malignancies. In one series, 35 of 90 AIDS patients required radiographic studies of the esophagus in a 3-year period.[71] In another series of AIDS patients, 27 of 57 patients undergoing routine upper endoscopy (48%) were found to have candidal esophagitis, although only 60% of those with documented esophagitis had symptoms.[86]

Differential diagnosis. Esophageal candidiasis is the commonest cause of dysphagia and odynophagia in patients with AIDS.[90] Other common esophageal disorders that may produce these symptoms include esophageal infections caused by cytomegalovirus,[104] herpes simplex, or, in rare cases, other opportunistic pathogens such as *Mycobacterium tuberculosis*[44] or *Cryptosporidium* organisms. HIV itself may be the cause of esophageal ulcers and odynophagia or dysphagia, particularly early in the course of the infection.[89]

Other HIV-related disorders that may result in pain or discomfort on swallowing include painful oral lesions and noninfectious disorders involving the pharynx or esophagus, including aphthous ulcers,[3] Kaposi's sarcoma,[83] squamous cell carcinoma,[36] and lymphoma.

The presence of oral candidiasis in patients with symptoms of esophagitis correlates well with the presence of candidal esophagitis (Figure 7-6). In one series, esophageal candidiasis was demonstrated by upper endoscopy in 88% of AIDS patients with oral candidiasis, regardless of symptoms.[86] However, either oral or esophageal candidiasis may occur alone. Pain on swallowing may be a clue to the presence of invasive infection.[45]

Diagnostic evaluation. Controversy exists regarding the optimum diagnostic workup for an HIV-infected patient with symptoms of dysphagia or odynophagia, specifically on the need for and timing of upper endoscopy.[95] Potential diagnostic strategies include upper endoscopy with biopsy as the initial diagnostic study; blind brushing of the esophagus through a nasogastric tube; barium radiography followed by endoscopy if the diagnosis is uncertain; and therapeutic trial of an antifungal medication such as ketoconazole or fluconazole, with radiographic or endoscopic investigation, or both, of patients who do not respond to empiric therapy.

In one large series in which double-contrast barium radiography was compared prospectively with upper endoscopy in HIV-infected patients who had a variety of upper gastrointestinal complaints, radiography had an overall sensitivity of only 31.1% and was particularly ineffective in detecting esophageal candidiasis (Figure 7-7).[25] In contrast, upper endoscopy was found to have a sensitivity of 97.5% in cases in which a histopathological diagnosis was confirmed. These data indicate that negative barium radiography cannot al-

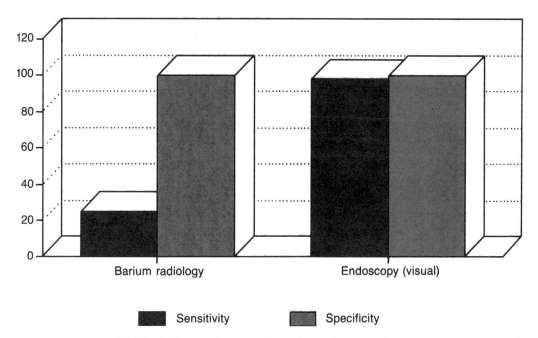

FIGURE 7-7. Yield of diagnostic procedures in patients with upper gastrointestinal complaints.

Data from Connolly GM et al: Investigation of upper gastrointestinal symptoms in patients with AIDS, *AIDS* 3(7):453-456, 1989.

ways exclude active esophagitis. In another prospective study, blind brushing of the esophagus through a nasogastric tube was found to have a sensitivity similar to upper endoscopy in the diagnosis of esophageal candidiasis in HIV-infected patients who complained of dysphagia or odynophagia.[13]

Despite endoscopy's excellent diagnostic results, not all patients may need to be subjected to the discomfort, potential morbidity, and cost of this procedure. Because of the high degree of correlation between oral and esophageal candidiasis, a therapeutic trial of antifungal therapy can be considered in patients with oral candidiasis and esophageal symptoms, with upper endoscopy reserved for those whose symptoms do not respond (Figure 7-8). Blind esophageal brushing, which potentially could be performed by the primary care physician, might provide a relatively safe and inexpensive alternative to endoscopy in some cases.[13]

Whenever empiric therapy for candidal esophagitis is initiated without histological confirmation of the diagnosis, it should be recalled that other HIV-related infections or malignancies may produce symptoms identical to those of esophageal candidiasis and may in fact coexist with it.

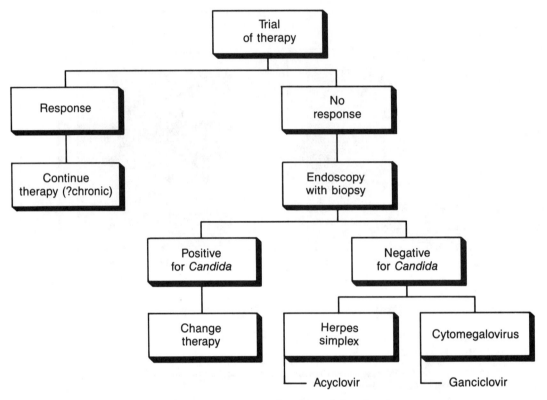

FIGURE 7-8. Evaluation of dysphagia.

Diarrhea
Incidence. Significant diarrhea occurs in more than 30% of AIDS patients[56] and also may be a prominent symptom at earlier stages of HIV infection.

Differential diagnosis. Persistent or recurrent diarrhea or diarrhea accompanied by fever, abdominal pain, or bloody stools should be evaluated thoroughly (Figure 7-9).

Among homosexual men[4] or patients from tropical or subtropical countries, diarrhea is frequently caused by intestinal parasites or bacteria that have no clear relationship to HIV infection. These parasites include *Giardia lamblia, Entamoeba histolytica,* and *Shigella* and *Campylobacter* species. HIV-related infections that produce diarrhea typically occur at advanced stages of the disease but may occur earlier. Important among these are infection with *Cryptosporidium* organisms, *Isospora belli,* and *Microsporidium* organisms. Cytomegalovirus and *Mycobacterium avium-intracellulare* may also cause diarrhea when they infect the bowel (Figure 7-10).

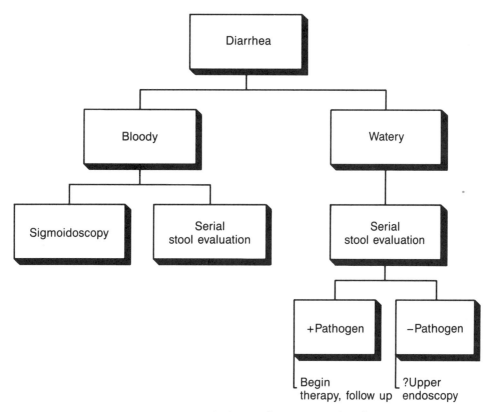

FIGURE 7-9. Evaluation of persistent diarrhea.

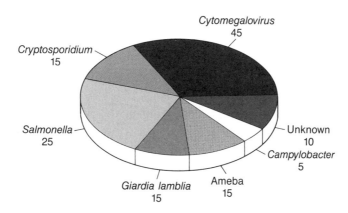

FIGURE 7-10. Intestinal pathogens in AIDS patients with diarrhea.

Data from Smith PD et al: Intestinal infections in patients with the acquired immunodeficiency syndrome (AIDS), *Ann Intern Med* 108:328-333, 1988.

In many HIV-positive patients with diarrhea, no intestinal pathogen is identified with routine tests. An enteropathy with characteristic pathological features[60] has been described in some of these cases.

Diarrhea may occur as a complication of therapy in patients receiving antibiotics for prophylaxis of *P. carinii* infection, or treatment of toxoplasmosis or other infections, or in those receiving the antiviral agent dideoxyinosine. Antibiotic-associated colitis caused by the toxin of *Clostridium difficile* also may be seen, particularly among patients receiving antibiotics.

Diagnostic evaluation. A thorough diagnostic workup of HIV-infected patients with diarrhea was found to yield a specific cause in 85% of cases in one study.[100] However, because several common causes of diarrhea, notably cytomegalovirus infection and cryptosporidiosis, are currently untreatable, it has been suggested that a limited diagnostic workup may be adequate in most cases.[56]

Stool specimens obtained on several days should be examined for parasites, including *Cryptosporidium* organisms, and cultured for routine pathogens. If the results of routine stool examinations and cultures are negative for pathogenic organisms, special cultures for viruses (e.g., cytomegalovirus) and mycobacteria (e.g., *M. avium-intracellulare*) should be considered. If no cause for the diarrhea is found, esophagogastroduodenoscopy to obtain both duodenal fluid and biopsies and colonoscopy with biopsy might yield the diagnosis.[100]

Management. Specific pathogens should be treated as outlined in Chapter 9. If a pathogen is identified for which no effective therapy is available (e.g., *Cryptosporidium*) or when diarrhea persists and no pathogen is identified, symptomatic therapy with antidiarrheal agents may be effective. Fluid losses may become severe and the risk of dehydration high, particularly in some cases of cryptosporidiosis or isosporiasis. Hospitalization for intravenous hydration is sometimes necessary.

Vomiting

Incidence. Nausea and vomiting are common symptoms in advanced HIV infection.[3]

Differential diagnosis. The differential diagnosis of recurrent vomiting in HIV-infected patients may include disorders involving the liver, gastrointestinal and biliary tracts, or central nervous system.

Diagnostic evaluation. Diagnostic evaluation of persistent vomiting should be guided by the immunological stage of HIV infection. Patients with CD4 lymphocyte counts under 200/mm^3 or with a history of AIDS-related opportunistic infections or malignancies are at high risk of opportunistic infections involving the gastrointestinal tract, liver, or central nervous system and should be evaluated with this in mind. Patients complaining of a persistent headache or presenting with a decreased level of consciousness should be evaluated thoroughly for signs of increased intracranial pressure. This evaluation may include brain imaging by computed tomography (CT) or magnetic resonance imaging (MRI) if an intracranial mass lesion cannot be excluded by history and physical examination.

The results of routine liver function tests and serum amylase determination are usually abnormal in patients with vomiting caused by hepatic, biliary, or pancreatic disorders.

Jaundice/hepatomegaly

Incidence. Despite the great variety of disorders associated with jaundice that may be seen in HIV-infected patients, it is an uncommon presenting complaint. Hepatomegaly may be present in most patients with AIDS[42] and is occasionally encountered at earlier stages of HIV infection.

Differential diagnosis. Causes of jaundice seen more frequently in HIV-infected patients include a number of disorders associated with intrahepatic or extrahepatic biliary obstruction and hepatocellular damage (Table 7-3).

Biliary obstruction. A syndrome of sclerosing cholangitis with stenosis of the common bile duct[76] and the papilla of Vater[96] in association with cytomegalovirus or cryptosporidial infection has been described in patients with AIDS. Acalculous cholecystitis associated with infections by *Campylobacter* organisms,[109] cytomegalovirus,[59] and *Candida* species[19] has also been reported. Kaposi's sarcoma and lymphoma involving lymph nodes adjacent to the liver may also cause biliary obstruction.

Hepatocellular dysfunction. Evidence of a prior hepatitis B infection is frequently found in HIV-infected patients with a history of homosexuality or intravenous drug use but appears to be no more common in these patients than in non-HIV–infected individuals with such histories. Severe chronic or

TABLE 7-3. Common hepatobiliary causes of jaundice in HIV-infected patients

Disorder	Cause
Sclerosing cholangitis	Cryptosporidiosis
	Cytomegaloviral infection
Common duct obstruction	Lymphoma
	Kaposi's sarcoma
Hepatocellular dysfunction	Drug toxicity
	Viral hepatitis

progressive hepatitis B is rare in HIV-infected patients.[94] Evidence exists that Hepatitis D, caused by superinfection with the delta virus in patients with prior hepatitis B infection, may be activated by HIV infection.[99]

A number of therapeutic agents commonly prescribed for HIV-infected patients are potentially toxic to the liver and may cause hepatitis. Among these are ketoconazole, zidovudine, trimethoprim-sulfamethoxazole, isoniazid, rifampin, and pyrazinamide.

Infection with opportunistic pathogens that commonly involve the liver in AIDS, including *Mycobacterium avium-intracellulare, Mycobacterium tuberculosis,* and *Histoplasma capsulatum,* is seldom associated with jaundice.

Diagnostic evaluation. The diagnostic evaluation of jaundice in HIV-infected patients should be directed at excluding extrahepatic biliary obstruction and hepatocellular disease due to reversible causes such as drug toxicity and treatable opportunistic infection (Figure 7-11). As in non-HIV-infected patients, significant elevation of transaminases or evidence of impaired hepatic synthetic function (decreased albumin, increased prothrombin time) suggests hepatocellular disease. Abdominal ultrasonograpy has proven to be effective in defining extrahepatic biliary obstruction.[47]

As discussed earlier in this chapter, liver biopsy may be of value in the diagnosis of occult opportunistic infection, particularly due to mycobacteria. Elevation of the alkaline phosphatase is often seen in such cases. Hepatic involvement by Kaposi's sarcoma or lymphoma may also be revealed by biopsy. Nonspecific abnormalities frequently seen in association with AIDS include steatosis, sinusoidal dilatation, and atrophy of hepatic parenchymal cells.[105]

Abdominal pain
Incidence. The incidence of abdominal pain as a presenting complaint in HIV-infected patients is unknown. Published studies of patients presenting with abdominal pain or intraabdominal pathology have focused on those with advanced HIV infection and AIDS (Figure 7-12). Less is known about the incidence and causes of abdominal pain in earlier stages of HIV infection. In one series of over 200 hospitalized AIDS patients, 12.3% reported abdominal pain for 2 or more days during their hospitalization.[5] In another series, 4.2% of over 900 consecutive hospitalized AIDS patients required abdominal surgical procedures including cholecystectomy, appendectomy, and exploratory laparotomy (Figure 7-13).[65]

Differential diagnosis. A variety of disorders associated with HIV infection may cause abdominal pain. Pain associated with diarrhea or vomiting may suggest an infectious enteritis such as that caused by cryptosporidiosis, *Isospora* infection, salmonellosis, or mycobacterial infection. Cryptosporidiosis

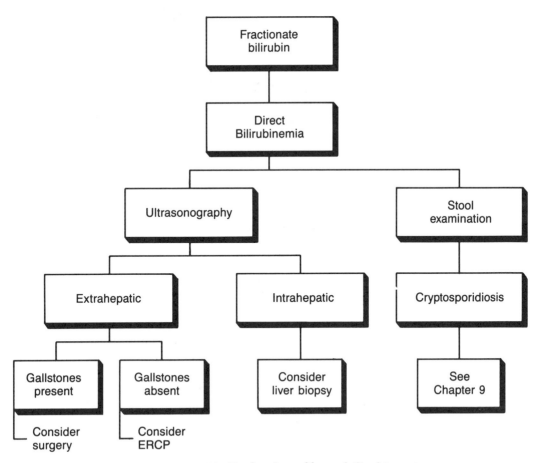

FIGURE 7-11. Evaluation of hyperbilirubinemia.

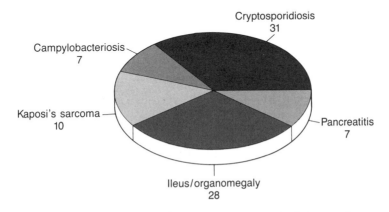

FIGURE 7-12. Disorders diagnosed in AIDS patients with abdominal pain.

Data from Barone JE et al: Abdominal pain in patients with acquired immune deficiency syndrome, *Ann Surg* 204(6):619-623, 1986.

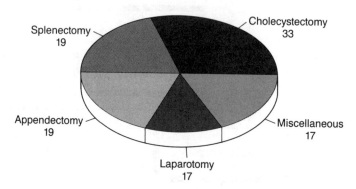

FIGURE 7-13. Abdominal surgical procedures performed on AIDS patients.

Data from LaRaja RD et al: The incidence of intra-abdominal surgery in acquired immunodeficiency syndrome: a statistical review of 904 patients, *Surgery* 105:175-179, 1989.

was the most common intestinal infection diagnosed in one large series of AIDS patients with abdominal pain, being seen in 31% of cases.[5] *Campylobacter* and *Giardia* infections were also seen. The pain associated with intestinal infections in these patients was most often diffuse. Diarrhea and hypoalbuminemia were seen in the majority of cases and over 40% of the patients complained of nausea and vomiting.

Pain localized to the right upper quadrant or more generalized throughout the abdomen may be caused by biliary tract disease associated with cryptosporidiosis, cytomegalovirus infection, or hepatitis caused by opportunistic infections (cytomegalovirus, mycobacterial infection, herpes simplex) or medications (ketoconazole, antituberculous therapy).

Generalized intraabdominal infection with cytomegalovirus, *Cryptococcus neoformans,* and *Mycobacterium avium-intracellulare* has been documented in AIDS patients having abdominal pain.[87] Diffuse abdominal pain with peritoneal signs should raise the possibility of peritonitis secondary to (1) bowel perforation caused by invasive infections or malignancies[87] or (2) direct involvement of the peritoneum by HIV-related infections such as tuberculosis,[7] toxoplasmosis,[54] or histoplasmosis.[1] HIV-infected patients receiving chronic ambulatory peritoneal dialysis appear to be at higher risk for bacterial and fungal peritonitis than other such patients.[32]

Midepigastric or left upper quadrant pain may signify pancreatitis related to biliary tract disease or to drug therapy, particularly with pentamidine or dideoxyinosine. Appendicitis with typical right-sided abdominal pain has been described in association with cytomegalovirus infection.[72] Nonspecific ileus and organomegaly may be seen in some patients with abdominal pain.[5]

Diagnostic evaluation. Diagnostic evaluation of abdominal pain in HIV-infected patients is not substantially different from that of abdominal pain seen in other settings. Symptoms suggesting ulcer disease should be investigated with radiographic studies or esophagogastroduodenoscopy. Pain localized to the right upper quadrant or left upper quadrant is best evaluated with imaging studies such as ultrasonography or CT. Liver function tests may help to distinguish biliary tract disease from hepatic parenchymal disorders. Patients with diarrhea accompanied by abdominal pain should undergo an evaluation comparable to that suggested for other patients with diarrhea (see above).

Since intraabdominal emergencies, particularly bowel perforation[31,65] and obstruction,[87] may occur in association with HIV-related infections and malignancies, it is extremely important that all patients with abdominal pain be evaluated carefully and followed closely for signs of peritonitis or obstruction. Emergency radiographic procedures and early surgical evaluation are indicated for patients in whom peritonitis or obstruction is suspected.

Gastrointestinal bleeding

Incidence. Bleeding is an uncommon manifestation of HIV-related gastrointestinal disorders.

Differential diagnosis. Causes of bleeding not related to HIV infection should be sought in HIV-infected patients with significant gastrointestinal blood loss. Potential HIV-associated causes of bleeding include esophagitis (caused by *Candida* organisms, herpes simplex virus, or cytomegalovirus); gastritis (cytomegalovirus); invasive infection of the small bowel (cytomegalovirus, *Salmonella*); colitis (cytomegalovirus); or Kaposi's sarcoma involving any segment of the gastrointestinal tract.

Diagnostic evaluation. The HIV-infected patient with gastrointestinal bleeding should be evaluated in the same fashion as other patients. Confirmed or suspected bleeding should be investigated with barium studies and with endoscopic procedures when indicated.

Splenomegaly

Incidence. Splenomegaly is a common manifestation of HIV infection in advanced stages of the disease. More than 70% of AIDS patients were found at autopsy to have enlarged spleens in one series.[105] A comparably high incidence of splenomegaly has been detected by CT[2] and on routine chest roentgenograms.[88] The incidence of splenomegaly in earlier stages of HIV infection is less clear.

Differential diagnosis. The cause of splenomegaly in HIV-infected patients is often obscure. The diagnostic evaluation should rule out treatable diseases that may manifest with splenomegaly.

Opportunistic infections. Opportunistic infections directly involving the spleen are most likely in patients with a prior history of AIDS or with an advanced degree of immunodeficiency (i.e., CD4 lymphocyte count under 200/ mm³). Infection with *Mycobacterium avium-intracellulare, Salmonella* organisms, and cytomegalovirus, as well as involvement with Kaposi's sarcoma, was seen in one series of patients undergoing splenectomy.[78] Cryptococcosis, histoplasmosis with splenic involvement,[105] and tuberculosis also have been described, as have a variety of less common infections.

AIDS-related malignancies. The spleen is a common site of involvement by metastatic Kaposi's sarcoma.[78,105] Involvement of the spleen by lymphoma may also occur[70a] but appears to be uncommon.[105]

Diagnostic evaluation. The optimum diagnostic approach to splenomegaly in HIV-infected patients is unknown. Large clinical series focusing on the causes of splenomegaly at various stages of HIV infection and the yield of various diagnostic tests are not available to guide the clinician. Because of this lack of clear data, it is probably best to approach treatment conservatively and attempt to identify a specific explanation in all patients. The wide variety of disorders that may involve the spleen and the frequency with which splenomegaly has been described in HIV-infected patients present obstacles to designing an effective workup. Patients with splenomegaly and unexplained fever, weight loss, or other signs that may represent a disseminated infection or malignancy should probably be evaluated more extensively than those with splenomegaly who do not have other signs or symptoms.

Even in otherwise asymptomatic patients, however, a careful effort should be made through the history, physical examination, routine laboratory data, and other diagnostic studies to establish a working diagnosis (i.e., nonspecific splenic enlargement caused by HIV infection itself or by a specific disorder unrelated to HIV infection, such as cirrhosis or portal hypertension).

Diagnostic studies of potential value in patients with splenomegaly include abdominal imaging (ultrasonography or CT) to evaluate for mass lesions or abscesses within the spleen and to identify other organ involvement, such as hepatomegaly or intraabdominal lymphadenopathy, that might provide a clue to the cause of the splenic enlargement. A thorough evaluation is important for other common sites of involvement by opportunistic infections and malignancies, including the respiratory and gastrointestinal tracts, the skin, the lymphatics, and the central nervous system. Blood cultures for pathogens known to disseminate to the spleen, particularly *Mycobacterium avium-intracellulare, Cryptococcus neoformans, Histoplasma capsulatum*, and cytomegalovirus, as well as routine bacteria, may be necessary. Biopsy of the liver or bone marrow, if feasible, may aid the clinician in excluding disseminated infection (mycobacterial or fungal) or malignancy (lymphoma) involving the spleen. Exploratory laparotomy may be necessary in rare cases of symptomatic patients in whom a definitive or reasonable working diagnosis cannot be made.

Management. Patients with hypersplenism resulting in pancytopenia or those with splenic abscesses may benefit from splenectomy.[78] Splenectomy must not be undertaken lightly, however, because of the risk of further significant impairment of the immune response, particularly to infection with encapsulated bacteria such as the *Pneumococcus* or *Haemophilus* species.

Musculoskeletal Signs

Joint pain and swelling

Incidence. Joint complaints are common among HIV-infected patients. In one series, 56 of 101 consecutive patients had nonspecific arthralgia or arthritis and an additional 12 had arthritis complicating psoriasis or Reiter's syndrome.[9] In this series 86% of the patients were in advanced stages of HIV infection.

Differential diagnosis. HIV-related opportunistic infections may cause arthritis by means of direct joint involvement, although this is quite rare. *Cryptococcus neoformans*,[91] *Sporothrix schenckii*,[73] and *Mycobacterium avium-intracellulare*[12] have been reported to cause septic arthritis in association with HIV infection.

Diagnostic evaluation. In general, patients with joint effusion should undergo diagnostic aspiration to exclude infectious causes. If no bacterial, mycobacterial, or fungal cause is identified in this manner, synovial biopsy, in consultation with a rheumatologist or orthopedist, may be appropriate in some patients. Blood tests that may aid in the diagnosis include VDRL, latex fixation, serum cryptococcal antigen, hepatitis B surface antigen, and tests for antinuclear antibodies.

Neurological Signs

Headache

Incidence. Headache is a common complaint among HIV-infected patients, although its exact incidence is unknown.

Differential diagnosis. The central nervous system (CNS) is a common site of involvement by HIV and various AIDS-related opportunistic infections and malignancies (Table 7-4). Cryptococcal meningitis and cerebral toxoplasmosis, the commonest of these infections, and non-Hodgkin's lymphoma, the commonest malignancy in these patients, are life-threatening disorders that may

TABLE 7-4. Common causes of cerebral dysfunction in HIV-infected patients

Infections	Cryptococcal meningitis
	Toxoplasma encephalitis
	HIV encephalopathy
	Progressive multifocal leukoencephalopathy
	Syphilis
	Tuberculous meningitis
Malignancy	Lymphoma
Metabolic	Hyponatremia
	Hypoglycemia*
	Uremia

*In patients receiving pentamidine therapy.

be accompanied by headache. Because headaches in HIV-infected patients often have organic causes, evaluation of this symptom poses a particularly difficult challenge to the primary care physician.

As with other clinical syndromes associated with HIV infection, the differential diagnosis of headache varies with the stage of HIV infection.

HIV itself may cause meningitis at the time of seroconversion or later in the course of infection. HIV meningitis may manifest as a self-limited process marked by fever, headache, and neck stiffness or as a chronic headache not associated with meningeal signs.[52] This syndrome is seldom associated with signs of encephalopathy, which often accompany opportunistic infections involving the central nervous system.

Late in the course of HIV infection, the opportunistic infections and malignancies are more prevalent, particularly if the CD4 lymphocyte count falls below $200/mm^3$ or if manifestations of full-blown AIDS occur. Cryptococcal meningitis typically manifests as a subacute illness marked by fever and headache and is rarely associated with focal neurological signs. However, in some cases cryptococcal infection may produce a more fulminant illness, with rapid progression to coma. Cerebral toxoplasmosis typically is accompanied by headache, a depressed level of consciousness, and/or focal neurological abnormalities of recent onset.

Two medications commonly given to HIV-infected patients also may cause headaches. A syndrome of fever, malaise, nausea, and headache has been described in patients receiving trimethoprim-sulfamethoxazole,[55] and headaches are a common side effect of zidovudine.[92]

Diagnostic evaluation. Because of the potentially life-threatening nature of the opportunistic infections and malignancies that may cause headache in HIV-infected patients, this symptom must always be evaluated carefully, particularly in patients with a prior diagnosis of AIDS or with CD4 lymphocyte counts below 200/mm³.

Diagnostic evaluation of a headache that lasts longer than several days or that progressively worsens should be directed at ruling out common CNS infections and malignancies associated with AIDS. Serum cryptococcal antigen is likely to be positive in patients with cryptococcal meningitis, and this test should be performed early in patients with headache. Prompt neurological evaluation and CT or MRI scans of the head are necessary to exclude cerebral toxoplasmosis and CNS lymphoma, even in patients without focal neurological deficits. A lumbar puncture should be performed on all patients with a persistent headache or other evidence of CNS infection when there is no suspicion of an expanding intracranial mass lesion.

Paresthesia/dysesthesia/weakness (peripheral neuropathy)

Incidence. Peripheral nerve disorders are seen in all stages of HIV infection and occur in 10% to 35% of patients with AIDS.[28,102] Among asymptomatic HIV-infected patients, a pattern of acute or chronic inflammatory polyneuropathy is seen most commonly.[67] Distal sensory neuropathy, with symptoms of painful or burning feet, is more characteristic of advanced HIV infection and AIDS.[67]

Diagnostic evaluation. Patients with inflammatory neuropathies typically seek care in an early, asymptomatic stage of HIV infection with progressive weakness, elevated cerebrospinal fluid protein, pleocytosis, and evidence of demyelination on nerve conduction studies.[26]

The diagnosis of distal sensory neuropathy usually may be made on clinical grounds, although characteristic findings may be seen on electrophysiological studies.[28,102] The combination of pain in the soles and absent or diminished ankle reflexes is characteristic,[28] and the syndrome typically occurs in patients with advanced immunodeficiency and systemic signs of illness.[102] Neurological consultation should be obtained in cases where spinal cord involvement cannot be excluded or when the cause of the symptoms is otherwise in doubt.

Management. Corticosteroids and plasmapheresis both have been used successfully to treat inflammatory polyneuropathy associated with HIV infection,[27] although the disorder may be self-limited. The decision to treat and the selection of therapeutic agents generally should be made with neurological consultation. Distal sensory neuropathy associated with AIDS may respond to tricyclic antidepressant agents.[28]

Seizure/focal neurological deficit

Focal neurological deficits. Most AIDS patients with focal intracerebral deficits are found to have *Toxoplasma* encephalitis or CNS lymphoma. A wide variety of other causes may be encountered, including tuberculous, *Listeria*, nocardial,

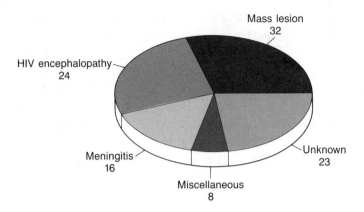

FIGURE 7-14. Etiology of new-onset seizures.

Data from Holtzman DM, Kaku DA, So YT: New-onset seizures associated with human immunodeficiency virus infection: causation and clinical features in 100 cases, *Am J Med* 87:173-177, 1989.

and fungal brain abscesses; neurosyphilis; herpes simplex encephalitis; and cerebrovascular accidents.

Seizures. Because CNS involvement by opportunistic infections and malignancies and HIV itself is common, seizures are a relatively common manifestation of HIV infection (Figure 7-14). In a retrospective review of more than 600 hospitalized patients at all stages of HIV infection, 76 (12%) were noted to have new-onset seizures.[111] Forty-six percent of these patients had single seizures, and 54% had recurrent seizures. Seizures were generalized in 94%.

Differential diagnosis. Approximately one third of HIV-infected patients with seizures are found to have an intracerebral mass lesion; 10% to 16% have meningitis, and 3% to 11% of cases have metabolic causes.[53,111]

Seizures have been reported to complicate 4% to 8% of cases of cryptococcal meningitis,[22,114] 14% to 23% of cases of cerebral toxoplasmosis,[24,110] and 17% of cases of primary CNS lymphoma (Table 7-5).[40] Less common HIV-related disorders may also be associated with seizures. Among these are CNS tuberculosis,[10] progressive multifocal leukoencephalopathy,[53] and CNS infection by herpes simplex or varicella zoster virus. Metabolic disturbances, including hyponatremia, renal insufficiency,[53] and hypoglycemia complicating pentamidine therapy, may also cause seizures.

The role of direct infection of the central nervous system by HIV in the pathogenesis of seizures has been emphasized in recent years as the impact of HIV infection on the brain has been more fully appreciated. Among patients having advanced HIV infection with dementia, 7% to 44% may have seizures,[80,101] and seizures may also complicate early HIV infection.[93] In recent

TABLE 7-5. Rate at which seizures complicate various disorders

Disorder	Incidence of seizures
Cerebral toxoplasmosis	14%-23%[24, 110]
CNS lymphoma	17%[40]
Cryptococcal meningitis	4%-8%[22, 114]
HIV encephalopathy	7%-44%[80, 101]

studies, 24% to 46% of new-onset seizures were attributed to HIV encephalopathy.[53,111]

Diagnostic evaluation. HIV-infected patients with new-onset seizures or focal neurological deficits, or both, should undergo a thorough evaluation for CNS infection and malignancy and metabolic derangements. Intracerebral mass lesions should be excluded through CT or MRI. Serological studies for *Toxoplasma gondii* and cryptococcal infection (see Chapter 5) may also provide important diagnostic information.

When intracranial lesions compatible with toxoplasmosis are demonstrated by imaging studies, empiric therapy may be justified.[24] A clinical and radiographic response to therapy with sulfadiazine and pyrimethamine strongly suggests toxoplasmosis and supports the diagnosis (Figure 7-15).

Tissue examination, by means of brain biopsy, provides the most definitive diagnostic information and may be necessary in some patients with intracerebral mass lesions.

Visual disturbances

Incidence. Loss of visual acuity is a common complaint among HIV-infected patients, particularly those in advanced stages of the disease.

Differential diagnosis. The eye is a major target organ for HIV and AIDS-associated opportunistic infections. The most serious of these disorders is cytomegalovirus (CMV) retinitis, which is also the most common cause of loss of vision in AIDS patients.[68] In one prospective series, 58% of patients with CMV retinitis initially had unilateral involvement.[46]

Other opportunistic infections that have involved the eye in HIV-infected patients include cryptococcal choroiditis,[15] herpes zoster keratitis,[33] and bacterial and mycobacterial endophthalmitis.[23] Syphilitic involvement of the eye has also been described in HIV-infected patients and has been reported as a cause of optic neuritis leading to blindness.[113]

Diagnostic evaluation. Because of the variety of disorders that may involve the eye in HIV-infected patients and the high risk of blindness from CMV retinitis, patients with visual complaints or decreased visual acuity should be

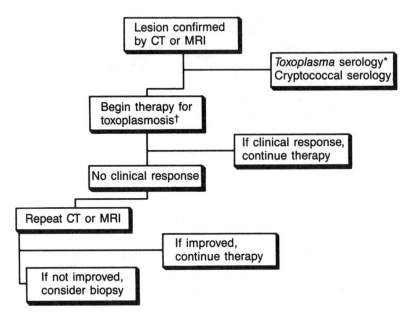

FIGURE 7-15. Evaluation and management of CNS mass lesion.

referred promptly for ophthalmological examination. Serum tests for syphilis, cryptococcal infection, and toxoplasmosis, as well as a CD4 lymphocyte count to establish the extent of immunodeficiency, may be useful adjunctive diagnostic tests.

REFERENCES

1. Alterman DD, Cho KC: Histoplasmosis involving the omentum in an AIDS patient: CT demonstration, *J Comput Assist Tomogr* 12(4):664-665, 1988.

2. Arrive L et al: Results of abdominal x-ray computed tomography in 25 patients with the acquired immunodeficiency syndrome, *J Radiol* 67:219-223, 1986.

3. Bach MC et al: Odynophagia from aphthous ulcers of the pharynx and esophagus in the acquired immunodeficiency syndrome (AIDS), *Ann Intern Med* 109(4):338-339, 1988.

4. Baker RW, Peppercorn MA: Gastrointestinal ailments of homosexual men, *Medicine* 61(6):390-404, 1982.

5. Barone JE et al: Abdominal pain in patients with acquired immune deficiency syndrome, *Ann Surg* 204(6):619-623, 1986.

6. Baum MK et al: Vitamin B_{12} and cognitive function in HIV infection. Paper presented at the Sixth International Conference on AIDS, San Francisco, June 22, 1990 (abstract).

7. Baumgartner DD et al.: Peritoneal dialysis-associated tuberculous peritonitis in an intravenous drug user with acquired immunodeficiency syndrome, *Am J Kidney Dis* 14(2):154-157, 1989.

8. Beach RS et al: Nutritional abnormalities in early HIV-1 infection. I.

Plasma vitamin levels. Paper presented at the Fifth International Conference on AIDS, Montreal, June 8, 1989 (abstract).

9. Berman A et al: Rheumatic manifestations of human immunodeficiency virus infection, *Am J Med* 85:59-64, 1988.

10. Bishburg E et al: Central nervous system tuberculosis with the acquired immunodeficiency syndrome and its related complex, *Ann Intern Med* 105:210-213, 1986.

11. Blatt S et al: Lipid abnormalities in HIV infection. Paper presented at the Sixth International Conference on AIDS, San Francisco, June 21, 1990 (abstract).

12. Blumenthal DR, Zucker JR, Hawkins CC: *Mycobacterium avium* complex–induced septic arthritis and osteomyelitis in a patient with the acquired immunodeficiency syndrome, *Arthritis Rheum* 33(5):757-758, 1990.

13. Bonacini M et al: Prospective evaluation of blind brushing of the esophagus for *Candida* esophagitis in patients with human immunodeficiency virus infection, *Am J Gastroenterol* 85(4):385-389, 1990.

14. Cappell MS, Schwartz MS, Biempica L: Clinical utility of liver biopsy in patients with serum antibodies to the human immunodeficiency virus, *Am J Med* 88:123-130, 1990.

15. Carney MD, Combs JL, Waschler W: Cryptococcal choroiditis, *Retina* 10(1):27-32, 1990.

16. Castella A et al: The bone marrow in AIDS: a histologic, hematologic, and microbiologic study, *Am J Clin Pathol* 84(4):425-432, 1985.

17. Centers for Disease Control: Classification system for human T-lymphotropic virus type III/lymphadenopathy virus infection, *MMWR* 35:334-339, 1986.

18. Centers for Disease Control: Diagnosis and management of mycobacterial infection and disease in persons with human immunodeficiency virus infection, *Ann Intern Med* 106:254-256, 1987.

19. Cervia JS, Murray HW: Fungal cholecystitis and AIDS, *J Infect Dis* 161:358, 1990.

20. Chaves RL et al: Lymphadenopathy and human immunodeficiency (HIV) infection in São Paulo, Brazil. Paper presented at the Fifth International Conference on AIDS, Montreal, June 5, 1989 (abstract).

21. Chlebowski R et al: Dietary intake, nutritional status, and immunologic function in patients with HIV infection. Paper presented at the Sixth International Conference on AIDS, San Francisco, June 21, 1990 (abstract).

22. Chuck SL, Sande MA: Infections with *Cryptococcus neoformans* in the acquired immunodeficiency syndrome, *N Engl J Med* 321(12):794-799, 1989.

23. Cohen JI, Saragas SJ: Endophthalmitis due to *Mycobacterium avium* in a patient with AIDS, *Ann Ophthalmol* 22:47-51, 1990.

24. Cohn JA et al: Evaluation of the policy of empiric treatment of suspected *Toxoplasma* encephalitis in patients with the acquired immunodeficiency syndrome, *Am J Med* 86:521-527, 1989.

25. Connolly GM et al: Investigation of upper gastrointestinal symptoms in patients with AIDS, *AIDS* 3(7):453-456, 1989.

26. Cornblath DR et al: Inflammatory demyelinating peripheral neuropathies associated with human T-cell lymphotropic virus type III infection, *Ann Neurol* 21(1):32-40, 1987.

27. Cornblath DR: Treatment of the neuromuscular complications of human immunodeficiency virus infection, *Ann Neurol* 23(suppl):S88-S91, 1988.

28. Cornblath DR, McArthur JC: Predominantly sensory neuropathy in patients with AIDS and AIDS-related complex, *Neurology* 38(5):794-796, 1988.

29. Davies SF, McKenna RW, Sarosi GA: Trephine biopsy of the bone marrow in disseminated histoplasmosis, *Am J Med* 67:617-622, 1979.

30. De La Rubia L et al: Isolation of *Toxoplasma gondii* in lymph nodes of patients with HIV infection and generalized lymphadenopathy. Paper presented at the Sixth International Conference on AIDS, San Francisco, June 21, 1990 (abstract).

31. DeRiso AJ et al: Multiple jejunal perforations secondary to cytomegalovirus in a patient with acquired immune deficiency syndrome: case report and review, *Dig Dis Sci* 34(4):623-629, 1989.

32. Dressler R, Peters AT, Lynn RI: Pseudomonal and candidal peritonitis as a complication of continuous ambulatory peritoneal dialysis in human immunodeficiency virus–infected patients, *Am J Med* 86:787-790, 1989.

33. Engstrom RE, Holland GN: Chronic herpes zoster virus keratitis associated with the acquired immunodeficiency syndrome, *Am J Ophthalmol* 105(5):556-558, 1988.

34. Fineman DS et al: Detection of abnormalities in febrile AIDS patients with In-111–labeled leukocyte and GA-67 scintigraphy, *Radiology* 170(3 pt 1):677-680, 1989.

35. Fordyce-Baum MK et al: Nutritional abnormalities in early HIV-1 infection. II. Trace elements. Paper presented at the Fifth International Conference on AIDS, Montreal, June 8, 1990 (abstracts).

36. Frager DH et al: Squamous cell carcinoma of the esophagus in patients with acquired immunodeficiency syndrome, *Gastrointest Radiol* 13(4):358-360, 1988.

37. Friedman H et al: Evolution of lymphadenopathy in HIV-1 seropositive homosexual men and involution among those who develop AIDS. Paper presented at the Sixth International Conference on AIDS, San Francisco, June 21, 1990 (abstract).

38. Gaines H et al: Clinical picture of primary HIV infection presenting as glandular fever–like illness, *Br Med J* 297:1363-1368, 1988.

39. Gardener TD et al: Disseminated *Mycobacterium avium-intracellulare* infection and red cell hypoplasia in patients with the acquired immune deficiency syndrome, *J Infect* 16(2):135-140, 1988.

40. Gill PS et al: Primary central nervous system lymphoma in homosexual men: clinical, immunologic, and pathologic features, *Am J Med* 78:742-748, 1985.

41. Gillin JS et al: Malabsorption and mucosal abnormalities of the small intestine in the acquired immunodeficiency syndrome, *Ann Intern Med* 102:619-622, 1985.

42. Glasgow BJ et al: Clinical and pathologic findings of the liver in the acquired immune deficiency syndrome (AIDS), *Am J Clin Pathol* 83:582-590, 1985.

43. Gluckman RJ, Rosner F, Guarneri JJ: The diagnostic utility of bone marrow aspiration and biopsy in patients with the acquired immunodeficiency syndrome, *J Natl Med Assoc* 81(2):119-125, 1989.

44. Goodman P et al: Mycobacterial esophagitis in AIDS, *Gastrointest Radiol* 14(2):103-105, 1989.

45. Gould E et al: Esophageal biopsy findings in the acquired immunodeficiency syndrome (AIDS): clinicopathologic correlation in 20 patients, *South Med J* 81(11):1392-1395, 1988.

46. Gross JG et al: Longitudinal study of cytomegalovirus retinitis in acquired immune deficiency syndrome, *Ophthalmology* 97(5):681-686, 1990.

47. Grumbach K et al: Hepatic and biliary tract abnormalities in patients

with AIDS: sonographic-pathologic correlation, *J Ultrasound Med* 8(5):247-254, 1989.

48. Grunfeld C et al: Hypertriglyceridemia in the acquired immunodeficiency syndrome, *Am J Med* 86:27-31, 1989.

49. Hecht SR et al: Unsuspected cardiac abnormalities in the acquired immune deficiency syndrome: an echocardiographic study, *Chest* 96:805-808, 1989.

50. Hewlett D et al: Lymphadenopathy in an inner-city population consisting principally of intravenous drug abusers with suspected acquired immunodeficiency syndrome, *Am Rev Respir Dis* 137(6):1275-1279, 1988.

51. Himelman RB et al: Cardiac manifestations of human immunodeficiency virus infection: a two-dimensional echocardiographic study, *J Am Coll Cardiol* 13:1030-1036, 1989.

52. Hollander H, Stringari S: Human immunodeficiency virus-associated meningitis: clinical course and correlations, *Am J Med* 83(5):813-816, 1987.

53. Holtzman DM, Kaku DA, So YT: New-onset seizures associated with human immunodeficiency virus infection: causation and clinical features in 100 cases, *Am J Med* 87:173-177, 1989.

54. Israelski DM et al: *Toxoplasma* peritonitis in a patient with acquired immunodeficiency syndrome, *Arch Intern Med* 148(7):1655-1657, 1988.

55. Jaffe HS et al: Complications of clotrimoxazole in the treatment of AIDS-associated *Pneumocystis carinii* in homosexual men, *Lancet* 2(8359):1109-1111, 1983.

56. Johanson JF, Sonnenberg A: Efficient management of diarrhea in the acquired immunodeficiency syndrome (AIDS): a medical decision analysis, *Ann Intern Med* 112:942-948, 1990.

57. Kaplan JE et al: Lymphadenopathy syndrome in homosexual men: evidence for continuing risk of developing the acquired immunodeficiency syndrome, *JAMA* 257(3):335-337, 1987.

58. Kauffman CA et al: Histoplasmosis in immunosuppressed patients, *Am J Med* 64:923-932, 1978.

59. Kavin H et al: Acalculous cholecystitis and cytomegalovirus infection in the acquired immunodeficiency syndrome, *Ann Intern Med* 104:53-54, 1986.

60. Kotler DP et al: Enteropathy associated with the acquired immunodeficiency syndrome, *Ann Intern Med* 101:421-428, 1984.

61. Kurtin PJ et al: Histoplasmosis in patients with acquired immunodeficiency syndrome: hematologic and bone marrow manifestations, *Am J Clin Pathol* 93(3):367-372, 1990.

62. Lahdevirta J et al: Elevated levels of circulating cachectin/tumor necrosis factor in patients with acquired immunodeficiency syndrome, *Am J Med* 85:289-291, 1988.

63. Lake-Bakaar G et al: Gastric secretory failure in patients with the acquired immunodeficiency syndrome (AIDS), *Ann Intern Med* 109:502-503, 1988.

64. Lang W et al: Clinical, immunologic and serologic findings in men at risk for acquired immunodeficiency syndrome: the San Francisco Men's Health Study, *JAMA* 257(3):326-330, 1987.

65. LaRaja RD et al: The incidence of intraabdominal surgery in acquired immunodeficiency syndrome: a statistical review of 904 patients, *Surgery* 105:175-179, 1989.

66. Lebovics E et al: The liver in the acquired immunodeficiency syndrome: a clinical and histological study, *Hepatology* 5(2):293-298, 1985.

67. Leger JM et al: The spectrum of polyneuropathies in patients infected with HIV, *J Neurol Neurosurg Psychiatry* 52(12):1369-1374, 1989.

68. Lehoang P et al: Foscarnet in the treatment of cytomegalovirus retinitis in acquired immune deficiency syndrome, *Ophthalmology* 96(6):865-873, 1989.

69. Levenson S et al: Abnormal pulmonary gallium accumulation in *P. carinii* pneumonia, *Radiology* 119:395-398, 1976.

70. Levin M et al: *Pneumocystis* pneumonia: importance of gallium scan for early diagnosis and description of a new immunoperoxidase technique to demonstrate *Pneumocystis carinii*, *Am Rev Respir Dis* 128:182-185, 1983.

70a. Levine AM et al: Development of B-cell lymphoma in homosexual men. Clinical and immunologic findings, *Ann Intern Med* 100:7-13, 1984.

71. Levine MS et al: Opportunistic esophagitis in AIDS: radiographic diagnosis, *Radiology* 165(3):815-820, 1987.

72. Lin J et al: Cytomegalovirus-associated appendicitis in a patient with the acquired immunodeficiency syndrome, *Am J Med* 89:377-379, 1990.

73. Lipstein-Kresch E et al: Disseminated *Sporothrix schenckii* infection with arthritis in a patient with acquired immunodeficiency syndrome, *J Rheumatol* 12(4):805-808, 1985.

74. Mantero-Atienza E et al: Vitamin B$_6$ and immune function in HIV infection. Paper presented at the Sixth International Conference on AIDS, San Francisco, June 21-24, 1990 (abstract).

75. Mantero-Atienza E et al: Nutritional knowledge, health beliefs and practices in the HIV-1 infected patient. Paper presented at the Fifth International Conference on AIDS, Montreal, June 8, 1989 (abstract).

76. Margulis SJ et al: Biliary tract obstruction in the acquired immuno-deficiency syndrome, *Ann Intern Med* 105:207-210, 1987.

77. Masur H et al: CD4 counts as predictors of opportunistic pneumonias in human immunodeficiency virus (HIV) infection, *Ann Intern Med* 111(3):223-231, 1989.

78. Mathew A et al: Splenectomy in patients with AIDS, *Am J Hematol* 32:184-189, 1989.

79. Miller B et al: The syndrome of unexplained generalized lymphadenopathy in young men in New York City: is it related to the acquired immune deficiency syndrome? *JAMA* 251(2):242-246, 1984.

80. Navia BA, Jordan BD, Price RW: The AIDS dementia complex. I. Clinical features, *Ann Neurol* 19:517-524, 1986.

81. O'Doherty MJ et al: Lymphatic scanning and HIV. Paper presented at the Sixth International Conference on AIDS, San Francisco, June 22, 1990 (abstract).

82. Parry GJ: Peripheral neuropathies associated with human immunodeficiency virus infection, *Ann Neurol* 23(suppl):S49-S53, 1988.

83. Patow CA et al: Pharyngeal obstruction by Kaposi's sarcoma in a homosexual male with acquired immune deficiency syndrome, *Otolaryngol Head Neck Surg* 92(6):713-716, 1984.

84. Pierce PF, DeYoung DR, Roberts GD: Mycobacteremia and the new blood culture systems, *Ann Intern Med* 99:786-789, 1983.

85. Podzamczer D et al: The value of gallium-67 scan in the diagnosis of lymphadenopathy in symptomatic HIV-infected patients. Paper presented at the Fifth International Conference on AIDS, Montreal, June 5, 1989 (abstract).

86. Porro GB, Parente F, Cernuschi M: The diagnosis of esophageal candidiasis in patients with acquired im-

mune deficiency syndrome: is endoscopy always necessary? *Am J Gastroenterol* 84(2):143-146, 1989.

87. Potter DA et al: Evaluation of abdominal pain in the AIDS patient, *Ann Surg* 199(3):332-339, 1984.

88. Pugh P, Brenner M, Milne EN: Splenic size on routine chest films in AIDS: diagnostic and prognostic significance, *J Thorac Imaging* 3(2):40-51, 1988.

89. Rabeneck L et al: Acute HIV infection presenting with painful swallowing and esophageal ulcers, *JAMA* 263(17):2318-2322, 1990.

90. Raufman JP: Odynophagia/dysphagia in AIDS, *Gastroenterol Clin North Am* 17(3):599-614, 1988.

91. Ricciardi DD et al: Cryptococcal arthritis in a patient with acquired immune deficiency syndrome: case report and review of the literature, *J Rheumatol* 13(2):455-458, 1986.

92. Richman DD, Andrews J, AZT Collaborative Working Group: Results of continued monitoring of participants in the placebo-controlled trial of zidovudine for serious human immunodeficiency virus infection, *Am J Med* 85(suppl 2a):208-213, 1988.

93. Rosenbaum GS, Klein NC, Cunha BA: Early seizures in patients with acquired immunodeficiency syndrome without mass lesions, *Heart Lung* 18:526-529, 1989.

94. Rustgi VK et al: Hepatitis B virus infection in the acquired immunodeficiency syndrome, *Ann Intern Med* 101:795-797, 1984.

95. San Roman AL et al: Dysphagia and the human immunodeficiency virus: endoscopy is not a first step, *Am J Gastroenterol* 84(11):1461-1462, 1989.

96. Schneiderman DJ, Cello JP, Laing FC: Papillary stenosis and sclerosing cholangitis in the acquired immunodeficiency syndrome, *Ann Intern Med* 106:546-549, 1987.

97. Schneiderman DJ et al: Hepatic dis-

ease in patients with the acquired immune deficiency syndrome, *Hepatology* 7(5):925-930, 1987.

98. Seaton T, Dworkin B, Wormser G: Dietary intake in AIDS, AIDS-related complex and asymptomatic seropositive HIV patients. Paper presented at the Sixth International Conference on AIDS, San Francisco, June 21, 1990 (abstract).

99. Shattock AG, Finlay H, Hillary IB: Possible reactivation of hepatitis D with chronic delta antigenaemia by human immunodeficiency virus, *Br Med J* 294:1656-1657, 1987.

100. Smith PD et al: Intestinal infections in patients with the acquired immunodeficiency syndrome (AIDS), *Ann Intern Med* 108:328-333, 1988.

101. Snider WD et al: Neurological complications of acquired immune deficiency syndrome: analysis of 50 patients, *Ann Neurol* 14:403-418, 1983.

102. So YT et al: Peripheral neuropathy associated with acquired immunodeficiency syndrome: prevalence and clinical features from a population-based survey, *Arch Neurol* 45(9):945-948, 1988.

103. Sorensen D et al: Serum copper and zinc levels predict progression to AIDS independently of CD4 level. Paper presented at the Sixth International Conference on AIDS, San Francisco, June 21, 1990 (abstract).

104. Teixidor HS et al: Cytomegalovirus infection of the alimentary canal: radiologic findings with pathologic correlation, *Radiology* 163(2):317-323, 1987.

105. Welch K et al: Autopsy findings in the acquired immune deficiency syndrome, *JAMA* 252(9):1152-1159, 1984.

106. Wheat J et al: The diagnostic laboratory tests for histoplasmosis: analysis of experience in a large urban outbreak, *Ann Intern Med* 97:680-685, 1982.

107. Wheat LJ, Kohler RB, Tewari RP: Di-

agnosis of disseminated histoplasmosis by detection of *Histoplasma capsulatum* antigen in serum and urine specimens, *N Engl J Med* 314(2):83-88, 1986.

108. Wheat LJ, Slama TG, Zeckel ML: Histoplasmosis in the acquired immune deficiency syndrome, *Am J Med* 78:203-210, 1985.

109. Wheeler AP, Gregg CR: *Campylobacter* bacteremia, cholecystitis and the acquired immunodeficiency syndrome, *Ann Intern Med* 105:804, 1986.

110. Wong B et al: Central nervous system toxoplasmosis in homosexual men and parenteral drug abusers, *Ann Intern Med* 100:36-42, 1984.

111. Wong MC, Suite ND, Labar DR: Seizures in human immunodeficiency virus infection, *Arch Neurol* 47:640-642, 1990.

112. Woods GL, Washington JA: Mycobacteria other than *Mycobacterium tuberculosis*: review of microbiologic and clinical aspects, *Rev Infect Dis* 9(2):275-294, 1987.

113. Zambrano W, Perez GM, Smith JL: Acute syphilitic blindness in AIDS, *J Clin Neuro Ophthalmol* 7(1):1-5, 1987.

114. Zuger A et al: Cryptococcal disease in patients with the acquired immunodeficiency syndrome: diagnostic features and outcome of treatment, *Ann Intern Med* 104:234-240, 1986.

CHAPTER 8

The Management of Minor Medical Problems Associated with HIV Infection

Oral candidiasis (thrush)
Seborrheic dermatitis
Dry skin
Fungal skin infections
Fungal nail infections

Molluscum contagiosum
Neuropathy
Chronic diarrhea
Anorexia

Infection with the human immunodeficiency virus (HIV) is associated with a large variety of non-life-threatening disorders that may be quite troubling to the patient. Because of the urgency of the more life-threatening infectious and neoplastic complications of AIDS, the therapy of such common HIV-related disorders as seborrheic dermatitis and sensory neuropathy has received relatively little attention in the medical literature. Nonetheless, the primary care physician caring for an HIV-infected patient is likely to be called upon to diagnose and treat a number of minor medical complaints.

Following is a discussion of common minor HIV-related disorders encountered in ambulatory practice. Those included are at least partly amenable to medical therapy and can often be managed with little or no diagnostic evaluation. Other common problems, such as headache, cough, fever, weight loss, and severe diarrhea, often represent serious infectious or neoplastic complications of AIDS. The diagnostic approach to these symptoms is reviewed in Chapter 7.

In some cases, complaints that are initially minor progress to devastating morbidity. This is especially true of neuropathy and diarrhea. Skin disorders such as seborrheic dermatitis or molluscum contagiosum may have severe cosmetic effects.

ORAL CANDIDIASIS (THRUSH)

Oral candidiasis is seen in more than 90% of AIDS patients.[23,32] Asymptomatic colonization of the oropharynx by *Candida albicans* is common even among patients without thrush[31] and is frequently present in homosexual men who are not HIV infected.[31] The onset of oral candidiasis has been predictive of progression to AIDS in longitudinal studies.[22]

The diagnosis of oral candidiasis is usually made clinically on the basis of characteristic white plaques on the palate, buccal mucosa, or tongue. Microscopic examination and culture of biopsy specimens or scrapings may be required to confirm the diagnosis in atypical cases. Symptoms are usually minimal, although extensive infection may be painful.

Several topical and systemic forms of therapy are effective for oral candidiasis, although comparative studies have not been done and most relevant clinical data come from series of cancer patients or patients with chronic mucocutaneous candidiasis. Relapse rates are high when therapy is discontinued, and the optimum long-term therapeutic regimens are unknown. Systemic therapy should be used if symptoms of esophagitis are present (see Chapter 9).

Nystatin, given as an oral suspension three or four times a day, usually is effective for mild to moderate infections. The patient should be instructed to hold the medication in the mouth for several minutes before swallowing.[24] Many patients find clotrimazole troches to be more palatable than nystatin, and they appear to be equally effective. Troches should be taken five times daily and allowed to dissolve in the mouth over 15 to 30 minutes.[26] Response rates of over 90% have been reported with this regimen.[37]

Oral therapy with ketoconazole[30] (200 to 400 mg daily) is generally effective in patients unresponsive to or intolerant of topical agents. Patients receiving ketoconazole chronically must be monitored carefully for hepatotoxicity. A newer oral antifungal compound, fluconazole (100 mg daily), is also quite effective. The results of trials comparing ketoconazole and fluconazole are not yet available.

SEBORRHEIC DERMATITIS

Seborrheic dermatitis is a chronic, inflammatory skin disorder commonly encountered in HIV-infected patients. Although the condition is diagnosed in 3% or less of the general population,[6] it was seen in more than 80% of AIDS patients and more than 40% of patients with AIDS-related complex (ARC) in one series.[19] The cause of seborrheic dermatitis is unknown, although the fungus *Pityrosporum orbiculare* appears to play a role.[11]

Seborrheic dermatitis typically appears as patches of erythema and scaling involving the scalp, eyebrows, nasal folds, and cheeks. The skin behind the ears, over the sternum, and in the genital region may also be involved. Although the condition poses no significant threat to health, patients are often distressed because of its cosmetic impact.

Topical therapy with corticosteroids (e.g., 1% hydrocortisone cream applied twice daily) may be effective. Topical or systemic antifungal therapy[11] (ketoconazole, 200 to 400 mg by mouth daily) may also be beneficial. The response to therapy usually is incomplete, and relapses are common.

DRY SKIN

Generalized dryness of the skin (xerosis, ichthyosis) was seen in 30% of patients with AIDS or ARC in one series[10] and can be a persistent source of discomfort. Typical manifestations are flaking, pain, and pruritus, which may be intense. All skin areas may be involved.

Patients should be instructed to use only soaps containing emollients. Liberal use of moisturing lotions or creams (e.g., Keri or Eucerin) usually provides substantial relief.

FUNGAL SKIN INFECTIONS

Cutaneous candidiasis and dermatophytosis were seen in 47% and 30%, respectively, of AIDS and ARC patients in one series.[10]

Candidiasis typically is characterized by erythema and pustules in the intertriginous areas. Infections with dermatophytes (*Trichophyton mentagrophytes, T. rubrum,* and *T. tonsurans; Microsporum canis* and *M. audouinii;* and *Epidermophyton floccosum*)[7] may manifest as tinea cruris, tinea capitis, or tinea corporis, or as psoriaform plaques. Fungal infection of the webs of the hands or feet occurs alone or may accompany onychomycosis. Tinea versicolor, caused by the nondermatophyte yeast *Pityrosporum orbiculare (Malassezia furfur),* is also commonly encountered in HIV-infected patients.[17]

The diagnosis of fungal skin infections can usually be confirmed by culture and by microscopic examination of scrapings after adding 10% potassium hydroxide.

Localized dermatophyte infections are best treated with topical agents. However, patients with nail (see below), hair, or widespread cutaneous involvement usually require oral antifungal therapy. Topical imidazole compounds such as clotrimazole and miconazole generally are effective against dermatophyte and candidal infections and tinea versicolor.[7] Therapy should be applied twice daily and continued for several weeks.

In extensive dermatophyte infections or when topical therapy fails, systemic therapy with oral griseofulvin (250 to 1,000 mg daily, depending on the preparation) may be effective. Therapy should be continued for several months. Published experience with griseofulvin therapy in the setting of HIV infection is limited, however. Infections caused by dermatophyte species unresponsive to griseofulvin[14,29] or by *Candida* or *Pityrosporum* species may respond to therapy with oral ketoconazole (200 mg daily),[2,16] although reports of severe hepatotoxicity during prolonged therapy have raised concerns.[33]

The investigational oral imidazole compound, itraconazole, has shown promise in the therapy of dermatophyte and candidal infections.[12]

Dermatological consultation should be considered in cases of widespread infection or when topical therapy is ineffective.

FUNGAL NAIL INFECTIONS

Fungal infection of the nails (onychomycosis) is commonly seen in HIV-infected patients. The involved nails typically become white and opaque and may subsequently become deformed and fragmented. The condition may be caused by *Candida albicans* or by dermatophytes, especially *Trichophyton rubrum*.[4,36]

Therapy of onychomycosis in HIV infection has not been thoroughly studied. In general, oral rather than topical agents are needed. Griseofulvin (10 mg/kg daily) traditionally has been the drug of choice in non-HIV-infected patients. However, data regarding toxicity in HIV-infected patients are unavailable and therapy must be continued for at least 6 months.

Two oral imidazoles, ketoconazole[9] and itraconazole, have been proven effective in the therapy of onychomycosis in studies of non-HIV-infected patients. Thirteen of 16 patients were cured by 3 months of therapy with ketoconazole (200 mg orally per day) after nail avulsion in one series.[21] Infections improved in over 50% of cases and were cured in 20% (toenail) and 43% (fingernail) in an open study of patients intolerant of griseofulvin.[29] Reports of severe[33] and fatal[5] hepatitis during therapy for onychomycosis have limited the use of ketoconazole for this infection in non-HIV-infected patients, however.

Itraconazole, which is currently investigational in the United States, has been shown to be highly effective in nail infections caused by *Candida albicans*[12] and to be superior to griseofulvin in onychomycosis caused by dermatophytes.[35]

MOLLUSCUM CONTAGIOSUM

Molluscum contagiosum is a skin infection caused by the molluscum contagiosum virus, a member of the poxvirus family.

It is thought to be transmitted by close contact, including sexual contact.

Typical lesions consist of umbilicated papules; they are most commonly seen in the genital area and may regress spontaneously in normal hosts.[28] Disseminated infection may be seen with HIV infection and other immunodeficiency states.[20]

In one series, 9% of patients with AIDS or ARC were found to have molluscum contagiosum.[10] Extragenital lesions are common in HIV-infected patients. The face is most frequently involved, although widespread dissemination may also be seen. The diagnosis should be confirmed by biopsy, since other AIDS-related skin disorders, particularly cryptococcosis,[25] may cause similar lesions.

Although molluscum contagiosum involves only the skin and does not pose a threat to survival, patients are often concerned about the cosmetic effect of facial lesions. Both cryotherapy and topical cantharidin may be effective for individual lesions, although attempts are often frustrated by continued dissemination. Dermatological consultation, especially for management of facial lesions, should be considered.

NEUROPATHY

Painful sensory neuropathy is a common problem for patients in advanced stages of HIV infection. Patients typically complain of pain or burning in the soles of the feet and lower legs. Analgesics and antiinflammatory agents seldom provide significant relief.

Distal sensory neuropathy associated with AIDS may respond to tricyclic antidepressant agents.[3] Low-dose therapy with amytriptyline (25 mg orally at bedtime) may provide partial relief of symptoms. The myelodepression often seen in advanced HIV infection may be exacerbated by this therapy, however, and particular caution should be used in patients receiving other marrow-toxic agents such as zidovudine or trimethoprim-sulfamethoxazole.

CHRONIC DIARRHEA

Diarrhea occurs in 30% to 60% of patients with AIDS.[15] In some cases diarrhea is associated with significant dehydration and malnutrition, whereas in others it persists for months or years without significant overall morbidity. Specific pathogens (e.g., *Cryptosporidium, Isospora, Salmonella,* and *Campylobacter* species; *Mycobacterium avium-intracellulare;* and cytomegalovirus) may be identified in 65% to 85% of cases.[15,27] Although systemic signs of infection may be present in these cases, it is often impossible to distinguish patients with identifiable infections from those with nonspecific diarrhea.

The approach to diagnosis and management of HIV-related diarrhea is controversial. Because of the poor response to therapy of several major AIDS-related intestinal pathogens (e.g., *Cryptosporidium*, cytomegalovirus, and *Mycobacterium avium-intracellulare*), symptomatic therapy with diphenoxylate hydrochloride may be more effective than specific antimicrobial therapy.[15]

Symptomatic therapy with either diphenoxylate hydrochloride with atropine (Lomotil) (two tablets four times daily) or loperamide (Imodium) (two capsules initially, followed by one capsule after each loose stool to a maximum of eight capsules daily) can be considered for patients with mild to moderate nonbloody diarrhea and no systemic signs of infection when no enteric pathogen has been identified on stool culture or daily stool examination for parasites for 3 days. It should be noted that antiperistaltic agents may precipitate toxic megacolon in patients with active colitis. Both diphenoxylate hydrochloride with atropine and loperamide should be avoided if pseudomembranous colitis is suspected; neither agent should be continued if diarrhea does not improve within several days or if abdominal distention, bloody stools, or systemic signs of infection occur. Diphenoxylate hydrochloride with atropine is contraindicated in patients with biliary obstruction.

ANOREXIA

HIV-infected patients frequently complain of loss of appetite. At advanced stages of symptomatic disease, anorexia is almost universal. Nonetheless, patients with recent loss of appetite, especially if accompanied by fever, should be evaluated for evidence of systemic infection or malignancy (see Chapter 7). Depression and gastrointestinal disorders may contribute to anorexia and should be excluded. Oral medications, particularly antibiotics and antifungal agents, which can be discontinued safely, should be. Liver function tests should be monitored for evidence of drug-induced hepatitis, particularly among patients receiving ketoconazole, trimethoprim-sulfamethoxazole, or antituberculous therapy.

Therapeutic options are limited. High-calorie food supplements may improve caloric intake but seldom relieve anorexia. Although some patients report weight gain when antiretroviral therapy is initiated,[8,18] this effect generally is short lived.

The synthetic progesterone megestrol acetate (Megace) has been shown to stimulate appetite and produce significant weight gain in patients with advanced cancer.[1] Preliminary results of megestrol therapy (80 mg by mouth four times daily) in AIDS patients have been encouraging but are limited.[34] The results are not yet available from controlled trials conducted by the AIDS Clinical Trials Group of the National Institute of Allergy and Infectious Disease.

REFERENCES

1. Bruera E et al: A controlled trial of megestrol acetate on appetite, caloric intake, nutritional status, and other symptoms in patients with advanced cancer, *Cancer* 66(6):1279-1282, 1990.
2. Cacciaglia GB, Tenczar AJ, Kanat IO: Pharmacologic review: a review of the literature of ketoconazole therapy in the treatment of tinea pedis and onychomycosis, *J Foot Surg* 23(5):420-423, 1984.
3. Cornblath DR, McArthur JC: Predominantly sensory neuropathy in patients with AIDS and AIDS-related complex, *Neurology* 38(5):794-796, 1988.
4. Dompmartin D et al: Onychomycosis and AIDS: clinical and laboratory findings in 62 patients, *Int J Dermatol* 29(5):337-339, 1990.
5. Duarte PA et al: Fatal hepatitis associated with ketoconazole therapy, *Arch Intern Med* 144(5):1069-1070, 1984.
6. Eisenstat BA, Wormser GP: Seborrheic dermatitis and butterfly rash in AIDS, *N Engl J Med* 311(3):189, 1984.
7. Feingold DS: What the infectious disease subspecialist should know about dermatophytes, *Curr Clin Top Infect Dis* 8:154-168, 1987.
8. Fischl MA et al: The efficacy of azidothymidine (AZT) in the treatment of patients with AIDS and AIDS-related complex: a double-blind, placebo-controlled trial, *N Engl J Med* 317(4):185-191, 1987.
9. Galimberti R et al: The activity of ketoconazole in the treatment of onychomycosis, *Rev Infect Dis* 2(4):596-598, 1980.
10. Goodman DS et al: Prevalence of cutaneous disease in patients with acquired immunodeficiency syndrome (AIDS) or AIDS-related complex, *J Am Acad Dermatol* 17(2 part 1):210-220, 1987.
11. Groisser D, Bottone EJ, Lebwohl M: Association of *Pityrosporum orbiculare*

(Malassezia furfur) with seborrheic dermatitis in patients with acquired immunodeficiency syndrome, *J Am Acad Dermatol* 20(5 part 1):770-773, 1989.
12. Hay RJ, Clayton YM: Treatment of chronic dermatophytosis and chronic oral candidiosis with itraconazole, *Rev Infect Dis* 9(suppl)1:S114-118, 1987.
13. Hay RJ et al: An evaluation of itraconazole in the management of onychomycosis, *Br J Dermatol* 119(3):359-366, 1988.
14. Hersle K, Mobacken H, Moberg S: Long-term ketoconazole treatment of chronic acral dermatophyte infections, *Int J Dermatol* 24(4):245-248, 1985.
15. Johanson JF, Sonnenberg A: Efficient management of diarrhea in acquired immunodeficiency syndrome (AIDS): a medical decision analysis, *Ann Intern Med* 112:942-948, 1990.
16. Jones HE: Consensus of the role and positioning of the imidazoles in the treatment of dermatophytosis, *Acta Derm Venereol Suppl* (Stockh) 121:139-146, 1986.
17. Kaplan MH et al: Dermatologic findings and manifestations of acquired immunodeficiency syndrome (AIDS), *J Am Acad Dermatol* 16:485-506, 1987.
18. Lambert JS et al: 2',3'-dideoxyinosine (DDI) in patients with the acquired immunodeficiency syndrome or AIDS-related complex: a phase I trial, *N Engl J Med* 322:1333-1340, 1990.
19. Mathes BM, Douglass MC: Seborrheic dermatitis in patients with acquired immunodeficiency syndrome, *J Am Acad Dermatol* 13(6):947-951, 1985.
20. Mayumi M et al: Selective immunoglobulin M deficiency associated with disseminated molluscum contagiosum, *Eur J Pediatr* 145:99-103, 1986.
21. Moncada B, Loredo CE, Isordia E: Treatment of onychomycosis with ketoconazole and nonsurgical avulsion of

the affected nail, *Cutis* 31(4):438-440, 1983.

22. Murray HW et al: Progression to AIDS in patients with lymphadenopathy or AIDS-related complex: reappraisal of risk and predictive factors, *Am J Med* 86(5):533-538, 1989.

23. Phelan JA et al: Oral findings in patients with acquired immunodeficiency syndrome, *Oral Surg Oral Med Oral Pathol* 64(1):50-56, 1987.

24. Quintiliani R et al: Treatment and prevention of oropharyngeal candidiasis, *Am J Med* 30:44-48, 1984.

25. Rico MJ, Penneys NS: Cutaneous *Cryptococcus* resembling molluscum contagiosum in a patient with AIDS, *Arch Dermatol* 121:901-902, 1985.

26. Shechtman LB et al: Clotrimazole treatment of oral candidiasis in patients with neoplastic disease, *Am J Med* 76:91-94, 1984.

27. Smith PD et al: Intestinal infections in patients with acquired immunodeficiency syndrome (AIDS): etiology and response to therapy, *Ann Intern Med* 108:328-333, 1988.

28. Steffen C, Markman JA: Spontaneous disappearance of molluscum contagiosum: report of a case, *Arch Dermatol* 116(8):923-924, 1980.

29. Svejgaard E: Oral ketoconazole as an alternative to griseofulvin in recalcitrant dermatophyte infections and on-

ychomycosis, *Acta Derm Venereol* (Stockh) 65(2):143-149, 1985.

30. Symoens J et al: An evaluation of two years of clinical experience with ketoconazole, *Rev Infect Dis* 2:674-682, 1980.

31. Torrsander J et al: Oral *Candida albicans* in HIV infection, *Scand J Infect Dis* 19(3):291-295, 1987.

32. Tukutuku K et al: Oral manifestations of AIDS in a heterosexual population in a Zaire hospital, *J Oral Pathol Med* 19(5):232-234, 1990.

33. Van Parys G et al: Ketoconazole-induced hepatitis: a case with definite cause-effect relationship, *Liver* 7(1):27-30, 1987.

34. Von Roenn JH et al: Megestrol acetate for treatment of cachexia associated with human immunodeficiency virus (HIV), *Ann Intern Med* 109:840-841, 1988.

35. Walsoe I, Stangerup M, Svejgaard E: Itraconazole in onychomycosis: open and double-blind studies, *Acta Derm Venereol* (Stockh) 70(2):137-140, 1990.

36. Weismann K, Knudsen EA, Pedersen C: White nails in AIDS/ARC due to *Trichophyton rubrum* infection, *Clin Exp Dermatol* 13(1):24-25, 1988.

37. Yap BS, Bodey GP: Oropharyngeal candidiasis treated with a troche form of clotrimazole, *Arch Intern Med* 139:656-657, 1979.

CHAPTER 9

The Treatment of Common HIV-Related Infections, Kaposi's Sarcoma, and Autoimmune Thrombocytopenia

Opportunistic infections
   Pneumocystis Carinii Pneumonia
   Toxoplasmosis
   Cryptococcosis
   Mycobacterium Avium-Intracellulare
     Infections
   Cryptosporidiosis
   Isosporiasis
   Cytomegalovirus (CMV) Infection

Herpes Simplex Virus
Candidiasis
Tuberculosis
Syphilis
Kaposi's Sarcoma
Autoimmune Thrombocytopenia
Drugs commonly used in the management of HIV-infected patients

An understanding of current approaches to diagnosis and management of common AIDS-related disorders is essential for the primary care physician caring for ambulatory HIV-infected patients. The need for hospitalization or subspecialty consultation cannot be adequately assessed without a working knowledge of the diagnostic procedures that may be required and the treatment options available. Continued ambulatory therapy after discharge from the hospital is indicated for most opportunistic infections.

The clinician should also recognize that HIV infection influences the clinical manifestations, natural history, and management of several disorders that are not numbered among the conventional AIDS-related opportunistic infections. Most important among these are tuberculosis and syphilis.

What follows is an overview of the diagnosis and management of common infectious complications of HIV infection, as well as Kaposi's sarcoma and autoimmune thrombocytopenia. Conventional approaches to management as well as selected therapies that are currently investigational are discussed. Brief summaries of clinical features and diagnostic criteria for each disorder are also given, although more detailed discussions of these aspects of each disorder are provided elsewhere in this book. Indications, common dosages, and side effects for drugs frequently used in the management of HIV-related infections are provided in the boxes at the end of the chapter.

Information concerning clinical trials of therapies for opportunistic infections and Kaposi's sarcoma can be obtained by contacting the National Institute of Allergy and Infectious Disease (NIAID). An informational telephone line (1-800-TRIALSA) is available for this purpose.

OPPORTUNISTIC INFECTIONS
Pneumocystis Carinii Pneumonia

Incidence. In the United States and other developed countries, pneumonia caused by *Pneumocystis carinii* is the initial opportunistic infection in approximately 60% of patients with AIDS, and it eventually occurs in more than 70% of patients.[62] As with other AIDS-related opportunistic infections, HIV-infected patients at greatest risk of developing *P. carinii* pneumonia (PCP) are those with a prior history of opportunistic infection or with a CD4 lymphocyte count below 200/mm^3.[78]

Clinical manifestations. A diagnosis of *Pneumocystis carinii* pneumonia should be considered in HIV-infected patients reporting new respiratory complaints. Fever, nonproductive cough, and dyspnea on exertion are the most frequent complaints in patients with PCP.[91] Symptoms may progress rapidly over a few days or gradually over weeks. In some cases the earliest clues to the diagnosis may be an unexplained fever or rising serum lactate dehydrogenase levels.[116] PCP may occur in patients receiving prophylaxis with any of the standard agents, including trimethoprim-sulfamethoxazole, pyrimethamine-sulfadoxine, dapsone, or pentamidine. The clinical and radiographic features of PCP may be altered in these patients, particularly those receiving aerosolized pentamidine.[57]

Extrapulmonary *Pneumocystis* infection[120] associated with nonspecific features and various sites of involvement, including the skin[29] and ear,[113] has been reported with increasing frequency, particularly among patients receiving aerosolized pentamidine (see below).

Diagnosis

Roentgenographic studies. A roentgenographic pattern of diffuse interstitial and alveolar infiltrates is suggestive but not diagnostic of PCP. Thoracic lymphadenopathy and pleural involvement are unusual. Atypical patterns, including localized infiltrates and cavity formation, may also be seen.

Radionuclide studies. Diffuse uptake on gallium scanning of the lungs is suggestive but not diagnostic of PCP.

Bronchoscopy. Cysts of *P. carinii* usually can be demonstrated in bronchoalveolar lavage or transbronchial biopsy specimens stained by the Giemsa or methenamine silver techniques. The definitive diagnosis of PCP is generally made in this manner. Examination of sputum specimens may also demonstrate the organism.

Conventional therapy. Confirmed or suspected PCP may be treated with either trimethoprim-sulfamethoxazole (20 mg/kg/day trimethoprim, 100 mg/kg/day sulfamethoxazole in a fixed combination given in four divided doses) or pentamidine isethionate (4 mg/kg in a single daily dose). Reported response rates have been in the range of 70% to 95%, depending on the severity of disease.[91] Prospective studies have failed to demonstrate a clear advantage of either pentamidine or trimethoprim-sulfamethoxazole in safety or efficacy.[112,138]

Side effects are commonly seen with both drugs. Rash and anemia were each seen in approximately 40% of patients receiving trimethoprim-sulfamethoxazole, whereas more than 60% of patients receiving pentamidine developed nephrotoxicity and approximately one fourth developed hypotension or hypoglycemia in one controlled study.[112] Many clinicians favor trimethoprim-sulfamethoxazole because toxicity is less often life threatening than that seen with pentamidine.

The optimum duration of therapy has not been determined through prospective studies, but retrospective data have suggested that AIDS-related PCP responds more slowly to antimicrobial therapy than does PCP occurring in other immunodeficiency states[64]; this has led to the common practice of continuing full-dose trimethoprim-sulfamethoxazole or pentamidine for approximately 21 days.

Alternative approaches to therapy

Oral trimethoprim-sulfamethoxazole. Patients with PCP generally should be hospitalized and treated with parenteral therapy. However, in one series,[82] oral trimethoprim-sulfamethoxazole (20 mg/kg trimethoprim and 100 mg/kg sulfamethoxazole, given in four divided doses) was effective in 90% of patients with initial episodes of mild to moderate PCP (Po$_2$ over 60 mm Hg). Oral therapy can be considered for compliant patients without gastrointestinal disease who can be closely monitored for respiratory symptoms.[65]

Dapsone-trimethoprim. Oral combined therapy with dapsone (100 mg/day) and trimethoprim (20 mg/kg/day) has been shown to be as effective as conventional therapy for mild to moderate PCP[71,82] and may have fewer side effects. As noted previously, however, oral therapy should be considered only for compliant patients without gastrointestinal disease whose respiratory status can be monitored closely.

Aerosolized pentamidine. Because of the significant toxicity of systemic therapy, aerosolized pentamidine, which is effective in prophylaxis for PCP, has been evaluated as therapy. In an early study, 13 of 15 patients with mild to moderate PCP (room air Po_2 over 50 mm Hg) were treated successfully with daily aerosolized pentamidine (600 mg via specific nebulizer) for 21 days.[88] The results of randomized trials have been discouraging, however. In one study, aerosolized pentamidine (600 mg daily) was associated with a lower response rate (53% versus 81%) and a higher relapse rate (24% versus 0) than reduced-dose systemic pentamidine (3 mg/kg daily) in patients with mild to moderate disease (Po_2 over 55 mm Hg)[27]; however, toxicity was not seen in this study among patients receiving aerosolized therapy, whereas 14% of patients receiving systemic therapy had major side effects. In another randomized trial, aerosolized pentamidine was shown to be effective only for patients with mild PCP (mean arterial Po_2 of 81 mm Hg).[51]

Although toxicity remains substantial with reduced-dose intravenous pentamidine (3 mg/kg/day), reported rates of major side effects are generally less than those seen with full-dose therapy (4 mg/kg/day). In view of its greater efficacy, therefore, reduced-dose intravenous therapy is probably preferable to aerosolized pentamidine for mild to moderate PCP.

Clindamycin-primaquine. Combination therapy with clindamycin (600 mg four times a day intravenously or 300 to 450 mg four times a day orally) and primaquine (15 mg base once a day orally) was shown to be effective in some patients who were unresponsive or intolerant to conventional therapy in one study.[121] The results of preliminary trials designed to further evaluate this therapy will probably be available in the next 2 to 3 years.

Trimetrexate-leucovorin. The antifolate drug trimetrexate, administered with leucovorin, was shown to be effective in approximately two thirds of cases either as initial therapy or as salvage therapy for patients failing conventional therapy.[2] The efficacy of trimetrexate currently is being evaluated in clinical trials.

Corticosteroids. Corticosteroids have improved the survival of patients with respiratory failure caused by PCP.[41,76] In one series,[41] the survival rate was 75% among patients with severe infection who received a regimen of methylprednisolone (40 mg intravenously four times a day) plus trimethoprim-sulfamethoxazole in standard doses; in contrast, the survival rate was 18% among patients receiving trimethoprim-sulfamethoxazole and a placebo.

In another controlled study, patients with moderate to severe PCP who received prednisone (40 mg twice daily) in addition to trimethoprim-sulfamethoxazole, trimethoprim-dapsone, or pentamidine had a substantially lower risk of respiratory failure than those receiving standard therapy alone.[11]

In 1990 a consensus panel of the National Institute of Allergy and Infectious Disease (NIAID) recommended that patients with PCP whose Po_2 was below 70 mm Hg or whose arterial-alveolar difference was greater than 35 mm Hg receive adjunctive corticosteroids within 72 hours of starting anti-*Pneumocystis* therapy. The panel recommended the following regimen: prednisone, 40 mg twice daily, days 1 through 5; 20 mg twice daily, days 6 through 10; and 20 mg once a day, days 11 through 21.

Prophylaxis/chronic suppressive therapy. HIV-infected patients who have had PCP and all those with a CD4 lymphocyte count under $200/mm^3$ should receive continuous prophylaxis.[21] See Chapter 6 for recommended regimens.

Toxoplasmosis

Incidence. Cerebral toxoplasmosis is the initial manifestation of AIDS in 2% of cases.[54]

Clinical manifestations. Toxoplasmosis typically manifests as an encephalitis that produces focal neurological deficits of sudden or gradual onset. Lethargy, confusion, and headache are other common symptoms.[92]

Diagnosis. Although the diagnosis of cerebral toxoplasmosis can be confirmed only by histological examination of brain tissue, the diagnosis is most often made on clinical and radiographic grounds because of the morbidity of brain biopsy.[24]

Typical findings of cerebral toxoplasmosis include multiple, bilateral ring-enhancing lesions demonstrated by computed tomography (CT) or magnetic resonance imaging (MRI). Solitary lesions also may be seen. Radiographic findings of cerebral lymphoma, cerebral tuberculosis, and, occasionally, other opportunistic infections may be indistinguishable from those of toxoplasmosis.

Blood tests for *Toxoplasma* antibody may be of value in patients with typical clinical and radiographic abnormalities, because cerebral toxoplasmosis is extremely unusual without serological evidence of the disease.

Therapy. Because of the morbidity of brain biopsy and the high frequency of toxoplasmosis in HIV-infected patients who have signs of focal encephalitis, the trend in recent years has been toward empirical therapy.[24]

The therapeutic regimen of choice for cerebral toxoplasmosis is a combination of sulfadiazine and pyrimethamine administered orally. The optimum duration of therapy has not been established. Relapse rates are high if therapy is discontinued, and it has become common practice to continue sulfadiazine and pyrimethamine indefinitely, although the most effective regimen for long-term suppressive therapy is not known. Pedrol and colleagues[96] reported no relapses among 14 patients receiving intermittent maintenance therapy (twice per week) with sulfadiazine and pyrimethamine. Many clinicians prefer to continue daily therapy, however.

Future directions in therapy. Preliminary clinical data suggest that combination therapy with clindamycin and pyrimethamine may represent an alternative to sulfadiazine in patients with sulfonamide hypersensitivity.[30,47,108,136] However, a relapse rate of 33% on therapy with clindamycin and pyrimethamine was reported in one small series,[72] suggesting that this regimen may be more effective for initial therapy than for maintenance. A pilot study of oral clindamycin and pyrimethamine, conducted by the AIDS Clinical Trials Group of the National Institute of Allergy and Infectious Disease, was in progress at the time of this writing.

Cryptococcosis

Incidence. The yeast *Cryptococcus neoformans* is the most common cause of meningitis in AIDS and may also cause infection of the respiratory tract and other extraneural sites. Cryptococcosis is the initial opportunistic infection in approximately 7% of AIDS cases.[16]

Clinical manifestations. Cryptococcal meningitis may present with subacute or acute manifestations. Fever and headache lasting from days to weeks are the most common presenting symptoms. Seizures and focal neurological abnormalities are unusual. Nuchal rigidity is seen only in the minority of cases.

Cryptococcal infection may involve sites outside the central nervous system, most often the respiratory tract or skin, although most patients have concomitant meningitis. Other sites of involvement include the myocardium,[13] pericardium,[114] lymph nodes, adrenal glands, spleen, kidneys,[44,95,106,135] prostate,[68,73] eyes,[14,74] placenta,[69] and thyroid.[77]

Interstitial infiltrates and hilar lymphadenopathy, either alone or in combination, are the radiographic patterns most often encountered in pulmonary cryptococcosis,[84] although mediastinal lymph node involvement,[122] empyema,[58,93,133] adult respiratory distress syndrome,[90] and nodules may also be seen.

Skin lesions mimicking molluscum contagiosum[26,107] and herpes simplex infection[10] have been described. Occasionally *Cryptococcus* has been isolated from oral lesions[45] and anal ulcerations.[127]

Diagnosis. The diagnosis of cryptococcal meningitis is confirmed by examination of the cerebrospinal fluid (CSF). India ink stain, cryptococcal antigen assay (serum and CSF), and culture are all positive in most cases. Extraneural infections may be diagnosed by biopsy of the affected organ (lung, skin), culture of blood or appropriate body fluid, or serum antigen assay.

Primary therapy. Amphotericin B, either alone or in combination with 5-flucytosine, is the established mode of therapy[5,126] for cryptococcal infection. The optimum duration of therapy in AIDS-related cases is unknown. Dismukes and colleagues[32] demonstrated that a 6-week course of therapy (amphotericin B, 0.3 mg/kg/day, and 5-flucytosine, 37.5 mg/kg every 6 hours) was associated with a lower relapse rate (16% versus 27%) than a 4-week regimen in a prospective study in which the minority of patients had AIDS. In general, therapy is continued until serum and CSF cryptococcal antigen levels fall significantly. Relapse rates in the range of 50% to 60% have been reported, however, even after prolonged courses of therapy.[63,144]

Fluconazole. Fluconazole, licensed in 1990, is a new antifungal triazole compound that can be administered orally and that attains high concentrations in the cerebrospinal fluid.[4] Early clinical data demonstrated higher rates of treatment failure with fluconazole (400 mg daily for 10 weeks) than with the combination of amphotericin B (0.7 mg/kg daily for 1 week, then three times a week for 9 weeks) and flucytosine (150 mg/kg daily in four divided doses).[69] The role of fluconazole in primary therapy has not yet been clearly defined.[42]

Suppressive therapy. Because of the high rate of relapse of cryptococcosis in AIDS, long-term suppressive therapy is advisable after primary therapy has been completed. None of seven patients relapsed while receiving suppressive therapy with weekly or twice-weekly amphotericin B infusions over follow-up periods ranging from 11 to 36 weeks in one series[144]; however, fatal relapse during similar therapy has been reported.

Two of 19 patients treated with daily oral fluconazole (50 to 200 mg) after primary therapy with amphotericin B (courses ranging from 20 to 257 days) relapsed during follow-up periods ranging from 3 to 21 months.[118] The results of additional clinical trials are pending.

Future directions in therapy. A related compound, itraconazole,[130] is active against the *Cryptococcus* organism and is under evaluation in human studies.

Mycobacterium Avium-Intracellulare Infections

Incidence. *Mycobacterium avium-intracellulare* (MAI) was isolated in 60% of AIDS cases in one autopsy series.[139] It is a common cause of disseminated infection in clinical reports.[48,141,142]

Clinical manifestations. Unlike typical tuberculosis, infection with MAI generally manifests in extrapulmonary sites. The symptoms of disseminated MAI infection usually are insidious. Unexplained fever, weight loss, diarrhea, or anemia should raise the suspicion of MAI involvement of the gastrointestinal tract, bone marrow, or liver particularly.

Diagnosis. The diagnosis of infection with MAI is most often made on the basis of histological examination and mycobacterial culture of tissue from sites such as liver or bone marrow. The organism may also be isolated from blood. The significance of MAI in respiratory secretions in the absence of progressive pulmonary disease is unclear. As with most mycobacterial infections, confirmation by culture may take several months.

Therapy. The optimum therapy of MAI has not been determined. Attempts at treatment are often frustrated by the organism's resistance to conventional antituberculous agents and by the advanced state of immunodeficiency usually present at the time of diagnosis.

Recent studies have suggested the efficacy of several multidrug regimens. Combined therapy with intravenous amikacin (7.5 mg/kg for 4 weeks), ciprofloxacin (750 mg twice a day), ethambutol (1,000 mg daily), and rifampin (600 mg daily) was associated with symptomatic improvement and suppression of cultures in one series.[22] A regimen of ansamycin (150 mg daily), isoniazid (300 mg daily), ethambutol (15 mg/kg daily), and clofazimine (100 mg daily) was associated with suppression of symptoms in all patients and clearance of mycobacteremia in 85% in another series.[1]

Future directions in therapy. The investigational macrolide antibiotic azithromycin has been shown to have activity against MAI.[7,53] It is unknown at present if this drug will prove clinically useful.

Cryptosporidiosis

Incidence. The protozoal parasite *Cryptosporidium* is a common cause of diarrhea in AIDS patients, although its exact incidence is unknown.

Clinical manifestations. Chronic, watery diarrhea is the most common clinical manifestation of cryptosporidial infection. Biliary tract involvement is also common and may be characterized by clinical or biochemical signs of common duct obstruction.

Diagnosis. The diagnosis of cryptosporidiosis is generally easily confirmed by examination of stool using special concentration techniques and the modified acid-fast stain. In rare instances the organism cannot be detected in stool but can be visualized on examination of small bowel secretions or biopsy specimens.

Therapy. Attempts to treat cryptosporidiosis with a variety of agents have been unsuccessful. Drugs used in the therapy of other protozoal infections (e.g., metronidazole, diiodohydroxyquin, tetracycline, chloroquine, primaquine, and quinacrine) are ineffective.[15]

Future directions in therapy

Diclazuril. On the basis of demonstrated efficacy against related organisms in animals,[128,129] the investigational anticoccidial drug diclazuril is being evaluated for therapy of cryptosporidiosis.

Bovine colostrum. Therapy of cryptosporidiosis using immunoglobulins derived from the colostrum of cows hyperimmunized against the *Cryptosporidium* organism has been shown to be effective in animals.[38] Preliminary reports have shown some efficacy of hyperimmune bovine colostrum therapy in AIDS-related cryptosporidiosis in humans.[94,124,125] The results of early clinical trials were not available at the time of this writing.

In related experimental strategies, an extract of lymph nodes[80] and oral bovine transfer factor from immunized cows[75] showed efficacy in preliminary human studies.

Spiramycin. The macrolide antibiotic spiramycin has been effective in the therapy of AIDS-related cryptosporidiosis in several uncontrolled studies.[89,101] Results have been equivocal in controlled trials in immunologically normal infants, however,[110,140] and treatment failures have been reported in AIDS patients.[98,143] The results of controlled trials should be available within the next few years.

Somatostatin. Somatostatin analogs have been used successfully to treat diarrhea related to cryptosporidiosis in AIDS in several reported cases.[23,28,59]

Isosporiasis

Incidence. Isosporiasis is a common cause of diarrhea in AIDS patients. Its exact incidence is unknown.

Clinical manifestations. Like cryptosporidiosis, isosporiasis typically is characterized by severe and persistent watery diarrhea.

Diagnosis. The diagnosis of *Isospora belli* infection can be confirmed in most cases by microscopic examination of stool or small bowel secretions.

Therapy. In contrast to cryptosporidiosis, isosporiasis typically responds well to therapy with trimethoprim-sulfamethoxazole.[137] Although the optimum treatment regimen is not known, one double-strength tablet (160 mg trimethoprim/800 mg sulfamethoxazole) is generally effective. Therapy may have to be continued for several weeks.[137] Pyrimethamine (75 mg daily) is also effective and may be used in cases of sulfa hypersensitivity.[134]

Cytomegalovirus (CMV) Infection

Incidence. Cytomegalovirus (CMV) has been the most common opportunistic pathogen identified in autopsies of AIDS patients in some series and is the most frequent cause of sight-threatening retinitis.

Clinical manifestations. Retinitis, esophagitis, and colitis are the most common specific clinical manifestations of CMV infection.

Diagnosis. The diagnosis of retinitis is strongly suggested by specific features of the fundoscopic examination. Ophthalmological consultation is advisable for confirmation of CMV retinitis. Endoscopic biopsy is usually required to confirm the diagnosis of esophageal or colonic involvement.

Therapy. The mainstay of therapy of serious infections caused by cytomegalovirus is ganciclovir (9-[1,3-dihydroxy-2-propoxymethyl] guanine), a derivative of the antiherpes drug acyclovir. Ganciclovir is effective in the therapy of retinitis, colitis, and, to a lesser extent, pneumonitis caused by CMV* and may prolong survival.[61] Ganciclovir-resistant CMV strains have been reported.[34]

Future directions in therapy. The pyrophosphate analogue Foscarnet may be effective in patients with retinitis[36,55] or pneumonia caused by CMV.[37] Clinical trials of this drug are in progress.

Herpes Simplex Virus

Incidence. Herpes simplex infections are seen in approximately 20% of patients with AIDS or ARC.[46]

Clinical manifestations. Herpes simplex infection typically manifests with painful ulcerations on the lips, in the mouth, or in the genital region. Disseminated cutaneous infection and, in rare cases, visceral disease may also occur.

Diagnosis. The diagnosis of herpes simplex infection often can be confirmed by culture or biopsy of lesions. Viral transport media, as well as laboratory facilities for viral culture, are required to isolate the virus. The lesions' response to antiviral chemotherapy may serve to confirm the diagnosis in some cases.

Therapy. Mucocutaneous herpes simplex infections generally respond to therapy with oral acyclovir (200 to 400 mg five times a day). Therapy should be continued until the lesions have resolved. For patients with gastrointestinal disease affecting absorption or for those with severe localized or disseminated cutaneous or visceral infection, parenteral acyclovir (5 mg/kg every 8 hours) is generally effective. Chronic suppressive therapy may be appropriate for patients with severe localized disease or frequent recurrences. The optimum dose for such long-term therapy in AIDS is unknown, although a regimen of 400 mg twice a day was found to be effective in preventing recurrences in normal hosts.[83]

Acyclovir-resistant herpes simplex isolates have been isolated from AIDS

*References 12, 25, 31, 39, 70, 79, 109.

patients.[9] The best approach to therapy of infection with resistant strains has not yet been determined, although trisodium phosphonoformate (foscarnet)[35,111] or continuous-infusion acyclovir[33] may be effective.

Candidiasis

Incidence. Oral candidiasis (thrush) occurred in more than 90% of patients with AIDS in one series[97] and more than 39% of symptomatic HIV-infected patients in another.[123] Candidiasis is the most frequent cause of esophagitis in HIV-infected patients[105] and was documented on routine endoscopic examination in approximately 50% of patients in one series.[100]

Clinical manifestations. Patients with candidal esophagitis typically have pain and discomfort on swallowing. Oral candidiasis with such symptoms is strongly associated with candidal infection of the esophagus.

Diagnosis. Oral candidiasis, which typically produces white plaques on the tongue, gingiva, and buccal mucosa, is most often diagnosed on clinical grounds. Distinguishing thrush from oral hairy leukoplakia occasionally may be difficult. Microscopic examination of scrapings may be necessary to confirm the diagnosis of candidiasis. Candidal esophagitis may be confirmed by esophagoscopy and biopsy, although a response of symptoms to empirical antifungal therapy allows a presumptive diagnosis in patients not undergoing this procedure.

Therapy. Candidal esophagitis typically responds promptly to systemic antifungal therapy with ketoconazole, fluconazole, or, in refractory cases, parenteral amphotericin B. Oral therapy with ketoconazole (200 to 400 mg daily) or fluconazole (200 mg in an initial dose, followed by 100 mg daily) is effective in most ambulatory patients.

Tuberculosis

Incidence. Beginning in 1986, after 30 years of steady decline, the incidence of tuberculosis in the United States began to rise.[20] This increase has been attributed in large part to increasing numbers of cases of active tuberculosis among HIV-infected individuals.[20,115]

Clinical manifestations. In most cases the clinical manifestations of tuberculosis in the HIV-infected individual are comparable to those in other patients. However, extrapulmonary infection (e.g., lymphatic and miliary) appears to be more common in HIV-related tuberculosis,[17] and distinctive pulmonary radiographic patterns, such as lower lobe involvement, are seen more frequently.[99] Cavitary disease may be less prevalent in HIV-related cases.[40]

Diagnosis. As in other patients, the diagnosis of tuberculosis in HIV-infected individuals is typically made on the basis of microscopic examination of respiratory secretions or tissue specimens stained with the acid-fast technique. Specific culture techniques are required to confirm the diagnosis of *Mycobacterium tuberculosis* infection, particularly in view of the high prevalence of atypical mycobacterial infections in these patients.

Therapy. The American Thoracic Society and the Centers for Disease Control have recommended the following treatment regimen for tuberculosis in which there is no proven or suspected isoniazid resistance[3]:

1. Isoniazid (300 mg orally), rifampin (600 mg orally), and pyrazinamide (15 to 30 mg/kg orally, to a maximum dosage of 2 g), for 2 months
2. Isoniazid and rifampin (in above dosages) for 4 more months

It has been suggested that therapy be continued for a minimum of 9 months, or 6 months after negative cultures have been obtained in HIV-infected patients.[17]

If isolated isoniazid resistance is documented, a regimen of isoniazid, rifampin, ethambutol, and, initially, pyrazinamide should be administered for a minimum of 12 months.[3]

Screening of HIV-infected individuals by means of tuberculin skin testing and therapy of those with positive skin tests without tuberculosis is discussed in Chapter 6.

Syphilis

Incidence. During the last half of the 1980s, the incidence of primary and secondary syphilis, as well as congenital infection, began increasing dramatically, particularly in areas with high seroprevalence of HIV infection.[18] It is unclear if a direct relationship exists between syphilis and HIV infection, although HIV-infected patients have been found to have a greater likelihood of previous syphilis in several series.[103,117]

Clinical manifestations. Although the clinical and laboratory features of syphilis in HIV-infected patients are usually similar to those in uninfected patients, in some cases the presentation of syphilis appears to be altered by concomitant HIV infection.[19,52] Progression of disease despite standard therapy[8,56] and false-negative serological tests[50] has been reported.

Diagnosis. It has been recommended that serological testing for syphilis (VDRL) be performed on all patients who acquired HIV infection through sexual contact or intravenous drug use.[19] Dark-field examination or direct fluorescent antibody staining of exudate from lesions should be performed when there is clinical suspicion of syphilis despite negative serological studies.[19]

Therapy. Early syphilis (primary, secondary, and early latent) should be treated as in non-HIV-infected patients; with benzathine penicillin 2.4 million units intramuscularly. VDRL tests should be done at intervals of 1, 2, and 3 months after treatment. If serological titers do not decrease (twofold by 3 months in primary syphilis, by 6 months in secondary syphilis), a lumbar puncture should be performed to exclude neurosyphilis.[19]

In cases of late latent syphilis or infection of unknown duration, the cerebrospinal fluid should be examined before therapy to exclude neurosyphilis. If there is no evidence of neurosyphilis, benzathine penicillin should be administered (2.4 million units intramuscularly weekly for 3 weeks). Patients with neurosyphilis, either symptomatic or asymptomatic, should receive intravenous therapy (aqueous penicillin G, 2 to 4 million units every 4 hours for 10 days).[19]

Tetracycline (500 mg orally, four times a day for 14 days) or doxycycline (100 mg two times a day for 14 days) should be used in the therapy of primary, secondary, or latent syphilis of less than 1 year's duration in cases of penicillin allergy. Tetracycline or doxycycline should be continued for 28 days in patients with late latent or tertiary syphilis who are unable to receive penicillin.

Kaposi's Sarcoma

Incidence. Kaposi's sarcoma has been reported in approximately 15% of AIDS cases in the United States.[6]

Clinical manifestations. Kaposi's sarcoma typically manifests as macular or nodular lesions, often purplish in color, on epidermal or mucosal surfaces. The mouth, face, trunk, and extremities are all frequently involved. There may be a single lesion or many. Visceral involvement is common, particularly of the lungs, lymph nodes, and gastrointestinal tract.

Diagnosis. Because several other AIDS-related skin disorders may resemble Kaposi's sarcoma, the diagnosis requires histological confirmation. Pulmonary involvement produces radiographic and clinical features comparable to *Pneumocystis carinii* pneumonia and other opportunistic infections.

Therapy. Limited Kaposi's sarcoma confined to the skin does not usually require specific therapy. Surgical excision or local irradiation may be used for cosmetic reasons, however. Widespread cutaneous or systemic (particularly pulmonary) Kaposi's sarcoma may require systemic therapy. Responses have been reported with α-interferon,[49,66,67] vincristine,[85] vinblastine,[131] or combination therapy with adriamycin, bleomycin, and vincristine, or bleomycin and vincristine.[43]

Future directions in therapy. A variety of regimens, using chemotherapeutic agents alone or combining AZT with interferons or chemotherapeutic regimens, are currently under evaluation for the therapy of Kaposi's sarcoma.

Autoimmune Thrombocytopenia

Incidence. Thrombocytopenia was found in 61% of AIDS patients in one series;[86] it may be caused by autoimmune mechanisms at all stages of HIV infection.[104]

Diagnosis. Examination of the bone marrow is required to distinguish autoimmune thrombocytopenia from depletion of megakaryocytes because of the effects of disseminated opportunistic infection (e.g., mycobacteriosis, histoplasmosis), drug toxicity, or HIV itself.

Therapy. No immediate therapy may be necessary for patients with no bleeding manifestations and platelet counts above 20,000/mm^3, since thrombocytopenia may resolve spontaneously.[132] Patients requiring therapy usually respond well to corticosteroids or to splenectomy,[132] although worsening of the immunodeficiency state obviously may result from these measures. Therapy with immunoglobulin, danazol, or cytotoxic agents such as vincristine is recommended in refractory cases.[104] The antiretroviral drug AZT has been shown to raise the platelet count in HIV-infected patients with and without autoimmune thrombocytopenia,[87] and it may have a role in therapy.[87,102,119] The means by which zidovudine elevates the platelet count currently is not clear.

DRUGS COMMONLY USED IN THE MANAGEMENT OF HIV-INFECTED PATIENTS

The following boxes provide a summary of indications, side effects, and dosage regimens of drugs commonly used in the treatment of ambulatory HIV-infected patients. The use of medications in pregnancy is discussed in Chapter 11. When dosage adjustment is required, the manufacturer's guidelines should be consulted.

Trimethoprim-Sulfamethoxazole[181]

Route of administration: Oral, intravenous
Indications: Therapy, primary or secondary prophylaxis of *Pneumocystis carinii* infection; therapy of isosporiasis, salmonellosis
Common side effects: Hypersensitivity reactions, Stevens-Johnson syndrome, photosensitivity, neutropenia
Usual adult dosage: Prophylaxis of *Pneumocystis carinii* infection—double-strength tablet (160 mg trimethoprim, 800 mg sulfamethoxazole) every other day to twice a day; treatment of *Pneumocystis carinii* infection—15 to 20 mg/kg trimethoprim, 75 to 100 mg/kg sulfamethoxazole daily in four divided doses
Dosage adjustments: Renal insufficiency

Sulfadiazine

Route of administration: Oral
Indications: Therapy (initial and suppressive) of toxoplasmosis, with pyrimethamine
Common side effects: Hypersensitivity reactions, Stevens-Johnson syndrome, photosensitivity, nephrolithiasis, bone marrow depression
Usual adult dosage: 2 to 6 g daily in four divided doses
Dosage adjustments: Renal insufficiency

Pyrimethamine

Route of administration: Oral
Indications: Toxoplasmosis (with sulfadiazine or clindamycin)
Side effects: Folate deficiency, pancytopenia, hypersensitivity reactions
Usual adult dosage: 25 to 75 mg a day orally with folinic acid, 5 to 15 mg a day orally
Dosage adjustments: No

Dapsone

Route of administration: Oral
Indications: Therapy (with trimethoprim) or primary or secondary prophylaxis of *Pneumocystis carinii* infection
Common side effects: Hypersensitivity reactions, blood dyscrasias
Usual adult dosage: 50 to 100 mg a day
Dosage adjustments: Renal insufficiency

Pentamidine

Route of administration: Aerosol, intramuscular, intravenous
Indications: Therapy (parenteral) or primary or secondary prophylaxis (parenteral or aerosolized) of *Pneumocystis carinii* infections
Common side effects: Systemic therapy—hypotension, hyperglycemia, hypoglycemia, renal insufficiency, bone marrow depression; aerosol therapy—bronchospasm
Usual adult dosage:
Pneumocystis carinii (therapy)—4 mg/kg a day intravenously for 14 to 21 days
Pneumocystis carinii pneumonia (prevention)—300 mg a month by aerosol
Dosage adjustments: Renal insufficiency

Ketoconazole

Route of administration: Oral
Indications: Oral, esophageal candidiasis; cutaneous fungal infections; suppressive therapy for histoplasmosis
Side effects: Gastrointestinal upset, hepatitis (occasionally severe), inhibition of glucocorticoid, and testosterone synthesis
Usual adult dosage: 200 to 400 mg orally every 12 to 24 hours
Dosage adjustments: No
Note: Requires acid gastric pH

Fluconazole

Route of administration: Oral, intravenous
Indications: Oral, esophageal candidiasis; chronic suppressive therapy of cryptococcal infection, including meningitis
Common side effects: Gastrointestinal upset occasionally is seen
Usual adult dosage: Oral or esophageal candidiasis—200 mg initial dose, followed by 100 mg daily; cryptococcosis or systemic candidiasis—400 mg initial dose, followed by 200 to 400 mg daily
Dosage adjustments: Renal insufficiency

Acyclovir

Route of administration: Topical, oral, intravenous
Indications: Therapy of mucocutaneous (oral, topical, intravenous) or systemic (intravenous) herpes simplex infections; long-term suppression of mucocutaneous herpes simplex infections; possible synergy with zidovudine; therapy of localized or disseminated varicella zoster infection
Common side effects: Headache, rash, nausea, diarrhea, and bone marrow depression; seizures and hepatic and renal toxicity are seen in rare cases
Usual adult dosage:
  Localized herpes simplex infection (genital): Topical—every 4 hours while awake; oral—200 mg every 4 hours while awake; intravenous—15 mg/kg/day in three divided doses
  Localized herpes simplex infection (oral): Oral—as above; intravenous—as above
  Generalized or visceral herpes simplex infection: Intravenous—as above
  Localized varicella zoster infection: Oral—800 mg every 4 hours while awake; intravenous—10 to 12 mg/kg every 8 hours
  Generalized or visceral varicella zoster infection: Intravenous—10 to 12 mg/kg every 8 hours
Dosage adjustments: Renal insufficiency

Ganciclovir

Route of administration: Intravenous
Indications: Therapy and long-term suppression of cytomegaloviral (CMV) retinitis; therapy of pneumonitis, esophagitis, and colitis caused by CMV
Common side effects: Bone marrow depression
Usual adult dosage: 5 mg/kg intravenously twice daily for 14 days, followed by 5 mg/kg intravenously once daily, indefinitely
Dosage adjustments: Renal insufficiency

Isoniazid

Route of administration: Oral
Indications: Single-drug therapy (prophylaxis) of tuberculin-positive patients; component of multidrug regimen in therapy of active mycobacterial infections
Side effects: Hepatitis, peripheral neuropathy, hypersensitivity reactions
Usual adult dosage: 300 mg per day orally
Dosage adjustments: Renal insufficiency

Rifampin

Route of administration: Oral
Indications: Component of multidrug regimen in therapy of active mycobacterial infection
Side effects: Hepatitis, hypersensitivity reactions, orange discoloration of urine and tears; accelerates metabolism of methadone (may cause withdrawal symptoms), corticosteroids, and oral hypoglycemic agents
Usual adult dosage: 600 mg per day orally
Dosage adjustments: None

Pyrazinamide

Route of administration: Oral
Indications: Component of multidrug regimen in therapy of active mycobacterial infections
Common side effects: Hepatitis, hyperuricemia
Usual adult dosage: 15 to 30 mg/kg per day orally (maximum daily dose: 2 g)
Dosage adjustments: Renal insufficiency

Zidovudine (AZT)

Route of administration: Oral, intravenous
Indications: Antiretroviral therapy of HIV-infected patients with CD4 lymphocyte count
    under 500/mm^3 (see Chapter 10)
Side effects: Bone marrow depression
Usual adult dosage: 100 mg orally every 4 hours while awake
Dosage adjustments: Renal insufficiency

REFERENCES

1. Agins BD et al: Effect of combined therapy with ansamycin, clofazimine, ethambutol, and isoniazid for *Mycobacterium avium* infection in patients with AIDS, *J Infect Dis* 159(4):784-787, 1989.

2. Allegra CJ et al: Trimetrexate for the treatment of *Pneumocystis carinii* pneumonia in patients with the acquired immunodeficiency syndrome, *N Engl J Med* 317:978-985, 1987.

3. American Thoracic Society: Treatment of tuberculosis and tuberculosis infection in adults and children, *Am Rev Respir Dis* 134:355-363, 1986.

4. Arndt CAS et al: Fluconazole penetration into cerebrospinal fluid: implications for treating fungal infections of the central nervous system, *J Infect Dis* 157(1):178-180, 1988.

5. Bennett JE et al: A comparison of amphotericin B alone and combined with flucytosine in the treatment of cryptococcal meningitis, *N Engl J Med* 301:126-131, 1979.

6. Beral V et al: Kaposi's sarcoma among persons with AIDS: a sexually transmitted infection? *Lancet* 335(8682):123-128, 1990.

7. Bermudez LE, Young LS: Activities of amikacin, roxithromycin, and azithromycin alone or in combination with tumor necrosis factor against *Mycobacterium avium* complex, *Antimicrob Agents Chemother* 32(8):1149-1153, 1988.

8. Berry CD et al: Neurologic relapse after benzathine penicillin therapy for secondary syphilis in a patient with HIV infection, *N Engl J Med* 316(25):1587-1589, 1987.

9. Birch CJ et al: Altered sensitivity to antiviral drugs of herpes simplex virus isolates from a patient with the acquired immunodeficiency syndrome, *J Infect Dis* 162(3):731-734, 1990.

10. Borton LK, Wintroub BU: Disseminated cryptococcosis presenting as herpetiform lesions in a homosexual man with the acquired immunodeficiency syndrome, *J Am Acad Dermatol* 10:387-390, 1984.

11. Bozzette SA et al: A controlled trial of early adjunctive treatment with corticosteroids for *Pneumocystis carinii* pneumonia in the acquired immunodeficiency syndrome, *N Engl J Med* 323:1451-1457, 1990.

12. Buhles WC et al: Ganciclovir treatment of life- or sight-threatening cytomegalovirus infection: experience in 314 immunocompromised patients, *Rev Infect Dis* 10(suppl 3): S495-506, 1988.

13. Cammarosano C, Lewis W: Cardiac lesions in acquired immune deficiency syndrome (AIDS), *J Am Coll Cardiol* 5:703-706, 1985.

14. Carney MD, Combs JL, Waschler W: Cryptococcal choroiditis, *Retina* 10(1):27-32, 1990.

15. Centers for Disease Control: Cryptosporidiosis: assessment of chemotherapy of males with acquired immune deficiency syndrome (AIDS), *MMWR* 31(44):589-592, 1982.

16. Centers for Disease Control: Acquired immunodeficiency syndrome: United States, *MMWR* 35:17-21, 1986.

17. Centers for Disease Control: Diagnosis and management of mycobacterial infection and disease in persons with human immunodeficiency virus infection, *Ann Intern Med* 106:254-256, 1987.

18. Centers for Disease Control: Syphilis and congenital syphilis—United States, *MMWR* 37(32):486-489, 1988.

19. Centers for Disease Control: Recommendations for diagnosing and treating syphilis in HIV-infected patients, *MMWR* 37(39):600-608, 1988.

20. Centers for Disease Control: A strategic plan for the elimination of tuberculosis in the United States, *MMWR* 38(S-5):1-25, 1989.

21. Centers for Disease Control: Guidelines for prophylaxis against *Pneumocystis carinii* pneumonia for persons infected with human immunodeficiency virus, *MMWR* 38(S-5):1-9, 1989.

22. Chiu J et al: Treatment of disseminated *Mycobacterium avium* complex infection in AIDS with amikacin, ethambutol, rifampin, and ciprofloxacin, *Ann Intern Med* 113:358-361, 1990.

23. Clotet B et al: Efficacy of the somatostatin analogue (SMS-201-995), Sandostatin, for cryptosporidial diarrhea in patients with AIDS, *AIDS* 3(12):857-858, 1989.

24. Cohn JA et al: Evaluation of the policy of empiric treatment of suspected *Toxoplasma* encephalitis in patients with the acquired immunodeficiency syndrome, *Am J Med* 86:521-527, 1989.

25. Collaborative DHPG Treatment Study Group: Treatment of serious cytomegalovirus infections with 9-(1,3-dihydroxy-2-propoxymethyl) guanine in patients with AIDS and other immunodeficiencies, *N Engl J Med* 314(13):801-805, 1986.

26. Concus AP et al: Cutaneous *Cryptococcosis* mimicking molluscum contagiosum in a patient with AIDS, *J Infect Dis* 158:897-898, 1988.

27. Conte JE et al: Intravenous or inhaled pentamidine for treating *Pneumocystis carinii* pneumonia in AIDS: a randomized trial, *Ann Intern Med* 113:203-209, 1990.

28. Cook DJ et al: Somatostatin treatment for cryptosporidial diarrhea in a patient with the acquired immunodeficiency syndrome (AIDS), *Ann Intern Med* 108(5):708-709, 1988.

29. Coulman CU, Greene I, Archibald RWR: Cutaneous pneumocystosis, *Ann Intern Med* 106:396-398, 1987.

30. Dannemann BR, Israelski DM, Remington JS: Treatment of toxoplasmic encephalitis with intravenous clindamycin, *Arch Intern Med* 148:2477-2482, 1988.

31. Dieterich DT et al: Ganciclovir treatment of gastrointestinal infections caused by cytomegalovirus in patients with AIDS, *Rev Infect Dis* 10(suppl 3):S532-537, 1988.

32. Dismukes WE et al: Treatment of cryptococcal meningitis with combination amphotericin B and flucytosine for four as compared with six weeks, *N Engl J Med* 317(6):334-341, 1987.

33. Engel JP et al: Treatment of resistant herpes simplex virus with continuous-infusion acyclovir, *JAMA* 263(12):1662-1664, 1990.

34. Erice A et al: Progressive disease due to ganciclovir-resistant cytomegalovirus in immunocompromised pa-

tients, *N Engl J Med* 320(5):289-293, 1989.

35. Erlich KS et al: Foscarnet therapy for severe acyclovir-resistant herpes simplex virus type 2 infections in patients with the acquired immunodeficiency syndrome (AIDS): an uncontrolled trial, *Ann Intern Med* 110(9):710-713, 1989.

36. Fanning MM et al: Foscarnet therapy of cytomegalovirus retinitis in AIDS, *J Acquir Immune Defic Syndr* 3:472-479, 1990.

37. Farthing C et al: Treatment of cytomegalovirus pneumonitis with foscarnet (trisodium phosphonoformate) in patients with AIDS, *J Med Virol* 22(2):157-162, 1987.

38. Fayer R, Guidry A, Blagburn BL: Immunotherapeutic efficacy of bovine colostral immunoglobulins from a hyperimmunized cow against cryptosporidiosis in neonatal mice, *Infect Immun* 58(9):2962-2965, 1990.

39. Felsenstein D et al: Treatment of cytomegalovirus retinitis with 9-(2-hydroxy-1-[hydroxymethyl]ethoxymethyl) guanine. *Ann Intern Med* 103:377-380, 1985.

40. Fournier AM et al: Tuberculosis and nontuberculosis mycobacteriosis in patients with AIDS, *Chest* 93(4):772-775, 1988.

41. Gagnon S et al: Corticosteroids as adjunctive therapy for severe *Pneumocystis carinii* pneumonia in the acquired immunodeficiency syndrome: a double-blind, placebo-controlled trial, *N Engl J Med* 323:1444-1450, 1990.

42. Galgiani JN: Fluconazole, a new antifungal agent, *Ann Intern Med* 113(3):177-179, 1990.

43. Gill PS et al: Pulmonary Kaposi's sarcoma: clinical findings and results of therapy, *Am J Med* 87:57-61, 1989.

44. Glasgow BJ et al: Adrenal pathology in the acquired immunodeficiency syndrome, *Am J Clin Pathol* 84:594-597, 1985.

45. Glick M et al: Oral manifestations of disseminated *Cryptococcus neoformans* in a patient with acquired immunodeficiency syndrome, *Oral Surg Oral Med Oral Pathol* 64(4):454-459, 1987.

46. Goodman DS et al: Prevalence of cutaneous disease in patients with acquired immunodeficiency syndrome (AIDS) or AIDS-related complex, *J Am Acad Dermatol* 17:210-220, 1987.

47. Grange et al: Successful therapy for *Toxoplasma gondii* myocarditis in acquired immunodeficiency syndrome, *Am Heart J* 120(2):443-444, 1990.

48. Greene JB et al: *Mycobacterium avium-intracellulare:* a cause of disseminated life-threatening infection in homosexuals and drug abusers, *Ann Intern Med* 97:539-546, 1982.

49. Groopman JE et al: Recombinant alpha-2 interferon therapy for Kaposi's sarcoma associated with the acquired immunodeficiency syndrome, *Ann Intern Med* 100:671-676, 1984.

50. Hicks CB et al: Seronegative secondary syphilis in a patient infected with the human immunodeficiency virus (HIV) with Kaposi sarcoma: a diagnostic dilemma, *Ann Intern Med* 107:492-495, 1987.

51. Hoo Soo GW, Mohsenifar Z, Meyer RD: Inhaled or intravenous pentamidine therapy for *Pneumocystis carinii* pneumonia in AIDS: a randomized trial, *Ann Intern Med* 113:195-202, 1990.

52. Hook EW: Syphilis and HIV infection, *J Infect Dis* 160(3):530-534, 1989.

53. Interlied CB et al: In vitro and in vivo activity of azithromycin (CP 62, 993) against the *Mycobacterium avium* complex, *J Infect Dis* 159(5):994-997, 1989.

54. Israelski DM, Remington JS: Toxoplasmic encephalitis in patients with AIDS, *Infect Dis Clin North Am* 2:429-445, 1988.

55. Jacobson MA, O'Donnell JJ, Mills J: Foscarnet treatment of cytomegalo-

virus retinitis in patients with the acquired immunodeficiency syndrome, *Antimicrob Agents Chemother* 33(5): 736-741, 1989.

56. Johns DR, Tierney M, Felsenstein D: Alteration in the natural history of neurosyphilis by concurrent infection with the human immunodeficiency virus, *N Engl J Med* 316:1569-1572, 1987.

57. Jules-Elysee KM et al: Aerosolized pentamidine: effect on diagnosis and presentation of *Pneumocystis carinii* pneumonia, *Ann Intern Med* 112(10):750-757, 1990.

58. Katz AS, Niesenbaum L, Mass B: Pleural effusion as the initial manifestation of disseminated cryptococcosis in acquired immune deficiency syndrome: diagnosis by pleural biopsy, *Chest* 96(2):440-441, 1989.

59. Katz MD, Erstad BL, Rose C: Treatment of severe *Cryptosporidium*-related diarrhea with octreotide in a patient with AIDS, *Drug Intell Clin Pharm* 22(2):134-136, 1988.

60. Kida M, Abramowsky CR, Santoscoy C: Cryptococcosis of the placenta in a woman with acquired immunodeficiency syndrome, *Hum Pathol* 20(9):920-921, 1989.

61. Kotler DP et al: Treatment of disseminated cytomegalovirus infection with 9-(1,3-dihydroxy-2-propoxymethyl) guanine: evidence of prolonged survival in patients with the acquired immunodeficiency syndrome, *AIDS Res Hum Retroviruses* 2(4):299-308, 1986.

62. Kovacs JA: Diagnosis, treatment and prevention of *Pneumocystis carinii* pneumonia in HIV-infected patients, *AIDS Updates* 2:1-12, 1989.

63. Kovacs JA et al: Cryptococcosis in the acquired immunodeficiency syndrome, *Ann Intern Med* 103:533-538, 1985.

64. Kovacs JA et al: *Pneumocystis carinii* pneumonia: a comparison between patients with the acquired immuno-deficiency syndrome and patients with other immunodeficiencies, *Ann Intern Med* 100:663-671, 1984.

65. Kovacs JA, Masur H: *Pneumocystis carinii* pneumonia: therapy and prophylaxis, *J Infect Dis* 158(1):254-259, 1988.

66. Krown SE et al: Kaposi's sarcoma and the acquired immune deficiency syndrome: treatment with recombinant interferon alpha and analysis of prognostic factors, *Cancer* 57(suppl 8):1662-1665, 1986.

67. Krown SE et al: Preliminary observations on the effect of recombinant leukocyte A interferon in homosexual men with Kaposi's sarcoma, *N Engl J Med* 308(18):1071-1076, 1983.

68. Larsen RA et al: Persistent *Cryptococcus neoformans* infection of the prostate after successful treatment of meningitis, *Ann Intern Med* 111:125-128, 1989.

69. Larsen RA, Leal MAE, Chan LS: Fluconazole compared with amphotericin B plus flucytosine for cryptococcal meningitis in AIDS: a randomized trial, *Ann Intern Med* 113:183-187, 1990.

70. Laskin OL et al: Ganciclovir for the treatment and suppression of serious infections caused by cytomegalovirus, *Am J Med* 83(2):201-207, 1987.

71. Leoung GS et al: Dapsone-trimethoprim for *Pneumocystis carinii* pneumonia in the acquired immunodeficiency syndrome, *Ann Intern Med* 105:45-48, 1986.

72. Leport C et al: An open study of the pyrimethamine-clindamycin combination in AIDS patients with brain toxoplasmosis, *J Infect Dis* 160(3): 557-558, 1989.

73. Lief M, Sarfarazi F: Prostatic cryptococcosis in acquired immune deficiency syndrome, *Urology* 28(4):318-319, 1986.

74. Lipson BK et al: Optic neuropathy associated with cryptococcal arach-

noiditis in AIDS patients, *Am J Ophthalmol* 107(5):523-527, 1989.

75. Louie E et al: Treatment of cryptosporidiosis with oral bovine transfer factor, *Clin Immunol Immunopathol* 44(3):329-334, 1987.

76. MacFadden DK et al: Corticosteroids as adjunctive therapy in treatment of *Pneumocystis carinii* pneumonia in patients with acquired immunodeficiency syndrome, *Lancet* 1:1477-1479, 1987.

77. Machac J, Nejatheim M, Goldsmith SJ: Gallium-67 citrate uptake in cryptococcal thyroiditis in a homosexual male, *J Nucl Med Allied Sci* 29(3):283-285, 1985.

78. Masur H et al: CD4 counts as predictors of opportunistic pneumonias in human immunodeficiency virus (HIV) infection, *Ann Intern Med* 111(3):223-231, 1989.

79. Masur H et al: Effect of 9-(1,3-dihydroxy-2-propoxymethyl) guanine on serious cytomegalovirus disease in eight immunosuppressed homosexual men, *Ann Intern Med* 104:41-44, 1986.

80. McMeeking A et al: A controlled trial of bovine dialyzable leukocyte extract for cryptosporidiosis in patients with AIDS, *J Infect Dis* 161(1):108-112, 1990.

81. The Medical Letter: Trimethoprim-sulfamethoxazole for treatment of urinary tract infections, *Med Lett Drugs Ther* 17(25):101-103, 1975.

82. Medina I et al: Oral therapy for *Pneumocystis carinii* in the acquired immunodeficiency syndrome: a controlled trial of trimethoprim-sulfamethoxazole versus trimethoprim-dapsone, *N Engl J Med* 323:776-782, 1990.

83. Mertz GJ et al: Long-term acyclovir suppression of frequently recurring genital herpes simplex virus infection: a multicenter, double-blind trial, *JAMA* 260(2):201-206, 1988.

84. Miller WT Jr, Edelman JM, Miller

WT: Cryptococcal pulmonary infection in patients with AIDS: radiographic appearance, *Radiology* 175 (3):725-728, 1990.

85. Mintzer DM et al: Treatment of Kaposi's sarcoma and thrombocytopenia with vincristine in patients with the acquired immunodeficiency syndrome, *Ann Intern Med* 102:200-202, 1985.

86. Mir N et al: HIV-disease and bone marrow changes: a study of 60 cases, *Eur J Haematol* 42(4):339-343, 1989.

87. Montaner JSG et al: The effect of zidovudine on platelet count in HIV-infected individuals, *J Acquir Immune Defic Syndr* 3:565-570, 1990.

88. Montgomery AB et al: Aerosolised pentamidine as sole therapy for *Pneumocystis carinii* pneumonia in patients with acquired immunodeficiency syndrome, *Lancet* 2:480-483, 1987.

89. Moskovitz BL, Stanton TL, Kusmierek JJ: Spiramycin therapy for cryptosporidial diarrhea in immunocompromised patients, *J Antimicrob Chemother* 22(suppl B):189-191, 1988.

90. Murray RJ et al: Recovery from cryptococcemia and the adult respiratory distress syndrome in the acquired-immunodeficiency syndrome, *Chest* 93:1304-1306, 1988.

91. Murray JF, Mills J: State of the art: pulmonary infectious complications of human immunodeficiency virus infection. II. *Am Rev Respir Dis* 141:1582-1598, 1990.

92. Navia BA et al: Cerebral toxoplasmosis complicating the acquired immune deficiency syndrome: clinical and neuropathological findings in 27 patients, *Ann Neurol* 19:224-238, 1986.

93. Newman TG et al: Pleural cryptococcosis in the acquired immune deficiency syndrome, *Chest* 91:459-461, 1987.

94. Nord J et al: Treatment with bovine

hyperimmune colostrum of crypto-sporidial diarrhea in AIDS patients, *AIDS* 4(6):581-584, 1990.

95. Pass HI et al: Thoracic manifestations of the acquired immunodeficiency syndrome, *J Thorac Cardiovasc Surg* 88:654-658, 1984.

96. Pedrol E et al: Central nervous system toxoplasmosis in AIDS patients: efficacy of an intermittent maintenance therapy, *AIDS* 4(6):511-517, 1990.

97. Phelan JA et al: Oral findings in patients with acquired immunodeficiency syndrome, *Oral Surg Oral Med Oral Pathol* 64(1):50-56, 1987.

98. Pilla AM, Rybak MJ, Chandrasekar PH: Spiramycin in the treatment of cryptosporidiosis, *Pharmacotherapy* 7(5):188-190, 1987.

99. Pitchenik AE, Rubinson HA: The radiographic appearance of tuberculosis in patients with the acquired immune deficiency syndrome (AIDS) and pre-AIDS, *Am Rev Respir Dis* 131:393-396, 1985.

100. Porro GB, Parente F, Cernuschi M: The diagnosis of esophageal candidiasis in patients with acquired immune deficiency syndrome: is endoscopy always necessary? *Am J Gastroenterol* 84(2):143-146, 1989.

101. Portnoy D et al: Treatment of intestinal cryptosporidiosis with spiramycin, *Ann Intern Med* 101:202-204, 1984.

102. Pottage JC et al: Treatment of human immunodeficiency virus–related thrombocytopenia with zidovudine, *JAMA* 260(20):3045-3050, 1988.

103. Quinn TC et al: Human immunodeficiency virus infection among patients attending clinics for sexually transmitted diseases, *N Engl J Med* 318:197-203, 1988.

104. Ratner L: Human immunodeficiency virus–associated autoimmune thrombocytopenic purpura: a review, *Am J Med* 86:194-198, 1989.

105. Raufman JP: Odynophagia/dyspha-gia in AIDS, *Gastroenterol Clin North Am* 17(3):599-614, 1988.

106. Reichert CM et al: Autopsy pathology in the acquired immunodeficiency syndrome, *Am J Pathol* 112:357-382, 1982.

107. Rico MJ, Pennys NS: Cutaneous cryptococcosis resembling molluscum contagiosum in a patient with AIDS, *Arch Dermatol* 121:901-902, 1985.

108. Rolston KV, Hoy J: Role of clindamycin in the treatment of central nervous system toxoplasmosis, *Am J Med* 83(3):551-554, 1987.

109. Rosecan LR et al: Antiviral therapy for cytomegalovirus retinitis in AIDS with dihydroxy propoxymethyl guanine, *Am J Ophthalmol* 101(4):405-418, 1986.

110. Saez-Llorens X et al: Spiramycin vs placebo for treatment of acute diarrhea caused by *Cryptosporidium*, *Pediatr Infect Dis J* 8(3):136-140, 1989.

111. Safrin S et al: Foscarnet therapy for acyclovir-resistant mucocutaneous herpes simplex virus infection in 26 AIDS patients: preliminary data, *J Infect Dis* 161:1078-1084, 1990.

112. Sattler FR et al: Trimethoprim-sulfamethoxazole compared with pentamidine for treatment of *Pneumocystis carinii* pneumonia in the acquired immunodeficiency syndrome: a prospective, noncrossover study, *Ann Intern Med* 109:280-287, 1988.

113. Schinella RA, Breda SD, Hammerschlag PE: Otic infection due to *Pneumocystis carinii* in an apparently healthy man with antibody to human immunodeficiency virus, *Ann Intern Med* 106(3):399-400, 1987.

114. Schuster M, Valentine F, Holzman R: Cryptococcal pericarditis in an intravenous drug abuser, *J Infect Dis* 152:842, 1985.

115. Selwyn PA et al: A prospective study of the risk of tuberculosis among intravenous drug users with human immunodeficiency virus infection, *N Engl J Med* 320(9):545-550, 1989.

116. Silverman BA, Rubinstein A: Serum lactate dehydrogenase levels in adults and children with acquired immune deficiency syndrome (AIDS) and AIDS-related complex: possible indicator of B cell lymphoprolifera-tion and disease activity: effect of in-travenous gammaglobulin on enzyme levels, *Am J Med* 78:728-736, 1985.

117. Simonsen JN et al: Human immu-nodeficiency virus infection among men with sexually transmitted dis-eases: experience from a center in Af-rica, *N Engl J Med* 319:274-278, 1988.

118. Sugar AM, Saunders C: Oral flucon-azole as suppressive therapy of dis-seminated cryptococcosis in patients with acquired immunodeficiency syndrome, *Am J Med* 85:481-489, 1988.

119. Swiss Group for Clinical Studies on the Acquired Immunodeficiency Syn-drome (AIDS): Zidovudine for the treatment of thrombocytopenia as-sociated with human immunodefi-ciency virus (HIV): a prospective study, *Ann Intern Med* 109:718-721, 1988.

120. Telzak EE et al: Extrapulmonary *Pneumocystis carinii* infections, *Rev Infect Dis* 12(3):380-386, 1990.

121. Toma E et al: Clindamycin with pri-maquine for *Pneumocystis carinii* pneumonia, *Lancet* 1:1046-1048, 1989.

122. Torres RA: Cryptococcal mediastini-tis mimicking lymphoma in the ac-quired immune deficiency syndrome, *Am J Med* 83(5):1004-1005, 1987.

123. Torrsander J et al: Oral *Candida al-bicans* in HIV infection, *Scand J Infect Dis* 19(3):291-295, 1987.

124. Tzipori S, Roberton D, Chapman C: Remission of diarrhea due to cryp-tosporidiosis in an immunodefi-cient child treated with hyperim-mune bovine colostrum, *Br Med J* 293(6557):1276-1277, 1986.

125. Ungar BL et al: Cessation of *Crypto-sporidium*-associated diarrhea in an acquired immunodeficiency syn-drome patient after treatment with hyperimmune bovine colostrum, *Gastroenterology* 98(2):486-489, 1990.

126. Utz JP et al: Therapy of cryptococ-cosis with a combination of flucyto-sine and amphotericin B, *J Infect Dis* 132:368-373, 1975.

127. Van Calck M et al: Cryptococcal anal ulceration in a patient with AIDS, *Am J Gastroenterol* 83(11):1306-1308, 1988.

128. Vanparijs O et al: Efficacy of dicla-zuril against turkey coccidiosis in dose-titration studies, *Avian Dis* 33(3):422-424, 1989.

129. Vanparijs O, Desplenter L, Mars-boom R: Efficacy of diclazuril in the control of intestinal coccidiosis in rabbits, *Vet Parasitol* 34(3):185-190, 1989.

130. Viviani MA et al: Itraconazole for cryptococcal infection in the ac-quired immunodeficiency syndrome, *Ann Intern Med* 106:166, 1987.

131. Volberding PA et al: Vinblastine ther-apy for Kaposi's sarcoma in the ac-quired immunodeficiency syndrome, *Ann Intern Med* 103:335-338, 1985.

132. Walsh C et al: Thrombocytopenia in homosexual patients: prognosis, re-sponse to therapy, and prevalence of antibody to the retrovirus associated with the acquired immunodeficiency syndrome, *Ann Intern Med* 103:542-545, 1985.

133. Wasser L, Talavera W: Pulmonary cryptococcosis in AIDS, *Chest* 92:692-695, 1987.

134. Weiss LM et al: *Isospora belli* infec-tion: treatment with pyrimethamine, *Ann Intern Med* 109:474-475, 1988.

135. Welch K et al: Autopsy findings in the acquired immunodeficiency syn-drome, *JAMA* 252:1152-1159, 1984.

136. Westblom TU, Belshe RB: Clinda-

mycin therapy of cerebral toxoplasmosis in an AIDS patient, *Scand J Infect Dis* 20(5):561-563, 1988.

137. Westerman C, Christensen RP: Chronic *Isospora belli* infection treated with co-trimoxazole, *Ann Intern Med* 91:413-414, 1979.

138. Wharton JM et al: Trimethoprim-sulfamethoxazole or pentamidine for *Pneumocystis carinii* pneumonia in the acquired immunodeficiency syndrome: a prospective randomized trial, *Ann Intern Med* 105:37-44, 1986.

139. Whimbey E, Kiehn TE, Armstrong D: Disseminated *Mycobacterium avium-intracellulare* disease: diagnosis and therapy, *Curr Clin Top Infect Dis* 7:112-133, 1986.

140. Wittenberg DF, Miller NM, Van den Ende J: Spiramycin is not effective in treating *Cryptosporidium* diarrhea in infants: results of a double-blind, randomized trial, *J Infect Dis* 159(1):131-132, 1989.

141. Wong B et al: Continuous high-grade *Mycobacterium avium-intracellulare* bacteremia in patients with the acquired immune deficiency syndrome, *Am J Med* 78:35-40, 1985.

142. Woods GL, Washington JA: Mycobacteria other than *Mycobacterium tuberculosis*: review of microbiologic and clinical aspects, *Rev Infect Dis* 9(2):275-294, 1987.

143. Woolf GM, Townsend M, Guyatt G: Treatment of cryptosporidiosis with spiramycin in AIDS: an "N of 1" trial, *J Clin Gastroenterol* 9(6):632-634, 1987.

144. Zuger A et al: Cryptococcal disease in patients with the acquired immunodeficiency syndrome: diagnostic features and outcome of treatment, *Ann Intern Med* 104:234-240, 1986.

CHAPTER 10

Overview of Antiretroviral Therapy

Before the AIDS epidemic and the discovery of the human immunodeficiency virus (HIV, HIV-1), antiviral therapy was in its infancy and no viral infection was considered curable. In research a greater emphasis had been placed on prevention, by means of vaccines. Childhood diseases, including polio, measles, mumps, and rubella were largely controlled by large-scale immunization programs, particularly in developed countries. Vaccination achieved its most spectacular victory in the worldwide eradication of smallpox.

In contrast to the success of vaccines, the development of antiviral drugs had been slow and frustrating. When the AIDS epidemic began, effective therapy was available for only a small number of viral infections. Among these were influenza, herpes simplex, and herpes zoster. Progress was impeded by the lack of in vitro systems by which new agents could be rapidly tested for antiviral activity. Because most common viral infections are self-limited diseases and not life threatening, antibacterial agents received greater attention in new-drug development.

Thus in the early 1980s, when the magnitude of the AIDS epidemic became apparent and its viral origin was recognized, the primitive status of antiviral chemotherapy presented a formidable obstacle to the development of effective means of treating and controlling the disease. The novel mode of replication shared by HIV and other retroviruses (i.e., reverse transcription of ribonucleic acid [RNA] into deoxyribonucleic acid [DNA]) further complicated the development of therapy. Existing antiviral compounds such as acyclovir and adenine arabinoside were ineffective against retroviruses, and there was no established therapeutic strategy available to guide the development of drugs active against these organisms, which were not previously known to cause human disease.

The immediacy of the epidemic ultimately necessitated changes in existing channels for the development, testing, licensing, and distribution of new drugs. By September 1986, zidovudine (AZT), a nucleoside analog capable of inhibiting the action of one of the unique enzymes of HIV, reverse transcriptase, was shown to have in vitro activity against the virus, to have clinical efficacy in patients with AIDS and advanced AIDS-related complex (ARC), and to have an acceptable level of toxicity. Zidovudine was made available to selected patients and ultimately licensed by the Food and Drug Administration in early 1987 for the treatment of HIV infection. It thus became the standard against which newer agents would be judged.

Chemically related compounds, such as dideoxycytidine (DDC) and dideoxyinosine (DDI), also shown to have in vitro efficacy, followed in clinical trials. Other potential therapies not directed at reverse transcriptase were simultaneously developed including soluble CD4, interferon-α, and chemical inhibitors of other important steps of viral replication.

These trials have been carried out at a number of medical centers across the United States under the auspices of the National Institutes of Health (NIH) by means of the AIDS Clinical Trials Group (ACTG) program. In addition, a program of expanded access was established to allow patients who were ineligible for established protocols to receive certain potentially effective drugs outside of randomized clinical trials.

Because of the large number of potentially active therapeutic agents and the difficulties of proving efficacy and safety and conducting large, well-constructed clinical trials,[20] progress in identifying additional effective drugs has been incremental as the epidemic has continued to expand. This tragic situation has led some patients to use untested compounds on the basis of insufficient evidence of efficacy and safety.

The AIDS epidemic has resulted in numerous clashes between various interests over a host of issues. The approach to development of treatments has caused perhaps the most controversy. The physician caring for HIV-infected patients must be aware not only of current treatment recommendations but also of the status of investigational protocols and the mechanism for enrolling patients in such trials.

The following is a summary of available information on the efficacy, safety, and availability of therapeutic agents for HIV infection at the time this book went to press. The role of specific agents may change rapidly, but therapeutic strategies and the means by which patients may gain access to therapy probably will change more slowly. The purpose of this chapter is not to summarize all potentially effective compounds but to emphasize current indications for antiretroviral therapy and review data about new potential therapies that have emerged from careful studies, both clinical and preclinical.

THE IDENTIFICATION AND TESTING OF ANTIVIRAL DRUGS

Shortly after the discovery of HIV-1, in vitro assays to identify compounds with antiviral activity were developed.[6] These techniques have facilitated the identification of potentially useful drugs in laboratory studies. Data on the safety and effectiveness of several drugs have emerged from controlled and uncontrolled studies. The validity of currently available data may be confirmed or refuted by future studies.

OVERVIEW OF CLINICAL TRIALS

What follows is an overview of clinical data gathered from studies of AZT and other antiviral compounds (see the boxes on p. 215). Only preliminary information was available on drugs other than AZT at the time of this writing. The results of several large clinical trials comparing several of these agents to AZT will be available within the next few years. Since the number of antiviral compounds under study is increasing steadily, updated information can be obtained through the hotline telephone numbers (pp. 219 and 222).

In evaluating reports about new antiviral drugs for HIV infection, the practitioner should distinguish between preclinical studies, preliminary clinical data, uncontrolled studies or case reports, and multicenter clinical trials. Large-scale, prospective clinical trials eventually will be needed to establish the relative efficacy and safety of various drugs and therapeutic strategies. During the first decade of the AIDS epidemic, particularly since the discovery of HIV, exaggerated claims of efficacy have been made for various compounds on the basis of uncontrolled studies or anecdotes. Patients should be cautioned about this phenomenon.

Antiviral Drugs with Clinical Efficacy Versus HIV

Nucleosides
    AZT[13,14,16,41,52]
    DDI[11,27]
    DDC[6,46]
Soluble CD4[21,45]
Interferon-α[28]

Major Side Effects of Nucleoside Drugs

AZT	Anemia, leukopenia
DDI	Peripheral neuropathy, pancreatitis
DDC	Peripheral neuropathy

NUCLEOSIDE ANALOGS

Nucleoside analogs, including 3'-azido-2',3'-dideoxythymidine (AZT, zidovudine), 2',3'-dideoxyinosine (DDI), 2',3'-dideoxycytidine (DDC), and 2',3'-dideoxyadenosine (DDA) were among the first compounds found to inhibit the replication of HIV-1.[5] The complete mechanism of action of these agents is not yet clear. After triphosphorylation inside the infected cell, each drug is capable of competitively inhibiting the binding of nucleotides to viral reverse transcriptase. Each may also cause chain termination after incorporation into viral DNA.[5]

AZT (zidovudine), the first of these compounds to undergo large-scale clinical trials, eventually was shown to have clinically significant antiviral activity in some categories of patients and was licensed for use. However, toxicity, most often in the form of bone marrow depression, was found to be substantial, especially in patients with advanced HIV infection. This finding, plus the observation that HIV may become resistant to AZT during prolonged therapy,[30,40] has helped to stimulate the search for other effective nucleoside compounds.

3'-Azido-2',3'-dideoxythymidine (AZT)

3'-Azido-2',3'-dideoxythymidine (AZT, zidovudine) was the first agent licensed for the treatment of HIV infection.

Mechanism of action. After conversion to a triphosphate form by the human host cell, zidovudine interferes with the action of the HIV enzyme reverse transcriptase and thus inhibits the replication of HIV.[20] Its action is by chain termination and competitive inhibition of nucleoside triphosphate compounds of the host cell.[20]

Effectiveness. The therapeutic efficacy of zidovudine was initially demonstrated in a blinded, randomized, placebo-controlled study involving patients with AIDS and advanced ARC.[13] Given in a dose of 250 mg every 4 hours, zidovudine therapy led to an improvement in survival and functional status and a decrease in the incidence and severity of opportunistic infections.[13] In some patients, particularly those with ARC at the time of enrollment, immunological parameters improved, including CD4 cell counts and skin test reactions. Survival in those receiving zidovudine was 84.5% and 57.6% at 12 and 21 months respectively, whereas survival in those receiving placebo was 36% at one year.[14]

Similar beneficial effects were observed in AIDS patients who received zidovudine after recovery from *Pneumocystis carinii* pneumonia by enrollment in a compassionate use program, before the drug was formally approved by the Food and Drug Administration.[10] Statistical evidence suggests that the wide availability of zidovudine after 1987 may have accounted for a lower than expected rate of increase in reported AIDS cases in the late 1980s.[17]

Subsequent studies conducted under the AIDS Clinical Trials Group (ACTG) program of the National Institute of Allergy and Infectious Diseases (NIAID) demonstrated that zidovudine in a dose of 200 mg every 4 hours slowed the progression to AIDS in patients with CD4 lymphocyte counts between 200/mm^3 and 500/mm^3, regardless of whether the patient had HIV-related symptoms.[16,52] Simultaneously, it was established that zidovudine was as effective in lower dose (100 mg five times a day) as in higher dose regimens among asymptomatic patients with CD4 lymphocyte counts under 500/mm^3.[52]

In early 1990, on the basis of these results, low-dose zidovudine therapy was recommended for all HIV-infected patients with CD4 lymphocyte counts below 500/mm^3 by the NIAID and was approved for this indication by the Food and Drug Administration.

Despite this approval, some experts remain uncertain that zidovudine confers significant therapeutic benefit for asymptomatic patients with CD4 lymphocyte counts between 200/mm^3 and 500/mm^3,[9] and concerns about long-term cumulative toxicity and viral resistance have been raised.[42] The results of additional prospective studies may soon address these concerns.

Toxicity. A variety of side effects have been described in patients receiving zidovudine.[41] Early side effects may include headache, nausea, myalgias, and insomnia. These symptoms usually can be managed symptomatically and often resolve within the few first days or weeks of therapy. The most serious side effects seen with zidovudine therapy have been hematological. Bone marrow depression, resulting in significant anemia, was seen in 24% of those receiving high-dose therapy (1,500 mg a day) in the initial clinical trials,[41] and 21% of patients required blood transfusions. Neutropenia was seen in 16%. A reduction in platelet counts of 50% or more was seen in 12% of patients. Hematological side effects were seen as early as 2 weeks after therapy began and became more frequent with continued therapy. Low CD4 lymphocyte counts, anemia, neutropenia, or vitamin B_{12} deficiency at the beginning of therapy were all associated with a higher incidence of hematological side effects. Current lower dose regimens (500 mg a day) have been associated with a substantially lower incidence of hematological side effects.[52]

Other side effects reported with zidovudine therapy have included darkening of the nails, rashes, Stevens-Johnson syndrome,[20] and myopathy.[18]

Indications. On the basis of available data from controlled trials, a panel sponsored by the National Institutes of Health (NIH) recommended that zidovudine therapy be initiated in HIV-infected patients with CD4 lymphocyte counts below 500/mm³ regardless of symptoms.[36]

Other potential uses of AZT

Neurological dysfunction. Zidovudine therapy resulted in improvement in acute confusional state and polyradiculopathy associated with HIV infection but had no effect on advanced encephalopathy or neuropathy in one small series.[12]

Thrombocytopenia. Zidovudine has been shown to increase the platelet count in HIV-infected patients with and without autoimmune thrombocytopenia.[35,39,49] Indications, as well as optimal dose and duration of such therapy, have not yet been determined.

Prophylaxis of HIV infection after exposure. On the basis of animal studies suggesting that zidovudine may be effective in preventing retroviral infection,[44,50] it has been suggested that postexposure prophylaxis be considered for health care workers who have been exposed by needle stick or other blood contact to blood or other body fluids of HIV-infected patients.[7] The effectiveness of this strategy has not been confirmed in human studies, however, and zidovudine failed to protect a patient who received an injection with a needle contaminated with blood from an HIV-infected patient in one report.[29]

Monitoring of patients receiving zidovudine (Figure 10-1). The medical follow-up of patients receiving zidovudine therapy is determined largely by clinical status. It is recommended that asymptomatic patients be reevaluated 2

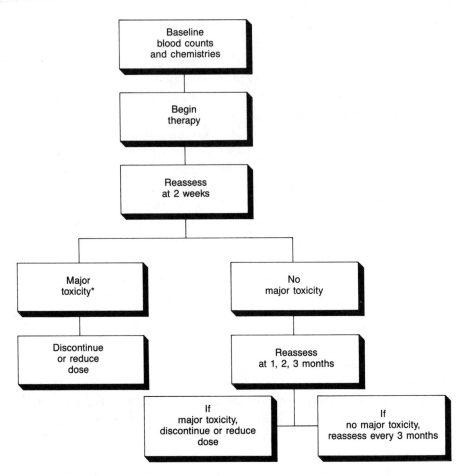

*Hgb<80 g/dL or granulocyte count< 750/mm³.

FIGURE 10-1. Recommended monitoring of patients receiving zidovudine.[36]

weeks after therapy is begun and at monthly intervals for the first 3 months for evidence of toxicity.[36] Baseline blood counts and chemistries should be obtained before therapy, and blood counts should be repeated monthly for the first 3 months. After 3 months of therapy, asymptomatic patients who do not manifest signs of drug toxicity may be reevaluated less frequently. It is recommended that the dose of zidovudine be reduced or therapy be discontinued if the hemoglobin level falls to less than 80 g/L or the granulocyte count falls to less than 750/mm³.[36] If therapy must be discontinued because of hematological toxicity, often it may be reinstituted at a lower dose after bone marrow recovery, although the minimal effective dose has not been determined.

Idiosyncratic reactions such as skin rashes, hepatitis, or myopathy also may necessitate discontinuation of zidovidine therapy.

2′,3′-Dideoxyinosine (DDI)

Clinical trials[8,27] of the purine nucleoside analog 2′,3′-dideoxyinosine (DDI, didanosine, Videx) were begun in 1989 on the basis of its demonstrated in vitro antiviral effect and its relative lack of hematological toxicity. Decreased levels of circulating p24 antigen and increased CD4 lymphocyte counts,[8] as well as some evidence of clinical benefit, were seen in these early studies.[11] A dose-related painful peripheral neuropathy and idiosyncratic pancreatitis[27] were the major side effects seen in the initial clinical trials. Elevations of transaminases, creatine phosphokinase, and urate, as well as cardiac conduction abnormalities, were each seen in a minority of patients.[8] Hematological toxicity was not seen in preliminary trials.

Multicenter clinical trials comparing DDI to AZT in patients with AIDS or ARC and comparing various doses of DDI among patients intolerant to AZT are under way. Information on trials conducted under the AIDS Clinical Trials Group (ACTG) program of the NIAID could be obtained at the time of this writing by calling 1-800-TRIALSA. Between 1989 and 1991 DDI was made available through an expanded access program to individuals who did not qualify for clinical trials. DDI was approved by the FDA and became available by prescription under the brand name Videx in October 1991. The drug should be considered for patients who are intolerant of zidovudine. The manufacturer's dosing guidelines should be consulted.

2′,3′-Dideoxycytidine (DDC)

Dideoxycytidine (DDC) is another nucleoside analog active against HIV that has undergone preliminary testing.[6] In vitro testing suggests that DDC may have a more potent antiviral effect than DDI or AZT[4] and, like DDI, may be active against viral strains resistant to AZT.[40]

Peripheral neuropathy was the most prominent toxicity of DDC in preliminary human studies.[33] In contrast to AZT, DDC did not appear to cause significant bone marrow depression in early trials.[33] Because of the contrast in toxicities between AZT and DDC, regimens in which the two drugs are alternated as a means of minimizing both peripheral neuropathy and bone marrow depression are under evaluation.[32,46]

Clinical trials comparing DDC to AZT are being conducted through the AIDS Clinical Trials Group (ACTG) program of the NIAID. Information on these trials could be obtained by calling 1-800-TRIALSA. An expanded access program through which DDC was made available to certain patients intolerant of AZT and DDI was in progress at the time of this writing. Information on enrollment in this program could be obtained by calling 1-800-332-2144.

OTHER ANTIVIRAL AND IMMUNOMODULATOR COMPOUNDS IN CLINICAL TRIALS
Soluble CD4

To cause infection, HIV must first bind to the surface of a target cell. The molecule to which the virus binds on the surface of the CD4 lymphocyte and certain other cells is designated CD4. It has been hypothesized that this molecule, in free form, could competitively inhibit the binding of HIV to cellular receptors and thus prevent infection. Preliminary trials employing recombinant soluble CD4 demonstrated antiviral activity at high doses[45] and little or no toxicity.[23,45]

The ultimate role that CD4 may have in the therapy of HIV infection was not clear from preliminary studies. Since the virus may invade cells not carrying the CD4 receptor molecule, soluble CD4 may not be suitable as a single therapeutic agent. The possibility exists that CD4 could be used to target infected cells for the delivery of antiviral drugs.[51]

Interferon-α

In a randomized, prospective study of asymptomatic HIV-infected patients with CD4 lymphocyte counts over $400/mm^3$, recombinant interferon-α administered subcutaneously (35 million units a day) significantly decreased the rate of viral isolation compared to placebo.[28]

An oral preparation of interferon-α produced symptomatic improvement and an increase in circulating CD4 lymphocyte accounts, according to preliminary reports from workers in Kenya.[2] Clinical trials of oral interferon-α were planned at the time of this writing.

Inosine Pranobex

In a placebo-controlled, multicenter Scandinavian study, therapy with inosine pranobex (isoprinosine), an immunomodulator compound, appeared to slow progression to AIDS among patients at all stages of HIV infection without improving immunological parameters.[37] However, the significance of these findings and the study design have been questioned.[26]

IMREG-1

IMREG-1, an immunomodular compound derived from leukocytes, was shown to decrease the rate of decline of CD4 cells in patients with ARC in a prospective study.[18a] The clinical significance of this effect is not yet clear.

Miscellaneous Agents

Several drugs that initially were felt to hold promise are currently thought to be ineffective. These include the compounds AL721, HPA23, and suramin. Other potential antiviral drugs under evaluation at the beginning of the 1990s included dextran sulfate, tricosanthin (compound Q), ribavirin, and ampligen.[20]

NEWER THERAPEUTIC STRATEGIES
Combination Therapy with Antiviral Agents

It has been suggested that therapeutic regimens consisting of several agents might have a synergistic antiviral effect.[22] Potential advantages of combination antiviral therapy include reduced toxicity as a result of a reduction in the dosage of individual agents, elimination or suppression of the emergence of resistant viral strains, and wider tissue distribution.[53] Antiviral drugs could also be combined with agents that reduce their toxicity or that suppress or eradicate opportunistic infections.[53]

Preliminary data have been gathered on several drug combinations.

AZT and interferon-α. Synergy between interferon-α and AZT has been demonstrated in vivo against a mouse retrovirus.[43] Preliminary human data indicated that AZT and interferon-α could be used safely in combination.[25]

AZT and acyclovir. In an uncontrolled trial of combination therapy with AZT (100 mg every 4 hours) and acyclovir (800 mg every 4 hours), all of the six patients with AIDS or ARC who were able to tolerate 10 weeks of therapy had significant increases in CD4, lymphocyte counts.[48] The significance of these preliminary data is unclear.

AZT and soluble CD4. Preliminary in vitro studies have indicated that AZT and soluble CD4 may act synergistically against HIV.[21]

Therapy with a three-drug combination of AZT, CD4, and interferon-α may hold promise.[22]

Adjuncts to Antiviral Therapy

Erythropoietin. Anemia is commonly seen in association with HIV infection, particularly in patients at advanced stages of disease. In some of these patients, circulating levels of erythropoietin are inappropriately low.[47] Such patients may be particularly prone to AZT-induced anemia. In a placebo-controlled trial, Fischl and colleagues demonstrated that recombinant human erythropoietin (100 U/kg three times a week) decreased the need for transfusions among AIDS patients receiving AZT when circulating levels of endogenous erythropoietin were below 500 IU/L.[15]

Recombinant human erythropoietin (epoetin alfa) was approved by the

Food and Drug Administration for the treatment of anemia associated with chronic renal failure in 1989.[31] Approval for use in AIDS patients was granted in early 1991.

Colony-stimulating factors. Leukopenia is commonly encountered during advanced stages of HIV infection and may limit the use of marrow-depressing drugs such as AZT. The hematopoietic hormones granulocyte-macrophage colony stimulating factor (GM-CSF) and granulocyte colony-stimulating factor (G-CSF) speed the maturation of myeloid precursor cells and stimulate the function of mature granulocytes and, in the case of GM-CSF, monocytes.[3,24,34] GM-CSF has been shown to raise the white blood cell count in HIV-infected patients with leukopenia.[19] A regimen of alternating recombinant GM-CSF and AZT caused less hematological toxicity than continuous therapy with AZT in one study.[38] Additional studies will be necessary to establish the role of these hormones in the management of HIV-infected patients.

ACCESS TO EXPERIMENTAL THERAPIES
Clinical Trials

Access to information on new agents. Information regarding experimental protocols conducted by the National Institutes of Health can be obtained through an information hotline of the National Institute of Allergy and Infectious Disease (1-800-TRIALSA). Protocol information may also be obtained through the AIDS/HIV Treatment Directory, published by the American Foundation for AIDS Research in New York.

The AIDS Clinical Trials Group. As of June 1990, 46 medical centers in the United States had been designated AIDS Clinical Trials Group (ACTG) centers. A variety of trials involving both antiretroviral agents and therapy for AIDS-related opportunistic infections and malignancies have been made available through this program. Information on the location of these centers and the availability of specific protocols may be obtained by contacting the National Institute of Allergy and Infectious Disease.

Expanded access programs. Certain investigational antiviral drugs have been made available to selected HIV-infected patients who do not qualify for controlled clinical trials. Such "parallel track" or "expanded access" programs have been the subject of controversy. Although potentially effective therapy has been made available quickly by this means, some have argued that these programs have reduced enrollment in clinical trials and thereby impeded drug evaluation.[1]

Community-based centers. A network of community-based clinical trials centers was established in the United States to increase access to treatment protocols. As of June 1990, there were 38 such units in 21 states, the District of Columbia, and Puerto Rico.[2]

EDUCATING THE PATIENT

Unfortunately, the first decade of the AIDS epidemic was frequently marked by confusion over therapy. Several drugs initially thought to hold promise on the basis of limited data eventually were shown to be ineffective. Concerns about the safety of zidovudine caused many patients to avoid this drug, which, when released, represented the only effective therapy available. A vigorous black market trade in unproven remedies arose. The widespread and often surreptitious use of such "alternate therapies" threatened the validity of clinical trials and in some cases encouraged an atmosphere of mistrust between patients and their physicians.

Under such circumstances, communicating accurate information about therapy may be difficult. In the context of a progressive, debilitating, and ultimately fatal disease, the time-consuming process of large-scale clinical trials may sometimes appear to be an unaffordable luxury to patient and practitioner alike. It may be difficult to explain to frightened patients why they should avoid unproven therapies.

HIV-infected patients represent a heterogeneous population that includes intravenous drug users with limited access to health care; homosexual men from a variety of cultural, ethnic, and socioeconomic backgrounds; and indigent women living in inner cities. Educating patients about appropriate therapy and providing up-to-date information about experimental drugs may be extremely difficult, particularly in the climate of uncertainty that has marked the epidemic since its inception. The practitioner must both provide care and act as advocate for the patient in a confusing atmosphere of new drugs, preliminary reports, misinformation, genuine breakthroughs, and, occasionally, false hope.

Before discussing therapeutic options with the patient, the practitioner should first identify indications for therapy on the basis of clinical and immunological parameters. In many cases the patient will meet indications for established antiviral drugs such as AZT but also qualify for one or more clinical trials involving new agents. The physician caring for HIV-infected patients should periodically request information about trials in progress locally. For federally sponsored studies in the ACTG program, such information may be obtained by contacting the National Institute of Allergy and Infectious Disease (1-800-TRIALSA).

Feelings of hopelessness are common among patients at all stages of infection. In addition to its medical benefits, antiviral therapy may provide a sense of purpose, optimism, and "fighting back." An honest discussion of the advantages and limitations of various treatments and a review of available options should take place early in the care of any HIV-infected patient. Such a discussion may serve to reassure the patient that potentially effective therapy is not being withheld.

The decision to participate in a clinical trial of a new drug should be individualized. In general, patients should be encouraged to enroll in federally sponsored randomized studies for which they qualify. Because effective antiviral therapy is generally available, however, many patients prefer receiving approved drugs to the uncertainty and potential inconvenience of a clinical trial protocol. Patients should be supported in their decisions regarding study participation if medically prudent and not be made to feel coerced.

Pending further developments in the therapy of HIV infection, the goal of the practitioner should be to provide one or more optimum alternatives to the patient and to maintain an atmosphere of trust and open discussion.

COMMON QUESTIONS PATIENTS ASK ABOUT THERAPY

1. IS AIDS CURABLE?
   Current antiviral drugs do not eradicate the AIDS virus from the body. However, the drugs that are effective appear to slow the rate at which the virus reproduces itself. By doing this, these drugs may help delay further damage to the immune system.

2. HOW WILL TAKING AN ANTIVIRAL DRUG HELP ME?
   Although available antiviral drugs do not cure HIV infection or prevent AIDS, it is hoped that by slowing the damage to the immune system, patients may have longer periods of good health and ultimately survive longer. AZT, the first drug approved for HIV infection, was shown to have these effects in clinical trials.

3. CAN I STILL SPREAD THE VIRUS IF I TAKE AN ANTIVIRAL DRUG?
   There is no evidence that taking an antiviral drug prevents you from spreading HIV infection to others through sexual contact or needle-sharing. You should always assume that you may spread the infection.

4. SHOULD OTHERS IN MY HOUSEHOLD TAKE THE DRUG TO PROTECT THEMSELVES FROM BECOMING INFECTED?
   You can only spread HIV infection to other members of your household through sex or sharing of needles. Nonsexual household contacts are not at risk of acquiring HIV infection from you. There is no definite evidence that taking an antiviral drug can protect a person from becoming infected with HIV.

5. WHAT HAPPENS IF I GET PREGNANT?

Women who are infected with HIV can transmit the virus to the fetus during pregnancy. The risk of this occurring appears to be approximately 30% (see Chapter 11). For this reason, HIV-infected women are advised to avoid pregnancy. The safety of most new drugs during pregnancy, including antiviral agents for HIV infection, has not been established. Clinical trials are under way to determine whether antiviral drugs such as zidovudine are safe and also whether they can help protect the fetus from becoming infected. Until the results of these studies are known, it should be assumed that new antiviral drugs might be harmful to the fetus and should only be taken during pregnancy if there is an immediate danger to the mother in avoiding them.

6. WHAT ABOUT SIDE EFFECTS?

By the time drugs are made available to patients, a great deal is known about their side effects. If you participate in an experimental study of a new drug, you should be checked frequently for such side effects. Since most antiviral drugs used in the treatment of HIV infection are new and have been given to a relatively small number of patients, side effects that had not been seen before may appear.

7. IS IT SAFE FOR ME TO POSTPONE THERAPY?

The damage to the immune system that is caused by the AIDS virus occurs gradually, over a period of years. Unless the immune system has been severely damaged already, there is probably no risk in delaying treatment for brief periods of time, such as several weeks. However, there is no known advantage to postponing therapy for most patients. Uncertainty about the risk of side effects is best dealt with by a more thorough explanation by the physician rather than by delay on the part of the patient.

8. ARE THERE NEWER DRUGS THAT ARE BETTER THAN THOSE NOW AVAILABLE?

Newer drugs for the treatment of HIV infection are being developed. It is hoped that some will be more effective than those currently available. Until studies comparing the new drugs to available treatments are carried out, however, it is impossible to know which drug is better and safer.

9. HOW WILL I FIND OUT ABOUT NEW DRUGS?

There are many sources of information about new drugs. Some are more reliable than others. Information about new drugs that are being studied and clinical trials can be obtained by contacting the National Institute of Allergy and Infectious Disease (1-800-TRIALSA). Throughout the history of the AIDS epidemic, misleading information and exaggerated claims have been disseminated about antiviral compounds and drugs to improve immune function. Patients and physicians should be skeptical about purported cures or breakthroughs that have not been reported through conventional medical professional channels such as peer-reviewed journals or recognized national or international meetings.

10. SHOULD I TAKE VITAMINS?

Some patients with HIV infection may be deficient in certain vitamins. However, it is not clear whether taking vitamins is necessary or beneficial. Some medications that are commonly given to HIV-infected patients, particularly trimethoprim-sulfamethoxazole, sulfadiazine, and pyrimethamine, may cause a relative deficiency of the vitamin folate. Therapy with folate or folinic acid may be advisable in patients receiving these drugs, particularly those with anemia or other manifestations of bone marrow depression.

11. SHOULD I TAKE BLACK MARKET DRUGS?

It is impossible to tell whether drugs that have not been thoroughly tested are effective or safe. Many drugs that initially appeared to be effective in small studies or individual patients have been shown to be ineffective. It is impossible to know if untested drugs interfere with the action of drugs that have been proven to be effective. If you choose to try an unproven drug, please inform your physician so that he or she can check for side effects.

12. WHAT IS A CLINICAL TRIAL?

A clinical trial is a program designed to test a drug. In most clinical trials, patients receive either the new drug or an older drug that is known to be effective. Neither the patients nor their physicians know which drug the patients are receiving (double-blinding). For a period of time which is predetermined, the patient is followed closely with repeated examinations and blood tests. At the end of the trial period, patients who received the new drug are compared to those receiving the older drug for signs of benefit or side effects. When there is no standard treatment to which a new drug can be compared, an inactive pill (placebo) may be given to some patients.

Patients who enroll in clinical trials must sign informed consent documents and must be told of the potential risks and benefits of participating. They must be informed if they may receive a placebo.

13. SHOULD I ENROLL IN A CLINICAL TRIAL?

The best therapy for HIV infection eventually will be determined through clinical trials. If more patients volunteer to participate in clinical trials, effective drugs may be identified sooner. An HIV-infected person should consider enrolling in clinical trials for which they are eligible if they understand that (1) the drug they receive may have greater, equal, or less efficacy than standard drugs, and (2) new drugs are more likely to have unexpected side effects than older drugs.

14. WILL THERE BE A CURE FOR AIDS?

It is not known if AIDS will eventually prove to be curable. It has been shown, however, that antiviral therapy can prolong the life of HIV-infected patients. This encouraging fact raises the possibility that overall survival may improve further with more effective drugs or treatment strategies. Since the discovery of HIV, efforts to find effective therapy have intensified steadily.

REFERENCES

1. AIDS Update 3(24):1-2, 1990.
2. American Foundation for AIDS Research: *AIDS/HIV Treatment Directory*, vol 4, New York, 1990, The Foundation.
3. Baldwin GC et al: Granulocyte-macrophage colony-stimulating factor enhances neutrophil function in acquired immunodeficiency syndrome patients, *Proc Natl Acad Sci USA* 85(8):2763-2767, 1988.
4. Broder S: Pharmacodynamics of 2',3'-dideoxycytidine: an inhibitor of human immunodeficiency virus, *Am J Med* 88:5B-2S-7S, 1990.
5. Broder S, et al: Antiretroviral therapy in AIDS, *Ann Intern Med* 113(8):604-618, 1990.
6. Broder S, Yarchoan R: Dideoxycytidine: current clinical experience and future prospects: a summary, *Am J Med* 88:5B-31S-33S, 1990.
7. Centers for Disease Control: Public Health Service statement on management of occupational exposure to human immunodeficiency virus, including considerations regarding zidovudine postexposure use, MMWR 39(RR-1):1-14, 1990.
8. Cooley TP et al: Once daily administration of 2',3'-dideoxyinosine (DDI) in patients with the acquired immunodeficiency syndrome or AIDS-related complex: results of a phase I trial, *N Engl J Med* 322(19):1340-1345, 1990.
9. Cotton P: Controversy continues as experts ponder zidovudine's role in early HIV infection, *JAMA* 263(12):1605, 1990.
10. Creagh-Kirk T et al: Survival experience among patients with AIDS receiving zidovudine: follow-up of patients in a compassionate plea program, *JAMA* 260(20):3009-3015, 1988.
11. Fauci AS: DDI: a good start, but still phase I, *N Engl J Med* 322(19):1386-1388, 1990.
12. Fiala M et al: Responses of neurologic complications of AIDS 3'-azido-3'-deoxythymidine and 9-(1,3-dihydroxy-2-propoxymethyl) guanine. I. Clinical features, *Rev Infect Dis* 10(2):250-256, 1988.
13. Fischl MA et al: The efficacy of azidothymidine (AZT) in the treatment of patients with AIDS and AIDS-related complex: a double-blind, placebo-controlled trial, *N Engl J Med* 317(4):185-191, 1987.
14. Fischl MA et al: Prolonged zidovudine therapy in patients with AIDS and advanced AIDS-related complex, *JAMA* 262:2405-2410, 1989.
15. Fischl M et al: Recombinant human erythropoietin for patients with AIDS treated with zidovudine, *N Engl J Med* 322(21):1488-1493, 1990.
16. Fischl MA et al: The safety and efficacy

of zidovudine (AZT) in the treatment of subjects with mildly symptomatic human immunodeficiency virus type 1 (HIV) infection: a double-blind, placebo-controlled trial, *Ann Intern Med* 112:727-737, 1990.

17. Gail MH, Rosenberg PS, Goedert JJ: Therapy may explain recent deficits in AIDS incidence, *J Acquir Immune Defic Syndr* 3:296-306, 1990.

18. Gertner E et al: Zidovudine-associated myopathy, *Am J Med* 86:814-818, 1989.

18a. Gottlieb MS et al: Response to treatment with the leukocyte-derived immunomodulator IMREG-1 in immunocompromised patients with AIDS-related complex. A multicenter, double-blind, placebo-controlled trial, *Ann Intern Med* 115:84-91, 1991.

19. Groopman JE: Granulocyte-macrophage colony-stimulating factor in human immunodeficiency virus disease, *Semin Hematol* 27(3 suppl 3):8-14, 1990.

20. Hirsch MS: Chemotherapy of human immunodeficiency virus infections: current practice and future prospects, *J Infect Dis* 161:845-857, 1990.

21. Johnson VA et al: Synergistic inhibition of human immunodeficiency virus type 1 (HIV-1) replication in vitro by recombinant soluble CD4 and 3'-azido-3'-deoxythymidine, *J Infect Dis* 159(5):837-844, 1989.

22. Johnson VA et al: Three-drug synergistic inhibition of HIV-1 replication in vitro by zidovudine, recombinant soluble CD4, and recombinant interferon-alpha A, *J Infect Dis* 161:1059-1067, 1990.

23. Kahn JO et al: The safety and pharmacokinetics of recombinant soluble CD4 (rCD4) in subjects with the acquired immunodeficiency syndrome (AIDS) and AIDS-related complex: a phase 1 study, *Ann Intern Med* 112(4):254-261, 1990.

24. Klingemann HG: Clinical applications of recombinant human colony-stimulating factors, *Can Med Assoc J* 140(2):137-142, 1989.

25. Krown SE et al: Interferon-alpha with zidovudine: safety, tolerance, and clinical and virologic effects in patients with Kaposi sarcoma associated with the acquired immunodeficiency syndrome (AIDS), *Ann Intern Med* 112(11):812-821, 1990.

26. Kweder SL, Schnur RA, Cooper EC: Inosine pranobex: is a single positive trial enough? *N Engl J Med* 322(25):1807-1809, 1990.

27. Lambert JS et al: 2'3'-Dideoxyinosine (DDI) in patients with the acquired immunodeficiency syndrome or AIDS-related complex, *N Engl J Med* 322(19):1333-1340, 1990.

28. Lane HC et al: Interferon-alpha in patients with asymptomatic human immunodeficiency (HIV) infection: a randomized, placebo-controlled trial, *Ann Intern Med* 112(11):805-811, 1990.

29. Lange JMA et al: Failure of zidovudine prophylaxis after accidental exposure to HIV-1, *N Engl J Med* 322:1375-1377, 1990.

30. Larder BA, Darby G, Richman DD: HIV with reduced sensitivity to zidovudine (AZT) isolated during prolonged therapy, *Science* 243:1731-1734, 1989.

31. The Medical Letter: Erythropoietin for anemia, *Med Lett Drugs Ther* 31:85-86, 1989.

32. Meng T, Fischl MA, Richman DD: AIDS Clinical Trials Group: phase I/II study of combination 2',3'-dideoxycytidine and zidovudine in patients with acquired immunodeficiency syndrome (AIDS) and advanced AIDS-related complex, *Am J Med* 88:5B-27S-30S, 1990.

33. Merigan TC et al: Safety and tolerance of dideoxycytidine as a single agent: results of early-phase studies in patients with acquired immunodefi-

ciency syndrome (AIDS) or advanced AIDS-related complex, *Am J Med* 88:5B-11S-15S, 1990.

34. Mitsuyasu RT, Golde DW: Potential role of granulocyte-macrophage colony-stimulating factor in patients with HIV infection, *Behring Inst Mitt* 83:139-144, 1988.

35. Montaner JSG et al: The effect of zidovudine on platelet count in HIV-infected individuals, *J Acquir Immun Defic Syndr* 3:565-570, 1990.

36. National Institutes of Health: Recommendations for zidovudine: early infection, *JAMA* 263(12):1606-1607, 1990.

37. Pedersen C et al: The efficacy of inosine pranobex in preventing the acquired immunodeficiency syndrome in patients with human immunodeficiency virus infection, *N Engl J Med* 322(25):1757-1763, 1990.

38. Pluda JM et al: Subcutaneous recombinant granulocyte-macrophage colony-stimulating factor used as a single agent and in an alternating regimen with azidothymidine in leukopenic patients with severe human immunodeficiency virus infection, *Blood* 76(3):463-472, 1990.

39. Pottage JC et al: Treatment of human immunodeficiency virus–related thrombocytopenia with zidovudine, *JAMA* 260(20):3045-3050, 1988.

40. Richman DD: Susceptibility to nucleoside analogues of zidovudine-resistant isolates of human immunodeficiency virus, *Am J Med* 88:5B-8S-15S, 1990.

41. Richman DD et al: The toxicity of azidothymidine (AZT) in the treatment of patients with AIDS and AIDS-related complex: a double-blind, placebo-controlled trial, *N Engl J Med* 317(4):192-197, 1987.

42. Ruedy J, Schechter M, Montaner JSG: Zidovudine for early human immunodeficiency (HIV) infection: who,

when, and how? *Ann Intern Med* 112(10):721-723, 1990.

43. Ruprecht RM et al: Interferon-alpha and 3'-azido-3'-deoxythymidine are highly synergistic in mice and prevent viremia after retrovirus exposure, *J Acquir Immun Defic Syndr* 3:591-600, 1990.

44. Ruprecht RM et al: Suppression of mouse viremia and retroviral disease by 3'-azido-3'-deoxythymidine, *Nature* 323:467-469, 1986.

45. Schooley RT et al: Recombinant soluble CD4 therapy in patients with the acquired immunodeficiency syndrome (AIDS) and AIDS-related complex: a phase I-II escalating dosage trial, *Ann Intern Med* 112(4):247-253, 1990.

46. Skowron G: Alternating and intermittent regimens of zidovudine (3'-azido'3'-deoxythymidine) and dideoxycytidine (2',3'-dideoxycytidine) in the treatment of patients with acquired immunodeficiency syndrome (AIDS) and AIDS-related complex, *Am J Med* 88:5B-20S-23S, 1990.

47. Spivak JL et al: Serum immunoreactive erythropoietin in HIV-infected patients, *JAMA* 261(21):3104-3107, 1989.

48. Surbone A et al: Treatment of the acquired immunodeficiency syndrome (AIDS) and AIDS-related complex with a regimen of 3'-azido-2',3'-dideoxythymidine (azidothymidine or zidovudine) and acyclovir: a pilot study, *Ann Intern Med* 108:534-540, 1988.

49. The Swiss Group for Clinical Studies on the Acquired Immunodeficiency Syndrome (AIDS): Zidovudine for the treatment of thrombocytopenia associated with human immunodeficiency virus (HIV): a prospective study, *Ann Intern Med* 109:718-721, 1988.

50. Tavares L et al: 3'-Azido-3'-deoxythymidine in feline leukemia virus–infected cats: a model of therapy and prophylaxis of AIDS, *Cancer Res* 47:3190-3194, 1987.

51. Tramont EC, Redfield RR: Soluble CD4: the first step, *Ann Intern Med* 112(40):241-242, 1990.

52. Volberding PA et al: Zidovudine in asymptomatic human immunodeficiency virus infection: a controlled trial in persons with fewer than 500 CD4-positive cells per cubic millimeter, *N Engl J Med* 322:941-949, 1990.

53. Yarchoan R, Mitsuya H, Broder S: Strategies for the combination therapy of HIV infection, *J Acquir Immun Defic Syndr* 3(suppl 2):S99-S103, 1990.

CHAPTER **11**

HIV Infection and Pregnancy

THE SCOPE OF HIV INFECTION AMONG WOMEN OF REPRODUCTIVE AGE

As the full extent of the worldwide epidemic caused by the human immuno-deficiency virus (HIV) has been recognized and patterns of infection within various groups have come into sharper focus, it has become apparent that women of reproductive age will bear an increasingly large share of the burden of acquired immunodeficiency syndrome (AIDS) for the foreseeable future. In countries where HIV infection is transmitted primarily by heterosexual contact (so-called pattern II countries), sexually active women have accounted for approximately half of reported cases of AIDS. Seroprevalence data gathered during the late 1980s from these countries, which include areas of Africa, the Caribbean, and South America, indicate that as many as 25% of young adults in some areas are infected.[39]

In the United States, where HIV transmission has occurred primarily among male homosexuals and intravenous drug users (pattern I), the proportion of AIDS cases among women of reproductive age has increased steadily over the first decade of the epidemic.[15] This trend has continued as the proportion of new AIDS cases among homosexual men has declined.[15]

Because of the potential for vertical transmission of HIV infection, increasing rates of infection among pregnant women have added the growing dimension of pediatric AIDS to the worldwide epidemic. The profound importance of infection with the human immunodeficiency virus (HIV) during pregnancy is illustrated by two facts: (1) most reported AIDS cases among women have occurred in those of childbearing age,[18] and (2) infection with HIV in women of childbearing age accounts for more than 80% of AIDS cases among children.[18]

The Incidence of AIDS in Women of Reproductive Age

Through October 1990, 14,816 cases of AIDS in women had been reported in the United States.[18] Of these cases 77% involved women between 20 and 44 years of age[18] (Figure 11-1). Surveillance statistics indicate that the proportion of AIDS cases in women rose from 7% before 1984 to 10% in 1988.[15] Between July 1990 and June 1991, 12.3% of adult AIDS cases occurred in women.[18] If trends seen over the first decade of the epidemic continue, by 1991 AIDS will have become one of the five most frequent causes of death among women between 15 and 44 years of age.[20]

The geographical distribution of AIDS cases among women in the United States parallels that of the general epidemic. From November 1989 to October 1990, the national incidence of AIDS in women was 4.3 per 100,000[19]; however, the District of Columbia, Florida, New York, New Jersey, and Puerto Rico all reported more than 10 cases per 100,000.[19]

The Prevalence of HIV Infection in Women of Reproductive Age

Because HIV-positive, asymptomatic women who may be unaware that they are infected can become pregnant and transmit the infection to the fetus, the

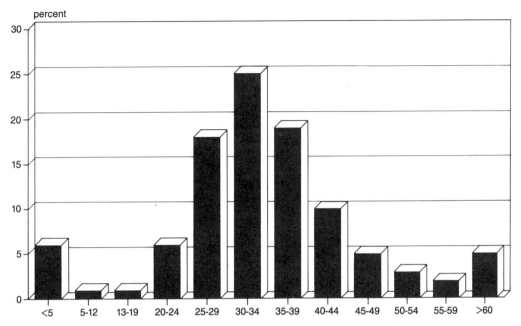

FIGURE 11-1. AIDS in U.S. women. Age distribution.
Based on data from CDC HIV/AIDS surveillance, May, 1991.

seroprevalence rate of HIV infection in women of reproductive age provides greater insight into the future of the epidemic than do AIDS incidence data. However, such seroprevalence data are largely unavailable. Demographic patterns in reported AIDS cases and routes of transmission indicate that seroprevalence varies greatly among geographical regions and ethnic groups.

Data gathered from HIV testing of applicants for military service have suggested some alarming trends. Although the prevalence of HIV infection among male applicants for service in the U.S. military is gradually falling, the prevalence among females has remained almost constant.[15] Although most AIDS cases still are seen in men, the prevalence of HIV infection among male and female teenagers applying for military service is approximately equal.[11]

The Prevalence of HIV Infection Among Pregnant Women

The prevalence of HIV infection among pregnant women in various parts of the United States has been measured in two ways, through prenatal screening of mothers and through testing of cord blood after delivery. These techniques have yielded comparable results.

The substantial impact of HIV infection in pregnancy in areas of high overall prevalence was reflected in a measured seroprevalence rate of 1.25% among newborns in New York City in 1988[50] and of 0.8% in inner-city hospitals in Massachusetts in 1987.[30] In prenatal screening studies of pregnant women, 0.28% of a population of inner-city women in Atlanta[38] and 0.5% of women in one series from Illinois[5] were HIV-infected. Other surveys reported during the late 1980s indicated a range of seroprevalence of 0 to 4.3%, with the highest rates reported from New York, Newark, and Miami.[15]

Broad-based seroprevalence data are currently being gathered in a national study that will further define geographical patterns of HIV infection among childbearing women.[52]

Risk Behavior Among Women

Of 4833 cases of AIDS in women reported in the United States between November 1989 and October 1990, intravenous drug use and heterosexual contact with risk-group males accounted for 48% and 34%, respectively.[18] Since the beginning of the epidemic, the proportion of cases among women attributed to intravenous drug use has fallen from 58% and the proportion resulting from heterosexual contact has risen from 16%[15] (Figure 11-2).

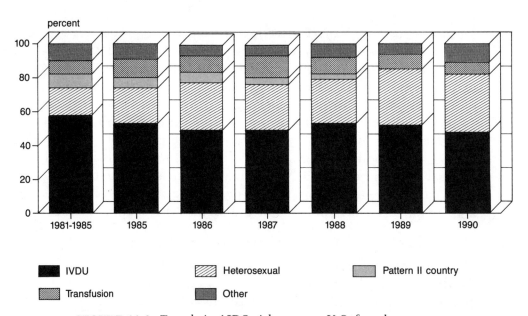

FIGURE 11-2. Trends in AIDS risk groups: U.S. females.

Based on data from CDC HIV/AIDS surveillance and MMWR 38(S-4):1-38, 1989.

Female HIV Infection and Pediatric AIDS

Shortly after the first cases of pediatric AIDS were described, it became apparent that children of mothers at risk for AIDS themselves were at highest risk.[3,70] As evidence for vertical transmission of HIV infection became stronger, a direct relationship between HIV infection among pregnant women and the epidemic of AIDS in children was recognized.

The important role of intravenous drug use in the pediatric AIDS epidemic has been established by epidemiological data. Through 1988 more than 70% of children who had acquired AIDS in the perinatal period were born to women who were either intravenous drug users or sexual partners of male intravenous drug users.[26]

THE IMPACT OF HIV INFECTION DURING PREGNANCY
Pregnancy Outcome

Asymptomatic HIV infection appears to have no substantial impact on fertility or on the rates of spontaneous abortion, stillbirth, or low birth weight.[64] However, premature labor complicated 35% of pregnancies among HIV-infected women in one series.[25]

The Risk of Acceleration of HIV Infection

Immunological alterations normally associated with pregnancy raise the theoretical possibility that the natural history of HIV infection could be accelerated in pregnant women. The CD4 lymphocyte count typically decreases progressively during pregnancy in both HIV-infected and noninfected women.[6] This count returns to normal at term in uninfected women, but HIV infection in pregnancy may be associated with persistent depletion of CD4 lymphocytes.[6]

Although AIDS has been reported among pregnant women,[29,57,71] retrospective data indicate that the incidence is low.[33] As in HIV-infected patients who are not pregnant, immunological parameters, particularly the CD4 lymphocyte count, correlate with the risk of progression to AIDS. In one prospective series, three of 16 women with CD4 lymphocyte counts under $300/mm^3$ during pregnancy developed opportunistic infections, whereas those with higher counts did not.[44]

INFECTION OF THE FETUS AND NEWBORN
The Risk of Transmission

Transmission of HIV from infected mother to fetus appears to occur in the minority of cases. It is not known what specific determinants (i.e., host or organism properties) dictate when and if such vertical transmission occurs. Although breast-feeding occasionally may be a route of transmission[69,72] and

TABLE 11-1.   Risk of transmission from infected mother to infant

Size of cohort	Rate of transmission
372	12.9%[23a]
230	25.2%[27]*
117	27%[7]
28	7.1%[46]
24	25%[31]†

*Estimated.
†Minimum rate of transmission.

infection during delivery has been postulated, the vast majority of cases of HIV infection among neonates appear to result from in utero transmission. This may occur whether the HIV-infected mother is symptomatic or asymptomatic.[85] An infected woman may or may not transmit infection to the fetus during successive pregnancies.[85]

It is not clear at which stage of pregnancy HIV transmission is most likely to occur, although fetal infection has been documented in first trimester[62] and second trimester[58] abortuses and may occur as early as 8 weeks of gestation.[65] Delivery by cesarean section does not eliminate the risk of transmission.[42]

Prospective studies have generally indicated that approximately one fourth to one third of children born to HIV-infected mothers will be infected.[4,7,27,31] However, transmission rates as low as 7%[46] and as high as 40%[32] have been reported (Table 11-1). Transmission rates appear to be comparable for all maternal risk groups.

The Effects of HIV Infection on the Fetus

Growth failure may be seen in 75% or more of infected infants.[23,40] It has been suggested that specific deformities, including microcephaly, ocular hypertelorism, prominent forehead, flat nasal bridge, long palpebral fissures, blue sclerae, and patulous lips may be associated with congenital infection.[40] However, the relationship of these features to HIV infection has been challenged.[23]

Pediatric HIV Infection

Through June 1991 3140 AIDS cases among children under 13 years of age had been reported in the United States.[18] Of these, 2645 (84%) were among children born to mothers known to be HIV-infected themselves or at high risk of infection[18] (Figure 11-3). The remaining cases occurred in children with hemophilia or other coagulation disorders (5%), other recipients of transfusions of blood or blood products (9%), and children of undetermined risk (2%).

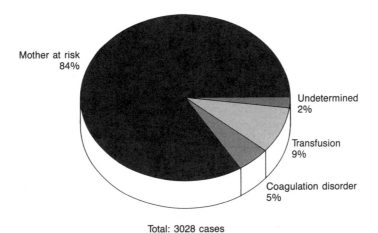

FIGURE 11-3. U.S. pediatric AIDS: risk categories.

Based on data from CDC: HIV/AIDS surveillance, May, 1991.

The racial distribution of pediatric AIDS cases reported from the United States through 1990 was black, 53%; Hispanic, 25%; white (non-Hispanic), 21%.[18] The male-to-female ratio was 1.16:1.[18]

The geographical distribution of the AIDS epidemic in children has paralleled that among adults in the United States. Through August 1990, 20% of all reported AIDS cases and 27% of pediatric cases had been reported from New York City.[49] Clusters of pediatric cases have been reported from metropolitan areas reporting large numbers of adult AIDS cases. These include Miami; Newark, New Jersey; Los Angeles; and San Francisco.[70]

The natural history of perinatally acquired AIDS differs from that of the adult disease. Whereas HIV-infected adults typically remain asymptomatic for several years after infection and AIDS-related disorders may not occur for 5 to 10 years, children who are born infected develop symptomatic disease at a median age of 8 months,[61] and 80% are symptomatic by 2 years of age.

THE ROLE OF EARLY SCREENING
Serological Screening of Mothers

If effective, screening programs designed to detect HIV infection among pregnant women would be expected to have a significant impact on the pediatric AIDS epidemic. HIV testing early in pregnancy would afford the opportunity for termination of the pregnancy if this is desired or, perhaps, for therapeutic interventions to prevent transmission to the fetus.

However, despite increasing recognition of the extent of the HIV epidemic among women of childbearing age, a number of technical obstacles to effective screening programs remain.[51] The social setting in which HIV infection occurs most commonly (i.e., drug abuse and poverty) has presented substantial logistical problems to the medical community.[37]

The U.S. Public Health Service has advised that all women at risk for HIV infection who are pregnant or who seek family planning services be counseled and offered HIV testing.[13] However, targeting only women who are aware that they are at risk for HIV infection may fail to identify a substantial proportion who are infected. In one series, 40% of HIV-infected pregnant women gave no history of risk behavior.[36] For this reason, screening programs based on routine HIV counseling and voluntary testing of all pregnant women may be more effective.[44]

Prenatal Screening for Fetal HIV Infection

In recent years the development of techniques to allow for prenatal diagnosis of fetal HIV infection has received increasing attention; however, reliable means of diagnosis based on viral studies have not been developed. Immunological testing of fetal blood, including lymphocyte subset analysis, failed to distinguish HIV-infected from uninfected fetuses in one series.[55]

Screening the Newborn for HIV Infection

Testing the newborn for HIV infection by means of standard antibody assays is complicated by the persistence of maternal antibodies for approximately 15 months,[12] resulting in uninfected infants initialing testing HIV antibody positive. Adding to the diagnostic confusion is the phenomenon of late seroconversion, such that some infected infants initially test HIV antibody negative.[8] In one reported case a child who tested HIV negative after 6 months developed detectable antibody at 22 months of age.[32]

Several diagnostic techniques may permit confirmation of HIV infection before 15 months of age in a child born to an infected mother. These techniques include detection of anti-HIV IgM antibodies,[32] IgG antibody against new HIV antigens,[32] p24 antigen,[32] and proviral DNA by the polymerase chain reaction (PCR)[22] and viral culture of peripheral blood mononuclear cells.[22] Unfortunately these techniques have not been standardized, are not generally available, and require the facilities of research laboratories.

Until precise techniques for early detection of HIV infection are developed further and become more widely available, the HIV status of asymptomatic infants born to infected mothers should be considered indeterminate for the first 18 months of life and definitive testing should be carried out after that age.

THE APPROACH TO COUNSELING
Routine HIV Testing and Counseling of Pregnant Women

Several approaches to screening for HIV infection in pregnancy have been proposed. Although it is generally agreed that women with a history of risk behavior should be urged to undergo voluntary testing and counseling, such directed screening may fail to identify significant numbers of women who are unaware of or unwilling to admit to possible HIV exposure. For this reason routine confidential testing has been advocated by some.[44]

All pregnant women should be questioned thoroughly about their potential HIV risk (see Chapter 4). Questioning should cover current or previous intravenous drug use, blood transfusions before 1985, and current or past sexual contact with males either known to be or suspected of being at high risk. Testing and counseling should be offered to and strongly advised for any woman who knows or suspects that she is at risk of infection.[13] Women with no apparent risk, particularly those with a history of several sexual partners, should be informed of the consequences of HIV infection in pregnancy and offered voluntary testing.

Women who have lived in countries of high HIV prevalence (i.e., Haiti, central Africa) or who have engaged in prostitution should be encouraged to undergo counseling and testing.

Advising HIV-Infected Women Who Want to Become Pregnant

Women who are known to be HIV infected should be advised to avoid pregnancy because of the high risk of perinatal transmission to their child. Those who give a history of definite or possible exposure to HIV should be counseled to postpone pregnancy until HIV infection has been ruled out. In some cases (i.e., when potential exposure has occurred within the preceding 6 months) serial testing over a period of 3 to 6 months may be required. Women who test negative and have continued to engage in risk behavior for several years should be informed that current tests may not detect infection for 6 months or more after exposure in some cases.[56]

Advising Pregnant HIV-Infected Women

The risk of transmission of HIV infection from mother to child during the perinatal period is approximately 1 in 3. Until reliable means of diagnosing fetal HIV infection early in pregancy are available, it must be assumed that all pregnancies of infected women carry an equal risk of transmission. It may be difficult for the asymptomatic HIV-infected mother to appreciate fully the impact of giving birth to an infected infant and the medical and social difficulties that she and her child may face. The practitioner should openly discuss these difficulties, including the following:

1. It is a near certainty that the infected mother will develop AIDS or other symptoms of HIV infection within the first few years of the child's life. It should be stressed that the mother's worsening health may create insurmountable emotional and financial problems in raising the child.

2. The possibility exists that carrying the pregnancy to term could accelerate the mother's HIV infection.

3. All HIV-infected infants will develop AIDS within several years, and AIDS is currently a uniformly fatal disease. Prospective data indicate that symptomatic disease appears at an average of 8 months and that nearly 80% of children become symptomatic within 2 years.[61] The pregnant woman should consider the emotional and financial implications of caring for a dying child while her own health may be deteriorating.

4. The safety of therapeutic agents currently used to manage HIV infection (e.g., antiretroviral and anti-*Pneumocystis* drugs) is unknown in pregnancy. Withholding these drugs out of concern for potential fetal toxicity may jeopardize the mother's health, whereas administering them may have deleterious effects on the fetus.

Despite the known high risk of fetal infection, HIV-infected pregnant women counseled about the risk often decline abortion on the basis of personal, religious, or family concerns.[63]

MEDICAL MANAGEMENT OF THE HIV-INFECTED PREGNANT WOMAN
Immunological Testing

Immunological staging, particularly lymphocyte subset analysis, has been demonstrated to correlate with the risk of opportunistic infection in HIV-infected pregnant women,[43] as it has in other patients.[16] See Chapter 6 for staging guidelines.

Immunization

Pneumococcal vaccine. Pneumococcal vaccine has been recommended for symptomatic HIV-infected patients[17] and can be given safely in pregnancy.[1]

Influenza vaccine. Symptomatic HIV-infected patients should be immunized against influenza.[14] Influenza vaccine is safe in pregnancy.[1]

Hepatitis B vaccine. Immunization against hepatitis B has been advised for nonimmune, HIV-infected patients.[28] The vaccine should be given to pregnant HIV-infected women at high risk of hepatitis B.

Tetanus and diphtheria vaccines. Vaccination against tetanus and diphtheria has been advised for nonimmune, HIV-infected individuals.[14] Pregnant women who have not been immunized should receive two doses of the combined vaccine, 4 to 8 weeks apart, during the second or third trimesters and a third dose 6 to 12 months later.[1] Booster doses are advised for individuals immunized more than 10 years previously.

Measles, mumps, and rubella (MMR) vaccines. Although the combined live virus vaccine MMR is recommended for unimmunized HIV-infected patients,[14] it should not be administered to women who are pregnant or likely to become pregnant within 3 months.[1] Immune globulin may be given to nonimmune, HIV-infected pregnant women after exposure to measles.[14]

Polio vaccine. It is recommended that the oral polio vaccine not be administered to HIV-infected patients.[14] The inactivated vaccine is recommended for patients who have not been immunized and may be administered in pregnancy.[1]

Varicella zoster immune globulin. Primary varicella infection may be particularly severe in pregnancy and in HIV-infected patients. Varicella zoster immune globulin (VZIG) may prevent or lessen the severity of varicella in a nonimmune patient. Children born to mothers with varicella beginning within 48 hours before delivery to 5 days after delivery should receive VZIG to prevent neonatal varicella.[1]

Antiretroviral Therapy

The safety and efficacy of zidovudine and other antiretroviral drugs in pregnancy is not yet known,[48] although zidovudine has been shown to cross the placenta and attain serum levels in the fetus comparable to those in the mother.[59] Despite this uncertainty, some authors have suggested that, for women requiring zidovudine, therapy be continued during pregnancy with close monitoring for maternal and fetal toxicity.[9] Current updated recommendations should be sought before such therapy is instituted.

Pneumocystis Carinii Prophylaxis

Prophylaxis against *Pneumocystis carinii* pneumonia (PCP) with either oral trimethoprim-sulfamethoxazole or aerosolized or systemic pentamidine can substantially reduce the incidence of this infection (see Chapter 6). Such prophylaxis has been recommended for AIDS patients with a previous diagnosis of PCP or for other HIV-infected patients with a CD4 lymphocyte count under $200/mm^3$ or less than 20% of the total lymphocyte count.[16]

Pentamidine. Little is known about the use of pentamidine in pregnancy. In vitro data suggest that small concentrations of the drug may reach the fetus.[24] Theoretical risks to the fetus have led some to recommend that pregnant health care workers avoid exposure to the drug.[21] Since serum levels of pentamidine are extremely low or undetectable after aerosol administration,[47] this technique may be preferable to the systemic route in pregnant women, although the preferred route of administration has not been established in clinical trials.

Trimethoprim-sulfamethoxazole. Trimethoprim in high doses may be teratogenic in animals. Since the drug is a folate antagonist and folate levels in pregnancy may be marginal, it should be avoided if possible.[34] Sulfonamides, including sulfamethoxazole, may also be teratogenic in animals. However, in a study of 90 HIV-negative women treated for bacteriuria during pregnancy with trimethoprim-sulfamethoxazole, no increase in congenital abnormalities over a placebo group was seen.[10] It is not known whether these data, derived from patients who received limited courses of therapy, may be applicable to HIV-infected patients receiving continuous therapy for the duration of the pregnancy.

Based on the lack of safety data, the Centers for Disease Control advises against using either pentamidine or trimethoprim-sulfamethoxazole in pregnancy[16] and recommends, instead, close monitoring for early clinical evidence of PCP. The effectiveness of this approach in preventing PCP mortality has not been established; however, the use of effective PCP prophylaxis (i.e., either trimethoprim-sulfamethoxazole or aerosolized pentamidine) may be justified in pregnant women at high risk and has been recommended by some authors.[45] However, potential risks and benefits should be discussed thoroughly with the mother before any therapy is instituted.

The Use of Other Common Therapeutic Agents in Pregnancy

Other drugs commonly given to HIV-infected patients include ketoconazole, fluconazole, acyclovir, isoniazid, rifampin, pyrazinamide, sulfadiazine, pyrimethamine, clindamycin, and amphotericin B. Only therapy necessary to treat or prevent relapse of a significant opportunistic infection should be given to HIV-infected pregnant women.

Following is a summary of the common indications in ambulatory patients of several frequently used drugs as well as their use in pregnancy:

Ketoconazole

Common indications. Ketoconazole is used to treat oral, esophageal, or cutaneous candidiasis, for maintenance therapy of disseminated histoplasmosis, and for dermatophyte infections.

Use in pregnancy. The safety of ketoconazole in pregnancy has not been established, and teratogenic effects have been seen in laboratory animals.[53] It is recommended that mothers do not breast-feed while taking the drug.[53]

Recommendation. Ketoconazole should not be used to treat non-life-threatening fungal infections during pregnancy. If possible, a nonabsorbable antifungal agent (e.g., Mycostatin) should be used to treat oral candidiasis.

Fluconazole

Common indications. Fluconazole is used to treat oral, esophageal, or cutaneous candidiasis, for dermatophyte infections, and for maintenance therapy of cryptococcosis.

Use in pregnancy. The safety of fluconazole in pregnancy has not been established.

Recommendations. Fluconazole should be use only to treat life-threatening fungal infections in pregnancy.

Acyclovir

Common indications. Acyclovir is used to treat localized or disseminated herpes simplex or herpes zoster infections.

Use in pregnancy. The safety of acyclovir in pregnancy has not been established, although teratogenicity has not been documented at therapeutic dosages.[41]

Recommendations. Acyclovir should be used only for life-threatening infections during pregnancy. Possible indications include invasive or disseminated cutaneous infections or any visceral infection caused by herpes simplex or herpes zoster, as well as localized herpes zoster in patients at high risk for dissemination. Topical acyclovir may provide an alternative for minor skin infections caused by herpes simplex, since systemic absorption appears to be minimal.[53]

Antituberculous therapy

Common indications. Antituberculous therapy is used for active tuberculosis or atypical mycobacterial infection; isoniazid prophylaxis against tuberculosis is used in some individuals with a positive tuberculin skin test.

Use in pregnancy. Teratogenic effects have not been attributed to isoniazid, rifampin, or ethambutol.[2] Streptomycin may cause congenital deafness. The safety of pyrazinamide, capreomycin, cycloserine, and ethionamide has not been established.[2]

Recommendations. Because active tuberculosis during pregnancy poses a substantial risk to both the mother and the fetus, it has been recommended that effective therapy be administered.[2] Isoniazid, rifampin and, if necessary, ethambutol are preferred because of their apparent safety. Breast-feeding is permissible for women receiving these drugs.[2] The relative risks and benefits of therapy for atypical mycobacterial infection in pregnancy have not been established.

Sulfadiazine

Common indications. Sulfadiazine is used for initial and maintenance therapy of cerebral toxoplasmosis (with pyrimethamine) and to treat isosporiasis.

Use in pregnancy. The safety of sulfadiazine in pregnancy has not been established. Sulfonamides have been teratogenic in animal studies. Sulfonamide antibiotics may replace bilirubin from albumin binding sites, causing jaundice. Infants born to mothers receiving sulfonamides may develop jaundice and in some cases kernicterus.

Recommendations. Because of the potential risk to the fetus, sulfadiazine should be administered during pregnancy only for life-threatening infections such as cerebral toxoplasmosis. This infection is often treated empirically with supportive radiographic and serological evidence (see Chapter 9).

Pyrimethamine

Common indications. Pyrimethamine is used for initial and maintenance therapy of cerebral toxoplasmosis (with sulfadiazine or clindamycin).

Use in pregnancy. Pyrimethamine may be teratogenic at high doses. It is recommended that folinic acid be administered concurrently in pregnant women.[54]

Recommendations. Pyrimethamine, usually in combination with sulfadiazine, is an essential component in the treatment of cerebral toxoplasmosis in AIDS, a life-threatening infection. Regimens that do not include pyrimethamine have not yet been shown to have equal efficacy. Since treatment of cerebral toxoplasmosis is often empiric, it is important that radiographic and serological studies support the diagnosis (see Chapter 9).

Clindamycin

Common indications. Clindamycin is used for initial or maintenance therapy of cerebral toxoplasmosis in sulfa-intolerant patients.

Use in pregnancy. Clindamycin is not known to be safe in pregnancy, although harmful effects have not been noted.[35] Small amounts may be secreted in breast milk.[66]

Recommendations. Clindamycin may provide an alternative to sulfadiazine in the treatment of cerebral toxoplasmosis (see Chapter 9), although its relative efficacy is under investigation.

Amphotericin B

Common indications. Amphotericin B is used for initial and maintenance therapy of cryptococcosis and for initial therapy of histoplasmosis and disseminated candidiasis.

Use in pregnancy. Amphotericin B crosses the placenta and its safety in pregnancy has not been established, although animal studies have not documented teratogenicity.

Recommendations. Amphotericin B should be used during pregnancy only to treat life-threatening systemic fungal infections such as cryptococcosis, histoplasmosis, and aspergillosis. Maintenance therapy with amphotericin B or fluconazole[67,68] may decrease the likelihood of clinical relapse in AIDS patients recovering from cryptococcal meningitis. The relative safety of continuing such therapy during pregnancy has not been established, although it is probably warranted in view of high relapse rates among patients not receiving such therapy.

Ganciclovir

Common indications. Ganciclovir is used to treat cytomegalovirus (CMV) infection, particularly retinitis, colitis, and esophagitis.

Use in pregnancy. The safety of ganciclovir in pregnancy has not been established.

Recommendations. Ganciclovir should be administered during pregnancy only for life- or sight-threatening cytomegalovirus infection.

SUMMARY

The incidence of AIDS and the prevalence of HIV infection are rising disproportionately fast among women of childbearing age. Minority women living in inner-city areas bear the greatest burden. As this trend continues and the pediatric AIDS epidemic expands, many critical questions must be answered:

What is the most effective means of screening this group?

Can fetal HIV infection be reliably diagnosed in utero?

Can antiretroviral therapy diminish the risk of mother-to-fetus transmission?

What forms of therapy are safe and effective in HIV-infected pregnant women?

Can we effectively and humanely respond to the medical and social needs of HIV-infected mothers and children?

REFERENCES

1. ACP Task Force on Adult Immunization and Infectious Diseases Society of America: Immunizations for special groups of patients. In *Guide for adult immunization*, ed 2, Philadelphia, 1990, American College of Physicians.
2. American Thoracic Society: Treatment of tuberculosis and tuberculosis infection in adults and children, *Am Rev Respir Dis* 134:355-363, 1986.
3. Amman AJ: The acquired immunodeficiency syndrome in infants and children, *Ann Intern Med* 103:734-737, 1985.
4. Andiman WA et al: Rate of transmission of human immunodeficiency virus type 1 infection from mother to child

and short-term outcome of neonatal infection: results of a prospective cohort study, *Am J Dis Child* 144(7):758-766, 1990.

5. Barton JJ et al: Prevalence of human immunodeficiency virus in a general prenatal population, *Am J Obstet Gynecol* 160(6):1316-1320, 1989.

6. Biggar RJ et al: Immunosuppression in pregnant women infected with human immunodeficiency virus. *Am J Obstet Gynecol* 161(5):1239-1244, 1989.

7. Blanche S et al: A prospective study of infants born to women seropositive for human immunodeficiency virus type 1: HIV Infection in Newborns, French Collaborative Study Group, *N Engl J Med* 320(25):1643-1648, 1989.

8. Borkowski W et al: Human immunodeficiency virus infections in infants negative for anti-HIV by enzyme linked immunoassay, *Lancet* 1:1168-1170, 1987.

9. Brown ZA, Watts DH: Antiviral therapy in pregnancy, *Clin Obstet Gynecol* 33(2):276-289, 1990.

10. Brumfitt W, Pursell R: Trimethoprim-sulfamethoxazole in the treatment of bacteriuria in women, *J Infect Dis* 128:S657-S663, 1973.

11. Burke DS et al: Human immunodeficiency virus infections in teenagers: seroprevalence among applicants for U.S. military service, *JAMA* 263 (15):2074-2077, 1990.

12. Centers for Disease Control: Revised case definition for acquired immunodeficiency syndrome, *MMWR* 36:142-145, 1987.

13. Centers for Disease Control: Public Health Service guidelines for counseling and antibody testing to prevent HIV infection and AIDS, *MMWR* 36:509-515, 1987.

14. Centers for Disease Control: Immunization of children infected with human immunodeficiency virus: supplementary ACIP statement, *MMWR* 37 (12):181-183, 1988.

15. Centers for Disease Control: AIDS and human virus infection in the United States: 1988 update, *MMWR* 38(S-4): 1-38, 1989.

16. Centers for Disease Control: Guidelines for prophylaxis against *Pneumocystis carinii* pneumonia for persons infected with human immunodeficiency virus, *MMWR* 38(S-5):1-9, 1989.

17. Centers for Disease Control: Recommendations of the immunization practices advisory committee: pneumococcal polysaccharide vaccine, *JAMA* 261(9):1265-1267, 1989.

18. Centers for Disease Control: HIV/AIDS surveillance, July, 1991.

19. Centers for Disease Control: AIDS in women: United States, *MMWR* 39(47):845-846, 1990.

20. Chu SY, Buehler JW, Berkelman RL: Impact of the human immunodeficiency virus epidemic on mortality in women of reproductive age: United States, *JAMA* 264(2):225-229, 1990.

21. Conover B et al: Aerosolized pentamidine and pregnancy, *Ann Intern Med* 108:927, 1988.

22. Edwards JR et al: Polymerase chain reaction compared with concurrent viral cultures for rapid identification of human immunodeficiency virus infection among high-risk infants and children, *J Pediatr* 115(2):200-203, 1989.

23. Embree JE et al: Lack of correlation of maternal human immunodeficiency virus infection with neonatal malformations, *Pediatr Infect Dis J* 8(10):700-704, 1989.

23a. European Collaborative Study: Children born to women with HIV-1 infection: natural history and risk of transmission, *Lancet* 337:253-260, 1991.

24. Fortunato SJ, Bawdon SE: Determination of pentamidine transfer in the in vitro perfused human cotyledon with high-performance liquid chromatography, *Am J Obstet Gynecol* 160(3):759-761, 1989.

25. Gloeb DJ, O'Sullivan MJ, Efantis J:

Human immunodeficiency virus infection in women. I. The effects of human immunodeficiency virus on pregnancy, *Am J Obstet Gynecol* 159(3):756-761, 1988.

26. Hahn RA et al: Prevalence of HIV infection among intravenous drug users in the United States, *JAMA* 261(18):2677-2684, 1989.

27. Halsey NA et al: Transmission of HIV-1 infections from mothers to infants in Haiti: impact on childhood mortality and malnutrition, *JAMA* 264(16):2088-2092, 1990.

28. Hibberd PL, Rubin RH: Approach to immunization in the immunosuppressed host, *Infect Dis Clin North Am* 4(1):123-142, 1990.

29. Hicks ML et al: Acquired immunodeficiency syndrome and *Pneumocystis carinii* infection in a pregnant woman, *Obstet Gynecol* 76(3 part 2):480-481, 1990.

30. Hoff R et al: Seroprevalence of human immunodeficiency virus among childbearing women: estimation by testing of blood of newborns, *N Engl J Med* 318:525-530, 1988.

31. Jason J, Evatt BL: Pregnancies in human immunodeficiency virus–infected sex partners of hemophiliac men: the Hemophilia AIDS Collaborative Study Group, *Am J Dis Child* 144(4):485-490, 1990.

32. Johnson JP et al: Natural history and serologic diagnosis of infants born to human immunodeficiency virus–infected women, *Am J Dis Child* 143:1147-1153, 1989.

33. Koonin LM et al: Pregnancy-associated deaths due to AIDS in the United States, *JAMA* 261(9):1306-1309, 1989.

34. Kucers A, Bennett N McK: Trimethoprim, cotrimoxazole (Co-T) and other trimethoprim combinations. In Kucers A, Bennett N McK, editors: *The use of antibiotics*, Philadelphia, 1987, JB Lippincott.

35. Kucers A, Bennett N McK: Lincomycin and clindamycin. In Kucers A, Bennett N McK, editors: *The use of antibiotics*, Philadelphia, 1987, JB Lippincott.

36. Landesman S et al: Serosurvey of human immunodeficiency virus infection in parturients: implications for human immunodeficiency virus testing programs of pregnant women, *JAMA* 258(19):2701-2703, 1987.

37. Landesman SH, Minkoff HL, Willoughby A: HIV disease in reproductive age women: a problem of the present, *JAMA* 261(9):1326-1327, 1989.

38. Lindsay MK et al: Routine antepartum human immunodeficiency virus infection screening in an inner-city population, *Obstet Gynecol* 74(3 part 1):289-294, 1989.

39. Mann JM, Chin J: AIDS: a global perspective, *N Engl J Med* 319(5): 302-303, 1988.

40. Marion RW et al: Human T-cell lymphotropic virus type III embryopathy: a new dysmorphic syndrome associated with intrauterine HTLV-III infection, *Am J Dis Child* 140:638-640, 1986.

41. Mertz GJ: Diagnosis and treatment of genital herpes infections, *Infect Dis Clin North Am* 1(2):341-366, 1987.

42. Minkoff H et al: Pregnancies resulting in infants with acquired immunodeficiency syndrome or AIDS-related complex, *Obstet Gynecol* 69(3 part 1):285-287, 1987.

43. Minkoff HL et al: Serious infections during pregnancy among women with advanced human immunodeficiency virus infection, *Am J Obstet Gynecol* 162(1):30-34, 1990.

44. Minkoff HL, Landesman SH: The case for routinely offering prenatal testing for human immunodeficiency virus, *Am J Obstet Gynecol* 159(4):793-796, 1988.

45. Mitchell JL et al: HIV infection in pregnancy: detection, counseling and care, *Pediatr AIDS HIV Inf* 1(5):78-82, 1990.

46. Mok JY et al: Vertical transmission of

HIV: a prospective study, *Arch Dis Child* 64(8):1140-1145, 1989.

47. Montgomery AB et al: Selective delivery of pentamidine to the lung by aerosol, *Am Rev Respir Dis* 137(2):477-478, 1988.

48. National Institutes of Health: State of the art conference on azidothymidine therapy for early HIV infection, *Am J Med* 89:335-344, 1990.

49. New York City Department of Health: AIDS surveillance update, Aug 29, 1990.

50. Novick LF et al: HIV seroprevalence in newborns in New York State, *JAMA* 261:1745-1750, 1989.

51. Ochs HD: The human immunodeficiency virus-infected infant: a diagnostic dilemma, *Am J Dis Child* 143:1138-1139, 1989.

52. Pappaioanou M et al: HIV seroprevalence surveys of childbearing women: objectives, methods, and uses of the data, *Public Health Rep* 105(2):147-152, 1990.

53. *Physicians' Desk Reference*, Oradell, NJ, 1988, Medical Economics Co, Inc.

54. *Physicians' Desk Reference*, Oradell, NJ, 1989, Medical Economics Co, Inc.

55. Plebani A et al: Prenatal immune status of fetuses of HIV-seropositive mothers, *Gynecol Obstet Invest* 29(2): 108-111, 1990.

56. Ranki A et al: Long latency precedes overt seroconversion in sexually transmitted human immunodeficiency virus infection, *Lancet* 2:589-593, 1987.

57. Rawlinson KF et al.: Disseminated Kaposi's sarcoma in pregnancy: a manifestation of acquired immune deficiency syndrome, *Obstet Gynecol* 63(suppl 3):2S-6S, 1984.

58. Schafer A et al: Proof of diaplacental transmission of HTLV-III/LAV before the 20th week of pregnancy, Geburtshilfe Frauenheilkd 46(2):88-89, 1986.

59. Schuman P et al: Pharmacokinetics of zidovudine during pregnancy. Paper presented at the Sixth International Conference on AIDS, San Francisco, June 22, 1990 (abstract).

60. Scott GB et al: Mothers of infants with the acquired immunodeficiency syndrome: evidence for both symptomatic and asymptomatic carriers, *JAMA* 253(3):363-366, 1985.

61. Scott GB et al: Survival in children with perinatally acquired human immunodeficiency virus type 1 infection, *N Engl J Med* 321(26):1791-1796, 1989.

62. Seidlin M et al: Maternal-fetal transmission of HTLV-III. Programs and abstracts of the Twenty-Sixth Interscience Conference on Antimicrobial Agents and Chemotherapy, New Orleans, October 1986.

63. Selwyn PA et al: Knowledge of HIV antibody status and decisions to continue or terminate pregnancy among intravenous drug users, *JAMA* 261(24):3567-3571, 1989.

64. Selwyn PA et al: Prospective study of human immunodeficiency virus infection and pregnancy outcomes in intravenous drug users, *JAMA* 261(9):1289-1294, 1989.

65. Sprecher S et al: Vertical transmission of HIV in a 15-week old fetus, *Lancet* 2:288-289, 1986.

66. Steen B, Rane A: Clindamycin passage into human milk, *Br J Clin Pharmacol* 13(5):661-664, 1982.

67. Stern JJ et al: Oral fluconazole therapy for patients with acquired immunodeficiency syndrome and cryptococcosis: experience with 22 patients, *Am J Med* 85:477-480, 1988.

68. Sugar AM, Saunders C: Oral fluconazole as suppressive therapy of disseminated cryptococcosis in patients with acquired immunodeficiency syndrome, Am J Med 85:481-489, 1988.

69. Thiry L et al: Isolation of AIDS virus from cell-free breast milk of three healthy virus carriers, *Lancet* 2:891-892, 1985.

70. Thomas PA et al: Unexplained immunodeficiency in children: a surveillance report, *JAMA* 252(5):639-644, 1984.

71. Wetli GV, Roldan EO, Fojaco RM: Listeriosis as a cause of maternal death: an obstetric complication of the acquired immunodeficiency syndrome (AIDS), *Am J Obstet Gynecol* 147:7-9, 1983.

72. Ziegler JB et al: Postnatal transmission of AIDS-associated retrovirus from mother to infant, *Lancet* 1:896-898, 1985.

CHAPTER **12**

The Coordination of Primary Care

General medical care of patients infected with the human immunodeficiency virus (HIV) has undergone a transformation since the first cases of AIDS were reported in 1981. AIDS initially was perceived as a rare disorder for which care was provided largely by physicians specializing in infectious diseases, clinical immunology, oncology, and dermatology. Since the full extent of the epidemic became obvious after the discovery of HIV, it has become clear that the relatively small numbers of clinicians specializing in AIDS would be unable to provide care for the hundreds of thousands of patients infected with the virus.[8,25]

The remarkably diverse manifestations of HIV infection have led to increasing involvement of other specialties and subspecialties, particularly ophthalmology, neurology, psychiatry, nephrology, and gastroenterology, in the care of these patients. As with other multisystem diseases, a need has arisen for primary care physicians who are knowledgeable about HIV infection and able and willing to provide general medical care and effective coordination of subspecialty involvement, particularly in the ambulatory setting.

Several studies have indicated that general primary care physicians have begun to respond to this need, but that incomplete knowledge of HIV infection[19] and negative attitudes toward the disease[29] may serve as obstacles to further involvement of this community of providers.

This chapter attempts to define the role of the primary care physician in the management of HIV-infected patients. In this discussion the term "primary care physician" may apply to both general internists and to subspecialists involved in the care of these patients. The means by which care is provided differs greatly, depending on the practice setting. The individual practitioner's ability to meet the complex medical and psychosocial needs of a large number of HIV-infected patients may be very limited. Nonetheless, the primary care physician can bring direction, organization, and common sense to long-term care that otherwise may become quite fragmentary because of the multisystem nature of HIV infection and the need for frequent involvement of subspecialists.

The role of other health care providers; practical concerns about infection control procedures, including recent recommendations for HIV screening of health care workers; and safeguards to patient confidentiality in the ambulatory setting are also discussed.

In the final section, issues of particular concern to academic ambulatory care and general internal medicine programs are discussed. Chief among these issues are systems of ambulatory care and the impact of the HIV/AIDS epidemic on medical education.

THE ROLE OF THE PRIMARY CARE PHYSICIAN

It is essential that a physician knowledgeable in the diagnosis and treatment of HIV-related disease be involved in the care of each patient. The specific goals of the primary physician should include the following:

1. Establishing a complete medical data base that includes the history, physical examination, and relevant laboratory data.

2. Classifying the HIV-positive patient according to the stage of the disease (e.g., AIDS, symptomatic HIV positive, asymptomatic) (see Chapter 2) and, on this basis, determining the need for prophylactic or antiretroviral therapy.
3. Providing ongoing care focused on monitoring for physical or laboratory evidence of HIV-related complications, periodic restaging of the disease, observing for evidence of drug toxicity, and general medical care.
4. Determining the need for subspecialty consultation and follow-up care.
5. Providing easy access to the health care system for patients and their family and loved ones.
6. Offering appropriate HIV screening for sexual partners and providing for support and counseling.
7. Assisting patients and their families and loved ones with decisions about home care, long-term hospitalization, and life-sustaining therapy.

THE GOALS OF AMBULATORY CARE

The primary goal of ambulatory care of HIV-infected patients is a consistent program of screening, testing, immunological staging, appropriate immunization, prophylaxis, therapy, and subspecialty consultation. Achieving this goal requires a logical and stepwise approach to HIV infection in all patients.

HIV Testing and Counseling

A mechanism by which blood may be tested for antibody to HIV infection should be established. Information about testing procedures may be obtained from local public health authorities or from the Centers for Disease Control. Only approved laboratories should be used. Staff members should be familiar with local regulations regarding informed consent and confidentiality of test results.

The physician providing primary care for adult patients should incorporate screening for HIV risk behavior into the routine medical history of all patients (Chapter 3). Patients with a history of intravenous drug use, male homosexuals, heterosexual partners of others at risk, and recipients of blood transfusions (particularly before 1985) should be strongly urged to undergo HIV testing. Any other patient who feels that he or she might be at risk for HIV infection should be made aware that testing is available.

Preventive Measures

Various immunizations, including vaccination against pneumococcal and *Haemophilus* infection, hepatitis B, influenza, and several other infections (see Chapter 6) should routinely be provided to HIV-infected patients.

A mechanism for administering aerosolized pentamidine for patients requiring prophylaxis against *Pneumocystis carinii* pneumonia[6] (see Chapter 6) should be established. Concerns have been expressed about the potential risk to health care workers administering this therapy, such as transmission of respiratory pathogens such as *Mycobacterium tuberculosis*[5] and possible toxicity of pentamidine itself after occupational exposure.[23] Until the risk to health care workers is better defined, aerosolized pentamidine should be administered in a well-ventilated room, and patients with symptoms of active respiratory disease should not receive aerosol treatment before undergoing a complete medical evaluation. Health care workers involved in administering aerosolized pentamidine should be screened periodically for tuberculosis by means of skin testing and chest roentgenogram when indicated.

During administration of aerosolized pentamidine, adequate staff should be available to observe patients for acute bronchospasm.

Antiretroviral Therapy

Programs of ambulatory care must have the capacity for monitoring for toxicity of antiretroviral therapy, as outlined in Chapter 10. This should include a mechanism for frequent return visits for patients beginning therapy with zidovudine or other antiviral drugs (see Chapters 6 and 10).

Experimental Protocols

Ambulatory care of patients enrolled in experimental treatment protocols may require frequent visits for clinical and laboratory reassessments and extensive documentation. Planning for the care of such patients should include projections of the expected number of eligible patients and a realistic review of facilities to assure that adequate follow-up can be provided. Establishing channels of referral among centers so that access to the widest variety of clinical trials can be offered should also be considered. Assigning specific protocol enrollment and organization to individual practitioners may be advisable.

Diagnostic Evaluations

Diagnostic evaluation of nonemergent symptoms can usually be conducted effectively in the ambulatory setting. The availability of routine radiographic and laboratory facilities can often permit the following HIV-related disorders to be diagnosed without hospitalization (see Chapters 7 to 9 for details of diagnostic and therapeutic approaches).

Intestinal infections

Disorders: Cryptosporidiosis, isosporiasis, salmonellosis, and candidal or cytomegaloviral esophagitis

Necessary tests and facilities: Diagnostic radiography (upper gastrointestinal series, barium enema), a diagnostic microbiological laboratory with the capacity for routine stool culture, ova, and parasites examination (including *Cryptosporidium* organisms and *Isospora belli*)

Possible additional requirements: Ambulatory gastroduodenoscopy and colonoscopy with biopsy capability, mycobacterial and viral culture facilities, and infectious disease consultation

Chronic fever and/or weight loss

Disorders: Disseminated mycobacterial infection, lymphoma, and intestinal malabsorption

Necessary tests and facilities: Diagnostic radiography, a microbiological laboratory with the capacity for routine mycobacterial, fungal, and viral cultures

Possible additional requirements: Radionuclide studies (gallium scanning), gastroenterological and hematological tests, infectious disease consultation, ambulatory liver biopsy, and bone marrow biopsy

Ocular disease

Disorder: Retinitis caused by cytomegalovirus or other opportunistic pathogens

Necessary tests and facilities: Ophthalmological consultation

Possible additional requirements: Neurological and infectious disease consultation

Nonacute respiratory syndromes

Disorders: Chronic cough, nodular lung lesions, pleural effusion

Necessary tests and facilities: Diagnostic radiography, including ambulatory computed tomography, gallium scanning, and a microbiological laboratory with the capacity for routine mycobacterial and fungal cultures

Possible additional requirements: Pulmonary, infectious disease, and thoracic surgical consultation; ambulatory bronchoscopy with biopsy; pulmonary function tests; and tomographic biopsy

Peripheral neuropathy

Necessary tests and facilities: Neurological consultation, electromyographic testing, and spine imaging studies (CT and/or MRI)

Skin disorders

Disorders: Kaposi's sarcoma; localized herpes zoster or herpes simplex infection; and minor disorders, including seborrheic dermatitis, dermatomycosis, onychomycosis, and molluscum contagiosum

Necessary tests and facilities: Microbiological laboratory with the capacity for routine mycobacterial, fungal, and viral culture and ambulatory biopsy capability

Possible additional requirements: Dermatological, surgical, and infectious disease consultation and cryotherapy capability

Oral disorders
Disorders: Candidiasis, hairy leukoplakia, and Kaposi's sarcoma
  Necessary tests and facilities: Microbiological laboratory with the capacity for routine mycobacterial, viral, and fungal culture
  Possible additional requirements: Dental, oral surgical, and infectious disease consultation and biopsy capability
Dementia
Necessary tests and facilities: Brain imaging studies (CT, MRI), cerebrospinal fluid examination, and laboratory facilities for syphilis serology and vitamin B_{12} and folate levels
  Possible additional requirements: Neurological and psychiatric consultation
Lymphadenopathy
Disorders: Nonspecific lymphadenopathy, lymphoma, and mycobacterial and fungal infections
  Necessary tests and facilities: Surgical consultation, ambulatory biopsy capability, and microbiological laboratory with capacity for routine mycobacterial, fungal, and viral cultures

Coordination of Inpatient and Outpatient Care

As HIV infection progresses into advanced symptomatic stages, the need for hospitalization arises more often. An involved primary care physician, familiar with the patient's prior medical and social history, can ensure that the goals of hospitalization remain focused and that diagnostic and therapeutic plans are carried out efficiently.

Patient Education

HIV-infected patients first coming to medical attention require substantial education about their disease. The natural history of HIV infection (Chapter 2) should be explained in terms of likely clinical events. Specific statements about prognosis rarely can be made with any accuracy, but the primary care physician should educate the patient about the need for ongoing care and the indications for prophylaxis and antiretroviral therapy. Education and often reeducation about routes of HIV transmission and the need for sexual abstinence are best provided in the ambulatory setting by the primary provider.

Emotional Support

The frightening specters of AIDS, progressive debilitation, social isolation, and death cause HIV-infected patients to turn to their physicians frequently for support and reassurance. Patients in the highest risk groups, intravenous drug users and male homosexuals, may be especially lacking in family and social support.

Entitlement Issues

The HIV epidemic has had its greatest impact on the poor. Many patients, particularly intravenous drug users and others living in inner cities, have no health insurance. Discrimination or lengthy hospitalization may result in loss of housing. Jobs may be lost for similar reasons, or a patient's symptoms may make it impossible to work. Home services may become vital for survival. For these reasons, issues of entitlement often become paramount.

THE ROLE OF THE SPECIALIST AND SUBSPECIALIST

Ready access to specialty and subspecialty consultants on an ambulatory basis may greatly facilitate the care of HIV-infected patients at all stages of the disease. Following are some specialties and subspecialties frequently consulted in the care of ambulatory patients.

Specialties

General surgery: Lymph node biopsy, skin biopsy, and interpreting abdominal complaints

Gynecology: Treatment and screening for sexually transmitted diseases, screening for cervical malignancy, birth control, safe sex counseling, and prenatal counseling

Ophthalmology: Evaluation of visual complaints and diagnosis, and follow-up of retinitis

Dermatology: Diagnosis and care of severe or life-threatening conditions

Neurology: Evaluation of peripheral neuropathy or cerebral disorders

Psychiatry: Evaluation and management of depression, dementia, and drug and alcohol addiction

Oral surgery: Diagnosis and management of oral infections and malignancies

Medical Subspecialties

Infectious diseases: Diagnosis and management of disseminated or life-threatening opportunistic infections; antiretroviral therapy in advanced HIV infection or in patients intolerant to conventional therapy; access to investigational protocols

Pulmonary diseases: Diagnosis and management of pulmonary infections and malignancies, bronchoscopy, percutaneous lung biopsy, or pleural biopsy

Hematology: Diagnosis and management of HIV-associated hematological disorders, including autoimmune thrombocytopenia, bone marrow depression, and lymphoma; diagnostic bone marrow biopsy for disseminated mycobacterial or fungal infection

Oncology: Diagnosis, staging, and management of Kaposi's sarcoma and lymphoma

Gastroenterology: Diagnostic evaluation and management of chronic diarrhea, malabsorption, esophagitis, gastrointestinal bleeding, rectal and perirectal infections and malignancies, and liver involvement by opportunistic infections, malignancies, or drug toxicity

Rheumatology: Evaluation and management of HIV-related musculoskeletal complaints

INTERACTION BETWEEN THE PRIMARY CARE PHYSICIAN AND CONSULTANTS
Asymptomatic Patients

What the primary care physician should provide. The general approach to treating the asymptomatic HIV-infected patient is reviewed in detail in Chapter 6. The most important step in the initial evaluation of such patients is clinical and immunological staging to determine the need for therapy. Decisions about the frequency of follow-up visits can be made more easily after staging has been completed. The patient should be alerted to early symptoms of disease and should be given specific instructions on what to do if such symptoms appear. Specifically, the patient should be particularly attentive to a new or persistent fever or cough, shortness of breath, headache, diarrhea, skin rash, pain on swallowing, or visual disturbance.

When subspecialty consultation should be sought. Subspecialty consultation generally is not needed for asymptomatic patients with a CD4 lymphocyte count over 200/mm^3 and no abnormalities on initial laboratory assessment. Exceptions include several symptoms and conditions that often present early in the natural history of HIV infection:

Dermatology consultation may be indicated for patients with severe skin manifestations of HIV infection that do not respond to standard treatment; such conditions may include seborrheic dermatitis, dermatomycosis, onychomycosis, xerosis, or localized herpes simplex or herpes zoster infection. Skin lesions of uncertain origin should be biopsied.

Patients with new-onset lymphadenopathy, whether generalized or localized, should be evaluated for biopsy.

Hematology consultation is advisable when evaluating patients with thrombocytopenia of unknown origin. Bone marrow biopsy and additional studies generally are necessary to confirm an autoimmune etiology.

Visual complaints at any stage of HIV infection should be evaluated promptly by an ophthalmologist.

Symptomatic Patients Without AIDS

What the primary care physician should provide. Evaluation of symptomatic HIV-infected patients is discussed in detail in Chapter 7. Because of the huge variety of disorders associated with HIV infection, symptomatic patients may seek care from specialists or from general primary care physicians. To avoid fragmentary care, however, it is important that one provider, whether specialist or generalist, who is familiar with the full range of HIV-related diseases coordinate the care of symptomatic patients.

As is discussed in Chapter 7, symptoms should be interpreted with a knowledge of the degree of immunodeficiency. Symptoms are relatively unlikely to represent life-threatening opportunistic infection in patients with CD4 lymphocyte counts above 200/mm³.

When subspecialty consultation should be sought. Consultation might be sought for many reasons. The immunological stage of HIV disease at which the patient seeks medical care largely dictates the differential diagnosis to be considered in symptomatic HIV-infected patients.

Patients with an advanced degree of immunodeficiency (i.e., CD4 lymphocyte count under 200/mm³) are at very high risk of developing opportunistic infections or malignancies, particularly those involving the respiratory or gastrointestinal tract and the central nervous system. In these cases prompt evaluation of new localizing symptoms may be lifesaving. Unexplained pulmonary infiltrates usually should prompt hospitalization for diagnostic studies, which often require pulmonary consultation. Similarly, focal neurological abnormalities usually justify hospitalization with urgent neurological consultation and evaluation. Gastrointestinal disorders, although less frequently life threatening, may necessitate endoscopic procedures and other services provided by subspecialists.

AIDS Patients

What the primary care physician should provide. The primary care physician should fully document the manner in which the diagnosis of AIDS was made. The patient's response to therapy for opportunistic infections or malignancies, adverse reactions to medications, and prior general medical care should be ascertained. All patients with a previous diagnosis of AIDS are candidates for both antiretroviral therapy and prophylaxis against *Pneumocystis carinii* pneumonia. Any such interventions should be carefully documented and recorded, along with adverse reactions.

The physical examination, medical history, and laboratory assessment should be directed toward eliciting signs and symptoms of potentially life-threatening opportunistic infections or malignancies. The general approaches to symptomatic patients and to AIDS-related disorders are reviewed in separate chapters.

When subspecialty consultation should be sought. The need for subspecialty consultation varies. In patients who have recovered fully from an opportunistic infection such as *Pneumocystis carinii* and are asymptomatic at the time of evaluation, involvement by subspecialists may be unnecessary. It should be kept in mind, however, that potentially serious disorders may present with few initial symptoms in AIDS patients. It is particularly important that a thorough evaluation for visual disturbances, neurological conditions, and respiratory disorders in particular be carried out before it is decided that consultation is not needed.

ACUTE HOSPITALIZATION

Emergency hospitalization is frequently necessary for HIV-infected patients at advanced stages of the disease. Common indications for acute hospitalization include progressive respiratory symptoms, focal neurological syndromes, progressive dementia or obtundation, severe dehydration caused by diarrhea, unexplained fever or headache, progressive leg weakness, and depression.

Several diagnostic studies commonly used in the evaluation of HIV-related diseases may necessitate hospitalization, including bronchoscopy, liver biopsy, lymph node biopsy, lumbar puncture, gastroduodenoscopy, colonoscopy, and exploratory laparotomy.

Opportunistic infections or malignancies requiring parenteral therapy (see Chapter 9) require hospitalization unless home infusion therapy can be provided efficiently and safely. In far-advanced disease, hospitalization for nutritional support or social service intervention may be necessary.

Malnutrition, particularly in the setting of intestinal malabsorption, may justify acute hospitalization for parenteral alimentation in advanced stages of HIV infection.

Many HIV-infected patients who live in inner cities are homeless. Acute hospitalization may be necessary for such patients while housing and home care options are explored. For patients with advanced, chronic, symptomatic infection, home services (e.g., visiting nurse, housekeeping) may be lifesaving.

INDICATIONS FOR HOME CARE

As the number of HIV-infected patients requiring hospitalization has grown, increasing emphasis has been placed on providing some services in the home that usually require hospitalization. Infusional therapy and enteral or parenteral nutrition may be administered in the home if adequate support personnel are available and if the patient can be hospitalized on short notice if necessary.

High-level home care is particularly appropriate for the patient who does not require hospitalization for diagnostic evaluation or nursing care but who must be maintained on continuous therapy with parenteral medications (e.g., ganciclovir) by means of an indwelling catheter.

Specific forms of therapy that could be provided at home include hyper-alimentation, parenteral therapy (amphotericin B and ganciclovir), and aero-solized pentamidine.

INDICATIONS FOR CHRONIC HOSPITALIZATION

The advanced stages of HIV infection may be characterized by progressive dementia, depression, immobilization, malnutrition requiring enteral or par-enteral nutritional support, and recurrent infections necessitating chronic in-fusional therapy. Such problems may become unmanageable despite adequate home care and may be rapidly devastating to the patient, family members, and other loved ones in the home. However, hospitalization in an acute care facility may not be appropriate for patients who do not require diagnostic evaluation or intensive nursing care. Long-term care facilities or hospices may be more appropriate for some patients.

As the HIV epidemic has progressed and the number of patients in all stages of the disease has continued to mount, the need for long-term institutional care for patients with advanced disease has become increasingly clear. But few appropriate facilities are available to provide this care, especially in areas where the disease is most prevalent. The decision to seek long-term hospital-ization should take into account the family's ability to provide supportive care in the home.

INFECTION CONTROL IN AMBULATORY CARE

Transmission of HIV infection from patients to health care workers after punc-ture wounds and exposure to blood or body fluid has been documented.[2,4,22] However, the likelihood of such transmission is small. Careful prospective studies have demonstrated that the risk of HIV infection after percutaneous exposure to the blood of an infected patient is approximately 0.3% to 0.4%.[13,20] Transmission by skin or mucous membrane exposure has not been documented in prospective studies, although there have been reports of such transmis-sion.[2,13,20]

Although the risk of transmission is small, many health care workers are very concerned about occupational exposure to HIV, and efforts have been made to establish strategies to diminish the incidence of needle-stick injuries and skin and mucous membrane exposure to the blood of infected patients.[3]

Unfortunately, there is little to suggest that educating staff members or improving needle disposal techniques has accomplished this.[16,17,27]

Relative Risk of HIV Transmission by Employment Category

Health care workers who have extensive contact with patients or blood, particularly nurses and laboratory technicians, are at the highest risk of sustaining needle-stick injuries,[15] although housekeeping personnel, respiratory therapists, physicians, and others exposed to blood or body fluids are also at risk. Needle-stick injuries are most likely to occur during the use of equipment requiring assembly, such as intravenous sets or vacuum tube phlebotomy sets, and result less frequently from the use of disposable syringes.[15]

The risk of transmission may be stratified by specific job titles and activities according to the likelihood of accidental needle-stick or skin or mucous membrane contact with blood.

Highest risk	Intermediate risk
Phlebotomist	Examiner having possible direct contact with mucous membranes or body fluid
Laboratory technician processing clinical specimens	
Nurse administering injections	Physician performing an invasive procedure (fiberoptic gastroduodenoscopy, colonoscopy, sigmoidoscopy, bronchoscopy, biopsy, dental care)
Custodial staff	

Lowest risk	No apparent risk*
Physician performing routine examination	Social work staff
Technician performing noninvasive procedure (e.g., roentgenogram, electrocardiogram)	Administrative, clerical, and secretarial staff
Physical therapist	Volunteers

*In performing normal duties.

Preventing HIV Transmission in the Health Care Setting

Currently recommended procedures to minimize the risk of HIV transmission during health care activities are based on two principles: Any patient, and therefore any clinical specimen, is potentially a source of HIV infection; and accidental injuries from needles and other sharp instruments pose the greatest risk of transmission.

Universal precautions. To minimize the risk of transmission of HIV and other bloodborne pathogens, it has been recommended that standard precautions be implemented. These so-called universal precautions include the following[3]:

1. Barrier precautions should be used when contact with blood or body fluids is anticipated. Gloves should be worn when touching body fluids,

performing venipuncture, or touching mucous membranes or broken skin and should be changed after each use. Masks or goggles should be worn during procedures when blood or body fluids are likely to become airborne droplets. Gowns should be worn when splashes of blood or body fluids are likely to occur.

2. Hands and other exposed areas of skin should be washed promptly after contact with blood or body fluids or after gloves are removed.
3. Needles and other sharp instruments used for drawing blood or obtaining specimens should not be recapped or otherwise manipulated but should be placed directly into puncture-resistant containers.
4. Mouthpieces and emergency ventilation equipment should be readily available to minimize the need for mouth-to-mouth resuscitation.
5. Health care workers with open skin lesions should avoid direct contact with patients or with equipment used in patient care.
6. Pregnant health care workers should observe universal precautions with particular care.

Precautions for invasive procedures. It is recommended that health care workers participating in invasive procedures (including surgery, angiographic or obstetrical procedures, or cutting of oral or perioral tissues) take specific precautions in addition to those outlined above.[3] These include:

1. Gloves and masks should be worn routinely.
2. Goggles or other protective eyewear should be worn if aerosolization of blood droplets, blood splashes, or the generation of bone chips is likely to result from the procedure.
3. Gowns or aprons should be worn when blood splashes are likely.
4. Gloves that are torn or punctured should be changed promptly.
5. Health care workers who provide dental care should routinely wear gloves. Masks and protective eyewear should be worn when droplets of blood or saliva are likely to be generated.

HIV testing of health care workers to prevent transmission to patients. Epidemiologic and virologic data suggesting that HIV infection had been transmitted from a dentist to several of his patients during dental procedures[7a] has led to great concern about the possible risk posed by HIV-infected health care workers. The means of potential transmission during dental procedures was not identified, however, and transmission of HIV to patients was not demonstrated in several studies of infected surgeons.[7b] Despite the apparent small risk of such transmission, the Centers for Disease Control recommended in 1991 that health care workers who perform exposure-prone invasive procedures be aware of their own HIV status and that infected workers not perform such procedures without the advice of a local expert review panel and without informing the patient of their HIV status.[7b]

Recommendations regarding testing of health care workers and restrictions on procedures that infected workers may perform are likely to change. Updated information should be sought.

Sterilization of instruments. Standard recommended procedures for sterilizing and disinfecting instruments are felt to be adequate to prevent HIV transmission.[3] Sterilization after each patient use is mandatory for instruments that come into contact with blood or sterile tissue. Instruments that come into contact with mucous membranes (e.g., endoscopes, bronchoscopes) should be cleaned thoroughly and then sterilized or subjected to high-level disinfection with approved agents after each patient use.

A variety of standard disinfectants have been shown to be effective against HIV.[21]

MANAGEMENT OF HEALTH CARE WORKERS EXPOSED TO HIV
Reassurance

Health care workers who believe that they may have been exposed to HIV through a needle-stick or other accident often become extremely fearful and anxious. They should be reassured that the risk of transmission is small and that appropriate testing and follow-up can reliably determine if they are infected.

HIV Testing of Health Care Workers after Possible Occupational Exposure

If the source patient is known to have AIDS or to be HIV infected or refuses to be tested, the health care worker should be offered HIV testing as soon after the incident as possible and at 6, 12, and 24 weeks after exposure.[7] Informed consent should be obtained from the health care worker before testing and counseling (Chapter 4) should be conducted before and after the test.

HIV Testing of Patients

When it is not known if the patient to whom the health care worker was exposed is HIV infected, testing should be offered to the patient and advised in accordance with local regulations governing informed consent and confidentiality. Repeat testing may be necessary for patients with a recent history of risk behavior (within 6 months) to exclude early infection.

Antiretroviral Therapy

As is discussed in Chapter 10, it has been suggested by some that administering AZT (azidothymidine, zidovudine) might prevent HIV infection in health care workers after exposure to the blood of an infected patient.[7,14] However, transmission of HIV despite such prophylaxis has been reported.[18] The optimum dose and duration of AZT therapy for postexposure prophylaxis is unknown.

Regimens of 200 mg by mouth, given five or six times a day for 4 or 6 weeks, have been commonly employed.[14] If postexposure prophylaxis is effective, it is likely that the level of protection conferred is greatest when prophylaxis is begun as soon after exposure as possible.

Documentation

The date, time, and circumstances of the exposure should be documented. If the health care worker elects to undergo evaluation and follow-up at the place of employment, the results of initial and subsequent HIV testing should be recorded confidentially.

CONFIDENTIALITY IN AMBULATORY CARE

All patients, including those seeking care in an ambulatory setting, are entitled to confidentiality of medical information. The specific laws governing confidentiality of HIV test results and related information vary among states[9] and are likely to change. Physicians, other health care workers, and support staff working with ambulatory HIV-infected patients must take all reasonable steps to prevent inappropriate disclosure of information. In general, staff members should be instructed not to release information likely to reveal that the patient is HIV infected without written authorization from the patient or someone legally permitted to act on the patient's behalf. Local regulations regarding exceptions to this principle may vary.

MODELS OF AMBULATORY CARE

Health care planners and others have debated the relative merits of various systems of care for HIV-infected patients. The potential and need for coordinated care of large numbers of ambulatory HIV-infected patients varies greatly among geographical regions. In areas of low HIV prevalence, a small number of private practitioners with appropriate access to subspecialty consultants may be able to provide an acceptable level of care. However, the complexity of HIV infection has led to a debate between those calling for centralization of AIDS treatment into regional facilities[1] and others favoring wider distribution of the responsibility for care.[10] In inner cities and other areas of high prevalence, dedicated outpatient units have arisen, particularly in conjunction with hospital-based academic ambulatory care programs.[26,28,31,34]

Several models of dedicated outpatient units have been proposed.[11,30]

Comprehensive Clinics

A health care team, consisting of a variety of professionals (e.g., physicians, nurses, social workers, individuals with specific training in HIV counseling, nutritionists, mental health professionals, and clerical support staff), provides comprehensive HIV-related care to patients at all stages of the disease. Specialty consultants (e.g., pulmonologists, gastroenterologists, dermatologists, oncologists, and infectious disease specialists) are available on site on a part-time basis.

Referral Clinics

A referral clinic is a dedicated outpatient unit designed to accept referrals of HIV-infected patients from general medical and specialty practitioners and clinics for the management of specific complications of HIV infection or enrollment in clinical treatment trials.

Expanded Primary Care Clinics

Appropriate subspecialty consultants (pulmonologists, oncologists, infectious disease specialists, and dermatologists) are available in a general medical clinic to assist in the management of HIV-related disorders.

THE ROLE OF OTHER HEALTH CARE PROFESSIONALS
Nurses

Nurses are well-suited to coordinate functions within an ambulatory care program for HIV-infected patients for several reasons:

1. They are often viewed by patients as being more accessible than physicians.
2. The traditional emphasis in nursing on the psychosocial needs of the patient allows the nurse in an ambulatory setting to provide both primary counseling and support to patients and their families and also to establish triage to social services, mental health resources, and other services available in the clinic and community.
3. Nurse clinicians may serve as primary providers for some patients.

Social Service Workers

Social service personnel are needed to assist indigent patients with entitlement issues and to facilitate arrangements for home care. If staffing permits, each patient should be followed up by an individual social worker or caseworker. Social workers who have received specific training may also provide family and individual counseling and organize and conduct support groups, drop-in centers, and other patient activities.

Dietary Personnel

Dietary staff may be needed to design diets for patients with specific HIV-related gastrointestinal and nutritional disorders such as protein-calorie malnutrition, malabsorption states, and chronic diarrhea.

Mental Health Professionals

The skills of psychologists, therapists, and other mental health professionals may be of great value in the ambulatory setting. Services may include individual diagnostic evaluations, individual and group therapy, family support and counseling, and counseling of staff members.

All professionals who work with HIV-infected patients should receive specific training in HIV testing and counseling procedures and should be familiar with routes of HIV transmission and basic approaches to therapy.

MEDICAL EDUCATION AND AIDS

The care of patients with AIDS and other HIV-related disorders has become a major component of residency training in areas of high prevalence. A survey conducted in 1989 indicated that in some training programs, more than 20% of hospital inpatients cared for by residents in internal medicine or family medicine had AIDS.[12] The impact of the epidemic on medical education is likely to become increasingly dramatic for the foreseeable future. In New York City, for example, it is expected that during the early 1990s between 25% and 50% of acute medical and surgical beds will be occupied by patients with HIV-related disease.[33]

The effect that the AIDS epidemic has had on medical education, although not established, has generally been regarded as negative. Many residents working with AIDS patients express fears of contagion[12] and feelings of frustration, depression, or exhaustion ("burnout"). These feelings, as well as antipathy toward homosexual men and intravenous drug users,[12] may cause some to try to avoid AIDS patients. AIDS often is cited as a partial explanation for the declining popularity of internal medicine postgraduate training among U.S. medical students in the late 1980s.

In the survey of residents cited above,[12] one third of the residents indicated that they would not or might not treat AIDS patients in their future practice if given a choice.

As the incidence of AIDS and HIV infection continues to rise and treatment options become more varied and complex, any widespread avoidance of AIDS care by physicians completing their training clearly will impede and complicate efforts to contain the epidemic and provide treatment for large numbers of infected individuals.

The extent to which changes in curriculum or clinical rotations could address the negative feelings held by some residents about caring for AIDS patients is not known. However, several strategies may be beneficial, primarily in the areas of ambulatory care and core curriculum.

1. *Greater emphasis should be put on ambulatory care.* In one series, 75% of

residents regarded training in ambulatory care of HIV-infected patients as a valuable educational experience.[12]

Caring for HIV-infected patients before the onset of life-threatening opportunistic infections or after recovery affords the resident several important opportunities, including:

Providing preventive and maintenance care: The availability of effective antiviral therapy and prophylaxis against *Pneumocystis carinii* pneumonia and other infections allows for an atmosphere of directed action and hopefulness. This is in contrast to the feelings of ineffectiveness and frustration often associated with caring for the terminally ill hospitalized patient.

Treating non-life-threatening disorders: Successful therapy of minor but troubling disorders such as seborrheic dermatitis or oral candidiasis (Chapter 8) also may provide the resident with a sense of effectiveness and allow for establishment of limited but attainable goals.

Establishing and maintaining an ongoing therapeutic relationship: Continuing involvement in the ambulatory care of HIV-infected patients allows the resident to experience the gratification inherent in the practice of primary care medicine. An awareness of the patient's home situation and social needs and an ability to assist in those areas when necessary may further reduce the resident's feelings of helplessness and may lead to a deemphasis of social stereotypes.

2. *The HIV core curriculum*. Providing a core curriculum of didactic sessions covering major microbiological, clinical, and social aspects of the HIV/AIDS epidemic[24] may enhance the educational value of AIDS care.

REFERENCES

1. Bennett CL et al: The relation between hospital experience and in-hospital mortality for patients with AIDS-related PCP, *JAMA* 261:2975-2979, 1989.
2. Centers for Disease Control: Update: human immunodeficiency virus infections in health care workers exposed to blood of infected patients, *MMWR* 36:285-289, 1987.
3. Centers for Disease Control: Recommendations for prevention of HIV transmission in health care settings, *MMWR* 36(2S):1S-18S, 1987.
4. Centers for Disease Control: Update: acquired immunodeficiency syndrome and human immunodeficiency virus infection among health care workers, *MMWR* 37:229-234, 1988.
5. Centers for Disease Control: *Mycobacterium tuberculosis* transmission in a health clinic: Florida, 1988, *MMWR* 38:256-264, 1989.
6. Centers for Disease Control: Guidelines for prophylaxis against *Pneumocystis carinii* pneumonia for persons infected with human immunodeficiency virus, *MMWR* 38(S-5):1-9, 1989.
7. Centers for Disease Control: Public Health Service statement on management of occupational exposure to human immunodeficiency virus, includ-

ing considerations regarding zidovudine postexposure use, *MMWR* 39(RR-1):1-13, 1990.

7a. Centers for Disease Control: Update: transmission of HIV infection during an invasive dental procedure—Florida, *MMWR* 40(2):21-33, 1991.

7b. Centers for Disease Control: Recommendations for preventing transmission of human immunodeficiency virus and hepatitis B virus to patients during exposure-prone invasive procedures, *MMWR* 40(RR-8):1-6, 1991.

8. Cotton DJ: The impact of AIDS on the medical care system, *JAMA* 260(4):519-523, 1988.

9. Gostin LO: Public health strategies for confronting AIDS: legislative and regulatory policy in the United States, *JAMA* 261(110):1621-1630, 1989.

10. Green J, Leigh MR, Passman LJ: AIDS treatment center: is the concept premature? *JAMA* 262:2537, 1989.

11. Greenfield S: Outpatient AIDS care, *Soc Gen Intern Med News* 13:3, 1990.

12. Hayward RA, Shapiro MF: A national study of AIDS and residency training: experiences, concerns and consequences, *Ann Intern Med* 114:23-32, 1991.

13. Henderson DK et al: Risk for occupational transmission of human immunodeficiency virus type 1 (HIV-1) associated with clinical exposures: a prospective evaluation, *Ann Intern Med* 113:740-746, 1990.

14. Henderson DK, Gerberding JL: Prophylactic zidovudine after occupational exposure to the human immunodeficiency virus: an interim analysis, *J Infect Dis* 160(2):321-327, 1989.

15. Jagger J et al: Rates of needle-stick injury caused by various devices in a university hospital, *N Engl J Med* 319:284-288, 1988.

16. Kelen GD et al: Human immunodeficiency virus infection in emergency department patients. Epidemiology, clinical presentations, and risk to

health care workers: the Johns Hopkins experience, *JAMA* 262:516-522, 1989.

17. Krasinski K, LaCouture R, Holzman RS: Effect of changing needle disposal systems on needle puncture injuries, *Infect Control* 8:59-62, 1987.

18. Lange JMA et al: Failure of zidovudine prophylaxis after accidental exposure to HIV-1, *N Engl J Med* 322(19):1375-1377, 1990.

19. Lewis CE, Freeman HE, Corey CR: AIDS-related competence of California's primary care physicians, *Am J Public Health* 77:795-799, 1987.

20. Marcus R: The Cooperative Needlestick Surveillance Group: Surveillance of health care workers exposed to blood from patients infected with the human immunodeficiency virus, *N Engl J Med* 319:1118-1123, 1988.

21. Martin LS, McDougal S, Loskoski SL: Disinfection and inactivation of the human T lymphotropic virus type III/lymphadenopathy–associated virus, *J Infect Dis* 152:400-403, 1985.

22. McCray E: The Cooperative Needlestick Surveillance Group: occupational risk of the acquired immunodeficiency syndrome among health care workers, *N Engl J Med* 314:1127-1132, 1986.

23. McDiarmid MA, Jacobson-Kram D: Aerosolised pentamidine and public health, *Lancet* 2:863, 1989.

24. Noble JT, Stearns NS, Wolff SM: Curriculum guidelines for AIDS education of primary care practitioners: outcome of an authority opinion survey, *Am J Prev Med* 6:42-50, 1990.

25. Northfelt DW, Hayward RA, Shapiro MF: The acquired immunodeficiency syndrome is a primary care disease, *Ann Intern Med* 108:773-775, 1988.

26. Pascarelli EF, Holtzworth BA: Developing an ambulatory care program for AIDS patients, *J Ambulatory Care Manage* 10:44-55, 1987.

27. Ribner BS et al: Impact of a rigid,

puncture-resistant container system upon needlestick injuries, *Infect Control* 8:63-66, 1987.

28. Selwyn PA et al: Primary care for patients with human immunodeficiency virus (HIV) infection in a methadone maintenance treatment program, *Ann Intern Med* 111:761-763, 1989.

29. Somogyi AA, Watson-Abady JA, Mandel FS: Attitudes toward the care of patients with acquired immunodeficiency syndrome: a survey of community internists, *Arch Intern Med* 150:50-53, 1990.

30. Turner B: Models of HIV ambulatory care: opportunities for SGIM, *Soc Gen Intern Med News* 13:2-4, 1990.

31. Volberding PA: Caring for the patient with AIDS: an integrated approach, *Infect Dis Clin North Am* 2:543-550, 1988.

32. Wallace MR, Harrelson WO: HIV seroconversion with progressive disease in health care worker after needlestick injury, *Lancet* 1:1454, 1988.

33. Weinberg DS, Murray HW: Coping with AIDS: the special problems of New York City, *N Engl J Med* 317:1469-1472, 1987.

34. Wofsy CB: AIDS care: providing care for the HIV-infected, *J Acquire Immune Defic Syndr* 1:274-283, 1988.

CHAPTER 13

Case Studies

This chapter consists of 12 cases illustrating situations commonly encountered in relation to HIV infection in the ambulatory setting. Each case description is followed by an analysis, which includes the following sections:

DIFFERENTIAL DIAGNOSIS: *general diagnostic considerations in the evaluation of the presenting complaint, as well as minor complaints and findings.*

ADDITIONAL INFORMATION NEEDED: *specific questions that the patient or family should be asked and previous laboratory data.*

LABORATORY STUDIES: *initial laboratory tests to be performed at the first encounter.*

OTHER DIAGNOSTIC STUDIES: *additional tests to be considered if the initial laboratory evaluation does not result in a diagnosis.*

THERAPEUTIC CONSIDERATIONS: *indications for therapy and prophylaxis.*

INDICATIONS FOR HOSPITALIZATION

COMMENT: *additional observations on specific issues raised by the case.*

CHAPTER REFERENCES: *chapters in which additional pertinent information can be located.*

CASE 1: General Medical Patient

A 30-year-old man requests a general medical evaluation. He has no current complaints.

PAST MEDICAL HISTORY

Asthma in childhood, usual childhood viral infections; appendectomy at age 19; denies smoking, alcohol, or drug use

MEDICATIONS

None

SOCIAL HISTORY

Unmarried, construction worker

PHYSICAL EXAMINATION

Vital signs: normal
Skin: normal
Lymphatics: normal
Head, eyes, ears, nose, and throat (HEENT): normal
Neck: normal
Chest: normal
Heart: normal
Abdomen: normal
Genitals: normal
Extremities: normal
Neurological examination: normal

DIFFERENTIAL DIAGNOSIS

All patients should be regarded as potentially infected with HIV until after thorough questioning about risk behavior and HIV antibody testing, if indicated.

ADDITIONAL INFORMATION NEEDED

The patient should be thoroughly questioned about HIV risk behavior: sexual contact with other men, prior intravenous drug use, heterosexual promiscuity, exposure to prostitutes, and blood transfusions. This information should be elicited regardless of marital status, standing in the community, and socioeconomic background.

LABORATORY STUDIES

If the patient admits to a history of risk behavior, he should be urged to undergo HIV testing. If the patient denies HIV risk behavior, he should be informed that confidential HIV testing is available if he desires it.

OTHER DIAGNOSTIC STUDIES

No other testing is necessary to define the HIV status of this patient.

THERAPEUTIC CONSIDERATIONS

Antiretroviral therapy and preventive measures, such as prophylaxis against Pneumocystis carinii *pneumonia, may be indicated if the patient is HIV infected.*

INDICATIONS FOR HOSPITALIZATION

None

COMMENT

A patient may be very reluctant to disclose current or prior HIV risk behavior. For this reason, a history of such behavior should be carefully sought in the general medical evaluation of any patient. Although the patient seeking a general medical evaluation who denies any prior HIV risk behavior is extremely unlikely to be infected, it should be noted that a substantial minority of HIV-infected patients initially deny such a history. All patients, regardless of prior history, should be made aware of the availability of HIV testing and should be counseled about routes of transmission and safe sexual practices.

CHAPTER REFERENCES

Chapters 3, 4, and 6

CASE 2: Asymptomatic HIV-Infected Patient, First Visit

A 25-year-old man has been referred for medical evaluation because he tested HIV positive after applying for life insurance.

PAST MEDICAL HISTORY

Two episodes of gonorrhea 1 and 4 years ago; herpes zoster 2 years ago; no history of smoking or alcohol or drug abuse

MEDICATIONS

None

SOCIAL HISTORY

Homosexual, sexually active since age 19; works as a waiter in a restaurant; unmarried

PHYSICAL EXAMINATION

Vital signs: normal
Skin: healed herpes zoster lesion, left side of chest
Lymphatics: bilateral, multiple, 1 to 2 cm posterior cervical lymph nodes
HEENT: white patches on sides of tongue
Neck: normal
Chest: normal
Heart: normal
Abdomen: normal
Genitals: normal
Extremities: normal
Neurological examination: normal

DIFFERENTIAL DIAGNOSIS

A major goal of the initial assessment of a patient who has tested positive for HIV is clinical and immunological staging. After evaluation, the patient should be classified according to staging criteria (Chapters 1 and 2).

ADDITIONAL INFORMATION NEEDED

The patient who appears to be asymptomatic should be specifically questioned about constitutional symptoms such as fever, anorexia, and weight loss and about such common early complaints as sustained diarrhea, lymphadenopathy, and mouth or skin lesions.

LABORATORY STUDIES

Complete blood count
Electrolytes; liver and renal function tests
Lymphocyte subset analysis (with CD4 and CD8 lymphocyte counts)
Urinalysis
Serological test for toxoplasmosis
Serological test for syphilis

OTHER DIAGNOSTIC STUDIES

Chest roentgenogram
Tuberculin skin test

THERAPEUTIC CONSIDERATIONS

Antiretroviral therapy: *The decision to initiate antiretroviral therapy should be based on the immunological stage of the disease (Chapter 10).*

Prophylaxis against Pneumocystis carinii *pneumonia: Prophylaxis should be initiated in all patients with a CD4 lymphocyte count below 200/mm³ (Chapters 6 and 9) regardless of clinical status.*

Immunizations: *All HIV-infected patients should receive immunizations, as discussed in Chapter 6.*

INDICATIONS FOR HOSPITALIZATION

None

COMMENT

An asymptomatic patient often comes to his first appointment with a great deal of anxiety and confusion. Some may react with profound pessimism and resignation whereas others may have unrealistic expectations. The patient should be supported in expressing his fears and goals. The natural history of HIV infection should be discussed (Chapter 2) and possible therapeutic options previewed.

A history of other sexually transmitted diseases, as in this case, is not unusual in HIV-infected homosexual men. White patches on the tongue may represent candidiasis or hairy leukoplakia and should be evaluated further.

As in case 1, routes of transmission and safe sexual practices should be reviewed carefully (Chapter 4). The patient should be asked to inform current and previous sexual partners of his HIV infection and suggest that they undergo testing. The patient should be asked at subsequent visits if he has informed such partners. Local regulations governing physician responsibility in informing contacts should be reviewed if necessary.

CHAPTER REFERENCES

Chapters 1, 2, 3, 4, 6, and 10

CASE 3: Early Symptomatic Patient, First Visit

A 42-year-old male homosexual who is HIV positive requests evaluation of mouth lesions.

PAST MEDICAL HISTORY

Found to be HIV infected 1 year ago; no significant past illnesses

MEDICATIONS

None

SOCIAL HISTORY

Works as a hospital social worker; no longer sexually active; lives alone

PHYSICAL EXAMINATION

Vital signs: normal
Skin: mild seborrheic dermatitis on face; onychomycosis on both hands
Lymphatics: normal
HEENT: painful ulcers on lips, buccal mucosa, and tongue
Chest: normal
Heart: normal
Abdomen: normal
Genitals: normal
Extremities: normal
Neurological examination: normal

DIFFERENTIAL DIAGNOSIS

Herpes simplex stomatitis is most likely, since lesions are painful and multiple; primary syphilis is unlikely but should be excluded; aphthous stomatitis and oral candidiasis should also be considered.

ADDITIONAL INFORMATION NEEDED

Prior clinical and immunological staging information should be reviewed. If lymphocyte subset analysis was not performed within the previous 3-6 months, it should be obtained. The patient should be questioned specifically about any prior history of mouth lesions and symptoms of esophagitis such as dysphagia or odynophagia.

LABORATORY STUDIES

Lymphocyte subset analysis (as indicated above)
Serological test for syphilis
Viral culture of scraping of lesion
Darkfield examination of scraping of lesion, if available

OTHER DIAGNOSTIC STUDIES

None necessary

THERAPEUTIC CONSIDERATIONS

Empiric therapy for herpes simplex stomatitis may be warranted (see Chapter 9), particularly if the patient is significantly immunodeficient (i.e., CD4 lymphocyte count is under $200/mm^3$).

INDICATIONS FOR HOSPITALIZATION

None

COMMENT

The overall approach to this patient should be similar to that for the asymptomatic patient (case 2).

Although the patient's employment as a hospital-based social worker is unlikely to be in jeopardy because he is HIV infected, local policies governing infected health care workers should be reviewed.

Job discrimination against HIV-infected individuals has been reported as a widespread problem. For this reason, unless regulations to the contrary are in effect, employers should not be informed that an employee is HIV infected without the employee's written informed permission.

CHAPTER REFERENCES

Chapters 5 through 10

CASE 4: AIDS Patient, First Visit After Hospitalization for Pneumocystis Carinii Pneumonia

A 35-year-old woman, a former intravenous drug user, seeks follow-up care; she recently was discharged from the hospital after a 3-week stay for Pneumocystis carinii *pneumonia.*

PAST MEDICAL HISTORY

Hepatitis 4 years previously, pneumococcal pneumonia 2 years previously

MEDICATIONS

None

SOCIAL HISTORY

Active intravenous drug user; separated from husband, and has two children with whom she lives

PHYSICAL EXAMINATION

Vital signs: normal
Skin: generalized xerosis
Lymphatics: bilateral, shotty anterior cervical lymphadenopathy
HEENT: moderate oral candidiasis
Chest: dry rales at bases
Heart: 2/6 systolic murmur

Abdomen: normal
Genitals: vaginal discharge
Extremities: normal
Neurological examination: normal

DIFFERENTIAL DIAGNOSIS

A diagnosis of AIDS can be made if the patient has no other known immuno-deficiency state and was not receiving immunosuppressive therapy at the time that Pneumocystis carinii *pneumonia (PCP) was diagnosed.*

ADDITIONAL INFORMATION NEEDED

The means by which the diagnosis of PCP was confirmed should be determined. Unless the organism was identified in respiratory secretions or on histological examination of lung tissue, the diagnosis should be considered presumptive.

The specifics of prior therapy should be determined. Hypersensitivity or other adverse reactions to standard therapy for PCP (i.e., pentamidine or trimethoprim-sulfamethoxazole) should be identified by history and documented.

Lymphocyte subset analysis and HIV testing are not necessary if the diagnosis of PCP was proven. These tests should be performed if the diagnosis was not confirmed.

LABORATORY STUDIES

Complete blood count
Electrolytes; liver and renal function tests
Urinalysis
Serological test for syphilis
Serological test for toxoplasmosis

OTHER DIAGNOSTIC STUDIES

Tuberculin skin test
Chest roentgenogram

THERAPEUTIC CONSIDERATIONS

Secondary prophylaxis against PCP (Chapters 6 and 9); antiretroviral therapy (Chapter 10); immunizations (Chapter 6); therapy for oral candidiasis (Chapter 8)

INDICATIONS FOR HOSPITALIZATION

Potential indications include increasing dyspnea, new pulmonary infiltrates, and manifestations of additional life-threatening opportunistic infections (e.g., new focal neurological signs, dehydrating diarrhea).

COMMENT

The goals of management of a patient with confirmed AIDS are to provide appropriate prophylaxis, immunizations, and antiretroviral therapy and to screen for early evidence of other AIDS-related opportunistic infections and malignancies. Follow-up appointments should be dictated by the patient's clinical status and guidelines for monitoring of antiretroviral therapy (Chapter 10).

Routes of HIV transmission and safe sexual practices should be discussed, and sexual abstinence should be advised. Clinical trials of antiretroviral agents, immunomodulators, and therapy for opportunistic infections for which the patient may qualify should be reviewed and discussed with her.

Arrangements should be made for HIV testing of her children, particularly those under 5 years of age, and discussion of current and former heterosexual partners should take place.

CHAPTER REFERENCES

Chapters 5 through 10

CASE 5: Pregnant HIV-Positive Patient

A 26-year-old woman requests a general medical evaluation. She is 16 weeks pregnant and, on the advice of her obstetrician, has undergone HIV testing. She has been told that the test was positive.

PAST MEDICAL HISTORY

Previously healthy; no apparent history of HIV risk behavior

MEDICATIONS

None

SOCIAL HISTORY

Schoolteacher; lives with husband; no children

PHYSICAL EXAMINATION

Vital signs: normal
Skin: normal
Lymphatics: normal
HEENT: normal
Neck: normal
Chest: normal
Heart: normal
Abdomen: uterus enlarged, consistent with dates

Genitals: normal
Extremities: normal
Neurological examination: normal

DIFFERENTIAL DIAGNOSIS

As in case 2, clinical and immunological staging should be carried out at the first visit. The patient should be questioned about constitutional symptoms including fever and anorexia, and other potential early symptoms of HIV infection such as oral or skin lesions, diarrhea, or lymph node enlargement.

ADDITIONAL INFORMATION NEEDED

The patient should be asked if her husband is aware of her HIV infection and if he has undergone HIV testing. Testing of the husband should be offered and carried out promptly if the patient is willing to inform him that she is infected. If the patient is unwilling to inform her husband, the physician should review local regulations governing disclosure of HIV information to sexual partners. If available, counseling should be offered to the patient and her husband.

LABORATORY STUDIES

Complete blood count
Electrolytes; liver and renal function tests
Lymphocyte subset analysis
Serological test for syphilis
Serological test for toxoplasmosis

OTHER DIAGNOSTIC STUDIES

None necessary if patient offers no symptoms and has received routine prenatal screening

THERAPEUTIC CONSIDERATIONS

Antiretroviral therapy: *The safety and effectiveness of antiretroviral therapy in pregnancy has not yet been defined (Chapter 11). If the pregnancy is terminated, indications for therapy as discussed in Chapter 10 should be followed.*

Prophylaxis against *Pneumocystis carinii* pneumonia: *Prophylaxis should be considered (see discussion, Chapter 11) for patients with a CD4 lymphocyte count below 200/mm³.*

Immunizations: *Immunizations should be provided as indicated in Chapter 11.*

INDICATIONS FOR HOSPITALIZATION

None unless termination of pregnancy is planned

COMMENT

The risk of transmission of HIV infection to the fetus is approximately 30% to 40%. The medical and social implications of this risk should be discussed thoroughly with the patient to help her decide if she wishes to continue the pregnancy. As discussed in Chapter 11, the certainty that an HIV-infected infant will develop AIDS within the first several years of life and the likelihood that the mother's health will fail within several years should be made clear. The mother's informed decision regarding continuation of the pregnancy should be respected.

CHAPTER REFERENCES

Chapters 10 and 11

CASE 6: Sexual Partner of an HIV-Positive Patient

A 28-year-old woman requests a general medical evaluation. Her husband of 3 years recently had told her that he tested HIV positive during an evaluation for life insurance. The patient has no medical complaints.

PAST MEDICAL HISTORY

Asthma in childhood

MEDICATIONS

None

SOCIAL HISTORY

Works as secretary; lives with husband and 6-month-old daughter

PHYSICAL EXAMINATION

Vital signs: normal
Skin: normal
Lymphatics: normal
HEENT: normal
Neck: normal
Chest: normal
Heart: normal
Abdomen: normal
Genitals: normal
Extremities: normal
Neurological examination:
   normal

DIFFERENTIAL DIAGNOSIS

The likelihood that the patient has become infected through sexual contact with her husband is impossible to estimate with precision. Studies of heterosexual partners of infected individuals indicate that the risk of transmission is in the range of 10% to 50% (Chapter 3). The risk for an individual couple is dictated in part by frequency of sexual contact, specific sexual practices, and the use of condoms. Individual host factors and determinants of viral infectivity, which currently are poorly understood, may also play important roles.

The patient's clinical status, including the apparent absence of HIV-related disorders and constitutional symptoms, is of no help in excluding HIV infection.

ADDITIONAL INFORMATION NEEDED

As in case 2, the patient should be carefully questioned about potential HIV-related symptoms. A past history of herpes zoster or recurrent bacterial pneumonia suggests HIV infection.

LABORATORY STUDIES

HIV antibody test
  Lymphocyte subset analysis may be obtained at the initial visit or deferred until it is determined whether the patient is HIV infected
  Routine laboratory tests (e.g., complete blood count, electrolytes, and hepatic and renal function tests) may be performed at the initial visit or deferred

OTHER DIAGNOSTIC STUDIES

None

THERAPEUTIC CONSIDERATIONS

None are necessary until the results of the HIV antibody test and, if that is positive, the results of the lymphocyte subset analysis are known.

INDICATIONS FOR HOSPITALIZATION

None

COMMENT

The patient is likely to be feeling great anxiety. She may be confused by a variety of emotions, including anger at her husband and anticipatory grief over his future death, fear that her child has become infected, and guilt. For these reasons it may be very difficult to help her understand the medical facts at the first visit. It is prudent to assume that HIV-related diseases and their treatment will have to be reviewed at subsequent visits. Although the practitioner should maintain an attitude of supportiveness, excessive reassurances are inappropriate and are likely to be met with disbelief. The importance of early testing and, if necessary, treatment should be emphasized.

Testing procedures for both the patient and her child should be explained (Chapters 3, 4, and 11) and the patient should be assured that testing will be done efficiently and confidentially. The need for repeated testing of the child should be explained thoroughly (Chapter 11).

The patient should be counseled about safe sexual practices, and sexual abstinence should be advised, at least until the results of the HIV testing are available.

CHAPTER REFERENCES

Chapters 3, 4, 6, and 11

CASE 7: Health Care Worker with a Needle-Stick Injury

A 29-year-old nurse requests evaluation after sticking herself with a needle while drawing blood from an HIV-infected patient. She has no medical complaints.

PAST MEDICAL HISTORY

Hepatitis 2 years previously

MEDICATIONS

None

SOCIAL HISTORY

Unmarried, sexually active; works on an inpatient medical unit

PHYSICAL EXAMINATION

Vital signs: normal
Skin: abrasions on both hands
Lymphatics: normal
HEENT: tonsils enlarged
Neck: normal
Chest: normal
Heart: normal
Abdomen: normal
Genitals: normal
Extremities: normal
Neurological examination: normal

DIFFERENTIAL DIAGNOSIS

The risk of transmission of HIV infection during such a needle-stick injury is 0.3% to 0.4% (Chapter 12). The possibility of transmission of hepatitis B virus (HBV) must also be considered.

ADDITIONAL INFORMATION NEEDED

The nurse should be questioned about the circumstances of the needle stick, including (1) the activity during which the injury occurred (e.g., blood drawing, recapping of needle, changing of intravenous tubing); (2) whether she was wearing gloves; (3) whether the injury was penetrating; (4) how promptly the injury was recognized; and (5) what she did immediately after the injury (e.g., washing, expressing blood).

Documentation that the source patient was HIV-infected should be sought. It also should be determined if the patient had a history of hepatitis B.

The nurse should be questioned about previous or current HIV risk behavior and previous needle-stick injuries or other work-related exposures to blood or other body fluids from patients known to be or suspected of being HIV infected. She should also be questioned about her own history of hepatitis, previous blood tests for hepatitis B, and previous vaccination against hepatitis B.

LABORATORY STUDIES

HIV antibody testing should be offered to the nurse and should be performed as soon after the injury as possible. Repeat testing should be performed at intervals of 6 weeks, 3 months, and 6 months.

The patient should be tested for HBV antigen and core and surface antibody unless this information is already available.

If the patient is known to be HBV antigen positive or if test results are not known, and the nurse has not received the hepatitis B vaccine previously or is not known to have detectable anti-HBV surface antibody, HBV antigen and core and surface antibody tests should be performed.

ADDITIONAL DIAGNOSTIC STUDIES

None indicated

THERAPEUTIC CONSIDERATIONS

The potential role of zidovudine (AZT) in postexposure prophylaxis of HIV infection for health care workers is discussed in Chapters 10 and 12.

If the nurse is not immune to hepatitis B (i.e., surface antibody negative) and the patient is HBV antigen positive, the nurse should receive hepatitis B immune globulin as well as the hepatitis B vaccine.

INDICATIONS FOR HOSPITALIZATION

None

COMMENT

The nurse should be informed that the risk of HIV transmission is small and she should receive appropriate counseling before and after HIV antibody testing if such testing is performed. Updated recommendations on postexposure prophylaxis with zidovudine or other antiretroviral agents should be reviewed. Such prophylaxis should be considered, particularly if the injury was severe, with massive blood exposure, or if the wound was neglected.

If the patient does not have documented HIV infection but is thought to be at risk, HIV testing should be performed in accordance with local regulations regarding informed consent and counseling before and after the test.

The nurse should be advised to report any febrile illnesses or syndromes compatible with acute retroviral infection (Chapter 2) during the period of follow-up testing and should be counseled regarding routes of HIV transmission and safe sex practices. Women should be counseled to defer pregnancy until the period of follow-up testing is completed.

The circumstances of the injury and subsequent testing and follow-up of the nurse should be documented, and her confidentiality should be protected. Universal precautions against HIV transmission in the health care setting should be reviewed (Chapter 12).

CHAPTER REFERENCES

Chapters 2, 10, and 12

CASE 8: Dementia

A 42-year-old man with a history of AIDS is brought in by his family because of his worsening forgetfulness.

PAST MEDICAL HISTORY

Pneumocystis carinii *pneumonia 2 years previously; candidal esophagitis 1 year previously; persistent diarrhea for 6 months*

MEDICATIONS

Zidovudine, trimethoprim-sulfamethoxazole

SOCIAL HISTORY

Homosexual, no longer sexually active; lives with parents; unemployed, former bookkeeper

PHYSICAL EXAMINATION

Vital signs: temperature (T), 100° F; blood pressure (BP), 100/60; heart rate (HR), 90; respirations (RR), 14
Skin: generalized xerosis
Lymphatics: normal
HEENT: white patches on sides of tongue; purple papular lesion; hard palate
Neck: normal
Chest: normal
Heart: normal
Abdomen: normal
Genitals: normal
Extremities: trace pedal edema
Neurological examination: decreased short-term memory, deep tendon reflexes at knees and ankles hyperactive

DIFFERENTIAL DIAGNOSIS

Probable AIDS dementia
Diagnoses to be excluded:
   Cerebral toxoplasmosis
   Cryptococcal meningitis
   Progressive multifocal leukoencephalopathy
   Central nervous system lymphoma
   Depression
   Disorder unrelated to HIV infection
   Oral hairy leukoplakia
   Probable oral Kaposi's sarcoma
   Generalized xerosis

ADDITIONAL INFORMATION NEEDED

The patient and his family should be questioned about the duration of the patient's forgetfulness. Because the patient had been a bookkeeper, his employment history might be particularly valuable. Gradual memory loss over a period of months to years is more suggestive of AIDS dementia than of a malignancy or an opportunistic infection of the central nervous system.

LABORATORY STUDIES

Complete blood count
Electrolytes; renal and hepatic function tests
Urinalysis
Serological test for syphilis

Serum toxoplasma antibody test
Chest roentgenogram
Serum levels of vitamin B_{12} and folic acid
Serum cryptococcal antigen
Brain imaging (computed tomography or magnetic resonance imaging)
Cerebrospinal fluid examination

OTHER DIAGNOSTIC STUDIES

Psychiatric evaluation
Electroencephalogram
Oral surgery consultation and biopsy of oral lesions

THERAPEUTIC CONSIDERATIONS

Therapy will be dictated by the results of the diagnostic evaluation. Patients found to have focal enhancing lesions on brain imaging studies should receive presumptive therapy for cerebral toxoplasmosis (Chapter 9). Brain biopsy should be considered in cases where confirmation of a specific diagnosis would likely lead to a meaningful change in therapy.

INDICATIONS FOR HOSPITALIZATION

Hospitalization of the AIDS patient with severe neurological impairment may be indicated for medical or social reasons.

Patients with new focal cerebral neurological deficits or evidence of spinal cord compression should be hospitalized for emergency diagnosis and therapy. New onset of seizures should also prompt hospitalization in most cases.

AIDS dementia may render the patient unable to care for himself. In advanced cases, 24-hour nursing care, intravenous hydration, and enteral feedings may be necessary.

COMMENT

It is unlikely that a reversible cause of the dementia described in this case will be found. If no definitive therapeutic options are found, the goals of management become (1) providing a supportive atmosphere for the patient in which nutritional needs and hygiene can be maintained; (2) providing professional home care when the family or other caregivers can no longer meet the patient's needs; and (3) offering emotional support to the family or caregivers and exploring their feelings and the patient's feelings about further medical care.

CHAPTER REFERENCES

Chapters 5, 7, and 9

CASE 9: Unexplained Fever

A 24-year-old man, a former intravenous drug user known to be HIV infected, seeks treatment with a 3-week history of daily fever to 102° F.

PAST MEDICAL HISTORY

Cerebral toxoplasmosis 6 months previously; oral candidiasis

MEDICATIONS

Sulfadiazine, pyrimethamine, ketoconazole, zidovudine

SOCIAL HISTORY

Unemployed and lives alone

PHYSICAL EXAMINATION

Vital signs: T, 101° F; BP, 120/70; HR, 96; RR, 12
Skin: perianal ulcers
Lymphatics: normal
HEENT: severe oral candidiasis
Neck: normal
Chest: normal
Heart: normal
Abdomen: liver palpable 10 cm below the right costal margin
Genitals: normal
Extremities: normal
Neurological examination: normal

DIFFERENTIAL DIAGNOSIS

Recurrence of cerebral toxoplasmosis
New opportunistic infection (e.g., disseminated mycobacterial infection, histo-
   plasmosis, cryptococcosis, Pneumocystis carinii *pneumonia)*
Drug fever (sulfadiazine most likely)

ADDITIONAL INFORMATION NEEDED

The patient should be questioned carefully about neurological symptoms, includ-
ing headache, focal weakness, and forgetfulness.

LABORATORY STUDIES

Complete blood count
Electrolytes; liver and renal function tests
Chest roentgenogram
Urinalysis

OTHER DIAGNOSTIC STUDIES

Routine cultures of blood, urine, and stool
Mycobacterial culture of blood
Gallium scan
Bone marrow biopsy and fungal and mycobacterial culture
Liver biopsy and fungal and mycobacterial culture

THERAPEUTIC CONSIDERATIONS

Therapy will be dictated by the results of the diagnostic evaluation.

Because mycobacterial infection commonly causes unexplained fever in HIV-infected patients and the results of mycobacterial cultures may not be known for weeks or months, presumptive therapy for tuberculosis may be indicated in some patients. Such therapy should be reserved for cases where fever is sustained for several weeks and no other diagnosis has been identified after extensive evaluation. If fever persists for more than several weeks after presumptive therapy is initiated, subsequent response is unlikely.

INDICATIONS FOR HOSPITALIZATION

Indications for hospitalization of the patient with unexplained fever include:
- *Development of symptoms of life-threatening infection, including hypotension, a new neurological disorder, severe or worsening respiratory symptoms, or de-hydrating diarrhea*
- *Performance of invasive diagnostic studies that are unavailable or inconvenient in an ambulatory setting*
- *Rapid performance of several diagnostic studies in a patient whose overall clinical status is worsening*
- *Observation of the fever pattern and exclusion of factitious fever when this is suspected*

COMMENT

Fever poses a common diagnostic dilemma in the ambulatory management of HIV-infected patients. In evaluating fever in a patient with AIDS, such as the one described, it is prudent to assume that new fever without obvious cause indicates a potentially life-threatening infection. Respiratory and central nervous system infections are the most dangerous and should be excluded.

Fever in HIV-infected patients who do not have AIDS or severe depression of the CD4 lymphocyte count (i.e., under 300/mm³) is often caused by disorders not directly related to HIV infection. It should be remembered that tuberculosis, pneumococcal pneumonia, Salmonella bacteremia, and several other life-threatening infections occur with greater frequency in HIV-infected patients at all stages of the disease.

CHAPTER REFERENCES

Chapters 5 and 7

CASE 10: Unexplained Weight Loss

A 35-year-old woman with HIV seeks treatment with a history of a 30-pound weight loss over 6 weeks.

PAST MEDICAL HISTORY

Oral candidiasis for 2 years; intermittent diarrhea for 6 months; no other prior illnesses

MEDICATIONS

Nystatin oral rinse

SOCIAL HISTORY

Housewife; lives with husband and children

PHYSICAL EXAMINATION

Vital signs: normal
Skin: extensive xerosis
Lymphatics: 3-cm lymph node in right posterior cervical area
HEENT: mild oral candidiasis
Neck: normal except for lymph node
Chest: normal
Heart: normal
Abdomen: normal
Genitals: normal
Extremities: normal
Neurological examination: normal

DIFFERENTIAL DIAGNOSIS

Decreased caloric intake
  Possible causes:
  esophagitis
  malabsorption
  dementia
  anorexia caused by medications or depression
  insufficent food available
Increased catabolism
  Possible causes:
  disease progression, occult infection, or malignancy

ADDITIONAL INFORMATION NEEDED

The patient should be questioned about changes in appetite, difficulty swallowing, nausea, vomiting, and diarrhea. Debilitated patients should be questioned carefully about their ability to obtain and prepare adequate amounts of food and the possible need for assistance.

Constitutional symptoms such as fever, night sweats, and chills should be sought. The mental status examination, including tests of short-term memory and other cognitive functions, should be reviewed.

DIAGNOSTIC STUDIES

Complete blood count
Electrolytes; hepatic and renal function tests
Prothrombin time
Biopsy of cervical lymph node

OTHER DIAGNOSTIC STUDIES

Malabsorption studies
Barium esophagram
Endoscopy
Stool examination for parasites
Stool culture
Psychiatric examination
If fever is present, the evaluation should proceed as in case 9.

THERAPEUTIC CONSIDERATIONS

Therapeutic options can be determined only after the diagnostic evaluation is complete. Oral nutritional supplements may be advisable, particularly in patients with reduced caloric intake but normal intestinal absorption.

Oral medications associated with nausea or anorexia (such as nystatin in this case) should be discontinued if possible.

INDICATIONS FOR HOSPITALIZATION

Potential indications for hospitalization include (1) invasive diagnostic procedures unavailable or inconvenient in the ambulatory setting; (2) rapid performance of several diagnostic procedures in the patient who is deteriorating clinically; and (3) enteral or parenteral nutritional therapy.

COMMENT

Weight loss is a common and often multifactorial problem in the HIV-infected patient, particularly at advanced stages of disease. In this case, the initial eval-

uation should focus on determining the cause of the cervical lymph node enlargement.

The impact of the patient's weight loss and possible progression of disease on her husband and children should be explored. If available, home assistance may be appropriate.

CHAPTER REFERENCE

Chapter 7

CASE 11: New-Onset Headache in an HIV-Positive Patient

An HIV-infected 36-year-old man seeks treatment with a 10-day history of constant headache.

PAST MEDICAL HISTORY

Found to be HIV positive 2 years previously

MEDICATIONS

Zidovudine

SOCIAL HISTORY

Homosexual; lives alone; works as an accountant

PHYSICAL EXAMINATION

Vital signs: T, 100° F; otherwise normal
Skin: tinea versicolor on back
Lymphatics: normal
HEENT: normal
Neck: slight nuchal rigidity
Chest: normal
Heart: normal
Abdomen: normal
Genitals: normal
Extremities: normal
Neurological examination: normal

DIFFERENTIAL DIAGNOSIS

The degree of immunodeficiency present at the time the patient is seen influences the differential diagnosis of headache.

In patients with moderate to severe impairment of cellular immunity (i.e., CD4

lymphocyte count below 300/mm³ within the previous 60 days), HIV-related opportunistic infections are common. Of those that affect the central nervous system,
cryptococcal meningitis is most likely to manifest with constant headache in the
absence of apparent focal cerebral deficits. Toxoplasmosis, tuberculous meningitis,
central nervous system lymphoma, and, less commonly, progressive multifocal
leukoencephalopathy should also be considered.

   If the CD4 lymphocyte count is over 300/mm³, more conventional causes of
headache are more likely. However, central nervous system lymphoma may
manifest earlier in the natural history of HIV infection than opportunistic infections.

   Zidovudine may cause headache, particularly in the initial stages of therapy.

ADDITIONAL INFORMATION NEEDED

The patient should be questioned carefully about symptoms of increased intracranial pressure, sinusitis, and dental and ear pain.

LABORATORY STUDIES

Lymphocyte subset analysis (if not performed within the preceding 60 days)
If CD4 lymphocyte count is under 300/mm³:
   Serum cryptococcal antigen
   Lumbar puncture, unless an expanding intracranial mass lesion suspected
   Brain imaging (computed tomography or magnetic resonance imaging)
If CD4 lymphocyte count is above 300/mm³:
   Brain imaging if focal neurological deficit or depressed sensorium is present
   Lumbar puncture if fever or meningeal signs are present

OTHER DIAGNOSTIC STUDIES

Dental, paranasal, and sinus roentgenograms

THERAPEUTIC CONSIDERATIONS

Patients found to have focal lesions on brain imaging should generally receive
presumptive therapy for cerebral toxoplasmosis. In other cases, therapy will be
guided by the results of the diagnostic evaluation. Zidovudine should be discontinued until evaluation is completed.

INDICATIONS FOR HOSPITALIZATION

The patient should be hospitalized if the headache is acute in onset and is accompanied by fever, depressed sensorium, seizure, focal neurological deficit, or
evidence of increased intracranial pressure. Hospitalization is also appropriate
if necessary diagnostic tests cannot be performed rapidly in the ambulatory
setting.

COMMENT

> *The sudden onset of severe or unremitting headache in an HIV-infected patient should be taken to indicate a potentially life-threatening opportunistic infection or malignancy. This is particularly true in patients at advanced stages of disease.*
>
> *Although non-life-threatening causes of headache are also seen (e.g., zidovu-dine therapy, tension headache), the practitioner should regard these as diagnoses of exclusion.*

CHAPTER REFERENCE

> *Chapters 5 and 7*

CASE 12: New-Onset Cough in an HIV-Positive Patient

> *A 42-year-old man with a history of AIDS seeks treatment with a 3-day history of cough.*

PAST MEDICAL HISTORY

> *Cryptococcal meningitis 1 year previously*

MEDICATIONS

> *Fluconazole*

SOCIAL HISTORY

> *Former intravenous drug user; works as a cook; unmarried and lives alone; non-smoker and has no history of alcohol abuse*

PHYSICAL EXAMINATION

> *Vital signs: T, 100.5° F; BP, 110/70; HR, 110; RR, 24*
> *Skin: 2-cm purple nodular lesion on right thigh*
> *Lymphatics: normal*
> *HEENT: normal*
> *Neck: normal*
> *Chest: dry rales at both lung bases*
> *Heart: normal*
> *Abdomen: spleen tip palpable 4 cm below the left costal margin*
> *Genitals: normal*
> *Extremities: normal*
> *Neurological examination: normal*

DIFFERENTIAL DIAGNOSIS

Pneumocystis carinii *pneumonia (PCP):*

*The patient who has a prior diagnosis of AIDS on the basis of cryptococcal
meningitis is receiving no prophylaxis and is at high risk of PCP*
Pulmonary cryptococcosis
Other opportunistic infection
Pulmonary Kaposi's sarcoma
Pulmonary tuberculosis
Bacterial pneumonia
Non-HIV-related respiratory infection

LABORATORY STUDIES

Complete blood count
Electrolytes; renal and hepatic function tests
Lactate dehydrogenase
Chest roentgenogram
Serum cryptococcal antigen

OTHER DIAGNOSTIC STUDIES

Gallium scan if chest roentgenogram is equivocal or negative
Arterial blood gas
Sputum acid-fast stain
Blood cultures
*Bronchoscopy with biopsy or bronchoalveolar lavage is indicated if unexplained
pulmonary infiltrates or masses are seen on the chest roentgenogram or if gal-
lium scanning documents diffuse pulmonary uptake*

THERAPEUTIC CONSIDERATIONS

*Definitive therapy will be dictated by the results of diagnostic studies. In general,
patients with diffuse pulmonary infiltrates of unknown cause should be treated
presumptively for PCP until the diagnostic evaluation has been completed.*

INDICATIONS FOR HOSPITALIZATION

*Diffuse pneumonia usually is an indication for acute hospitalization so that
respiratory parameters can be monitored and diagnostic studies can be obtained
rapidly.*

*In cases where symptoms are not progressing rapidly, the blood oxygenation
on inspired room air is acceptable (e.g., Po_2 over 80 mm Hg), and the diagnosis
of PCP can be confirmed promptly without hospitalization, ambulatory therapy
with frequent monitoring can be considered. Only patients with a history of
compliance with medications and with medical follow-up should be considered
candidates for ambulatory therapy.*

Patients with symptoms of bacteremia (shaking chills, hypotension) should be hospitalized.

COMMENT

New respiratory symptoms in an HIV-infected patient should be regarded as potentially life threatening. This is especially true if the patient has a prior diagnosis of AIDS, as in this case, or is severely immunodeficient on the basis of lymphocyte subset analysis (i.e., CD4 lymphocyte count under $200/mm^3$).

CHAPTER REFERENCES

Chapters 5 and 7

Index

*Italicized page numbers indicate illustrations.

ISBN 0-8016-3159-9

9 780801 631597

90000>